A TEXTBOOK OF
MEDICAL CONDITIONS FOR
PHYSIOTHERAPISTS

A TEXTBOOK OF
MEDICAL CONDITIONS
FOR
PHYSIOTHERAPISTS

by

JOAN E. CASH

B.A., M.C.S.P. (Teacher's Certificates)

with a foreword by

FRANK D. HOWITT

C.V.O., M.A., M.D., F.R.C.P.

FABER AND FABER LIMITED

24 Russell Square

London

First published in mcmli
by Faber and Faber Limited
24 Russell Square London W.C.1
Second impression November mcmli
Third impression July mcmliv
Second edition mcmlvii
Reprinted mcmlix and mcmlxii
Printed in Great Britain by
Purnell and Sons Limited
Paulton (Somerset) and London

FOREWORD

by the late F. D. Howitt, C.V.O., M.A., M.D., F.R.C.P.

Physician, with charge of Physical Medicine, Middlesex Hospital
Honorary Consultant in Physical Medicine to the Army
Senior Physician to the Arthur Stanley Institute for Rheumatic Diseases

It gives me particular pleasure to write a short foreword to this book, partly because I have read it with great interest, and partly because I am convinced that it supplies a long-felt need.

The face of medicine in this country has changed considerably in recent years, mainly as the result of dire necessity imposed upon us by two World Wars. It has become less departmentalised, and has assumed a more purposeful character. We have come to realise that the achievement and maintenance of health, the conduct of serious disease and injury, and the rehabilitation and revocation of disabled persons are, none of them, a one-man job. Success can only be achieved by team-work, and in this team there are no two members more important than the doctor and the physiotherapist. Each has his separate functions to fulfil, yet neither can fulfil it adequately unless he works in harmony with the other.

I suspect that Miss Cash had some difficulty in selecting the title for her book. It would manifestly be an impertinence for a doctor to write a textbook on physiotherapy for doctors, although there is great need for such a work. For it is most important that before prescribing the various forms of physical treatment, a medical man should be fully conversant with their uses and abuses, actions and reactions, indications and contra-indications. He should also realise the difficulties which beset the physiotherapist, when faced with an incorrect or inadequate prescription. It would be equally presumptuous for a physiotherapist to attempt to write a textbook on medicine for physiotherapists. Yet it is vital that the physiotherapist should appreciate the problems which the doctor has to face when assessing the likely value of physiotherapy in conjunction with other medical measures; its effect upon the constitutional and psychological condition of the patient; its prospects and sometimes its dangers. All physical treatments, whether preventive, corrective or remedial should be welded into a general and

7

organised scheme. These are the points which Miss Cash has so admirably stressed from the viewpoint of the physiotherapist.

The author has aimed at simplicity, both in the general lay-out and in the description of the various medical conditions. The rationale for treatment has been fully explained in each instance, and there is a refreshing freedom from extravagant claims. It is up-to-date, and should serve equally as a work of reference for the qualified physiotherapist and for the senior student preparing for her Diploma.

FRANK HOWITT

PREFACE

In writing this book the author has not attempted to teach any new material but rather to explain in detail some of the medical conditions most often seen in a department of physical medicine. It is, therefore, a book for students of physiotherapy, and it is hoped that with a better understanding of the changes occurring in these conditions the physical treatment may be carried out with a greater degree of intelligence, interest and improved efficiency.

The subject matter covers many medical conditions, but it was felt that a chapter on physical treatment in the surgical group of respiratory conditions should be included, as many chest conditions alternate between surgical and medical treatment and the physiotherapist is required to treat cases throughout both stages.

Each chapter, as well as describing medical conditions, is followed by a short outline dealing with the broad principles of treatment of these conditions by physical measures. In certain of these diseases there is little information available about the physical treatment, and so to fill in this gap a fuller account has been given.

PREFACE TO THE SECOND EDITION

Considerable revision of this book has been undertaken partly because of the rapid advances in physiology, medicine and physiotherapy, and partly because of the many helpful criticisms and suggestions made by my colleagues and friends.

The section dealing with Rheumatic Affections has been completely re-written with a greater emphasis on the part which the physiotherapist can play in the rehabilitation of the patient. Considerable alteration has been made in the chapters dealing with neurological disorders. The description of the motor and sensory systems has been omitted, due to the fact that the knowledge of the central nervous system is developing so rapidly that whatever is written now will probably be out of date by the time the book is in the hands of the reader. A number of new methods of physical treatment for disorders of the locomotor system have been mentioned. No detail of these has been given as they are still not universally used, but it is hoped that sufficient has been said to stimulate students' interest in these methods. Since physiotherapy is rarely ordered in the treatment of diseases of the abdominal viscera and peritoneum this section has been omitted.

I would like particularly to thank Dr. A. G. W. Whitfield, of the United Birmingham Hospitals, for reading the section on Rheumatic Affections and giving many helpful suggestions; Dr. E. R. Bickerstaff of the Midland Centre for Neuro-Surgery, who helped me so much with Part IV, and Miss B. Chatwin, Principal of the School of Physiotherapy, The Queen Elizabeth Hospital, who drew the additional figures and read and corrected the text.

I value this opportunity of expressing my sincere thanks to my colleagues on the School Staff, who have not only helped me with their criticisms, but have done much of my work while I have been revising this book.

I am glad also to express my thanks to Miss M. Harris who has patiently typed and re-typed the chapters, and to Miss P. Jean Cunningham of Faber and Faber Ltd., without whose help I am sure this second edition would never have been completed.

J.E.C.

Birmingham, 1956.

ACKNOWLEDGMENTS

I should like to express a very deep debt of gratitude to Dr. A. C. Boyle, M.D., M.R.C.P., D.Phys.Med., who gave up so much of his valuable time to read and criticise these chapters. Without his help this book would never have been completed.

My special thanks are also due to Miss G. E. Bristow, M.C.S.P., who read many of the chapters, gave much valuable help and advice and inspired me to continue.

The section on electrical tests was written by Miss B. Chatwin, M.C.S.P. I am glad to take this opportunity of expressing my appreciation both for the article and for much help and many suggestions given during the writing of this book.

I should also like to give my warmest thanks to Mr. Dee, Clinical Photographer to the Queen Elizabeth Hospital, Birmingham, for the photographs; to Mr. W. J. Pardoe of the Anatomy department of the Birmingham Medical School, who drew the illustration 11a, and to Miss M. Everall, M.C.S.P., for all the other drawings.

Many standard textbooks and articles have been consulted during the preparation of the book. It would be impracticable to mention each one in the text, but a list of those most frequently referred to has been added at the end of the work.

Finally these acknowledgments would be incomplete without a very sincere word of thanks to the publishers, Messrs. Faber and Faber, Limited, who have shown great consideration and kindness and given me much help.

CONTENTS

Part I

PATHOLOGICAL CHANGES

Part II

RHEUMATIC AFFECTIONS

CONTENTS

Part III

DISEASES OF THE
RESPIRATORY SYSTEM

Part IV

DISORDERS OF THE
NERVOUS SYSTEM

CONTENTS

Part V

DISEASES OF THE
CARDIO-VASCULAR SYSTEM

Part VI

SOME COMMON DISEASES OF THE
SKIN AND ITS APPENDAGES   365

15

ILLUSTRATIONS

PLATES

ILLUSTRATIONS

FIGURES IN TEXT

PART ONE

PATHOLOGICAL CHANGES

Chapter I

DEGENERATION. INFLAMMATION.
REPAIR

Pathology is the study of the changes in tissues consequent upon disease. Disease manifests itself at some stage in its development by the appearance of signs and symptoms produced as a result of disturbance of function. Each specific cell has its own special function to perform in order that the various activities of the body can be carried on normally. Changes occurring in any group of cells are liable to produce alteration in function of those cells. It is true that changes cannot always be discovered, and a patient may die of an acute poison although showing no changes in the post-mortem examination. In many cases in which pain is the main symptom no organic lesion is apparent, but it is probable that the changes are too minute to be detected by present-day methods.

The changes which occur in human tissues are of two main types: those which are the direct result of damage—degenerative changes, and those whose purpose is to remove the irritant and repair the damage—reparative or reactive changes.

DEGENERATIVE CHANGES

It often happens in the body that, owing to some injury, cells and fibres degenerate and are replaced by a less specialised type. This is shown in ischaemia of muscle, where the muscle fibres are replaced by fibrous tissue. Such alteration in tissue invariably results in impaired function. Thus a fibrosed muscle no longer has the property of contractibility, and its power of conferring movement on the part is therefore lost.

Different types of degeneration occur, the commonest being: cloudy or parenchymatous, fatty degeneration, and necrosis and gangrene.

Cloudy degeneration. Two characteristic features are present in this type. The cell is swollen and numerous small granules appear in the cytoplasm. As a result of the swelling of each cell the whole organ appears to be slightly larger and becomes pale due to the pressure of the swollen cells on the blood vessels. The presence of abnormal granules indicates disturbance in the metabolism of the cell.

Cloudy degeneration is nearly always the result of the action of toxins on the cell.

Fatty degeneration. Interference with the blood supply of cells, or chemical and bacterial toxins tend to bring about this type of degeneration. Part of the cytoplasm disappears and droplets of fat are deposited in its place. The presence of fat interferes with the proper functioning of the cell. The cells which are most commonly affected are those with a secreting function, with the result that the amount of secretion will be diminished. The cells of the heart may also be affected, producing reduction of the force of the contraction of the affected cells, the heart's action consequently being impaired.

Necrosis and gangrene are terms applied to the death of cells while they are part of the living body. Once dead, they must inevitably cease to function. The presence of groups of dead cells leads to changes in the surrounding tissues. The area around becomes invaded by leucocytes from the blood vessels. These cells break down and absorb the dead tissue, leaving cystic cavities. Not only do leucocytes invade the area in large numbers, but other tissue cells multiply and a fibrous capsule tends to form around the necrosed area.

Many factors may cause death of cells, the most outstanding feature being a deprivation of blood so that the cells die because they receive insufficient oxygen and nutriment. Toxins, indirectly, have the same effect because they often act on the blood vessels, causing a clotting of the blood and so cutting off the nutrition to the cells. Trauma may actually destroy the cells, while physical and chemical agents may have the same effects.

A necrosed area no longer having a blood supply, quickly tends to become invaded by bacteria. The speed with which this occurs is significant and will depend upon the amount of fluid in the part. If the area of necrosis is relatively free from fluid the growth of bacteria will be slow. The area gradually shrinks in size and becomes black in colour because the haemoglobin of the red blood corpuscles is broken up when these cells are liberated by the disintegration of the vessels. Its pigments are therefore freed, causing staining of the tissues. Gradually a line of demarcation, consisting of inflammatory granulation tissue, appears between the dead and living tissue and eventually the dead area completely disappears. This type of gangrene is known as dry gangrene.

If the necrosis occurs in an area rich in fluid, as, for example, in a part from which the arterial supply is suddenly cut off, then the growth of bacteria is favoured. The bacteria act on the dead tissue, breaking down the proteins and, in the process, liberating gases which not only give rise to the characteristic foul odour but also accumulate in the tissues, causing a condition of emphysema. One great danger of this moist gangrene is absorption of toxins into the blood stream, with consequent severe toxaemia and death.

Gangrene may be met with in diabetes, where not only are the arteries narrowed as a result of atheromatous patches, but also the excess sugar in the tissues is particularly conducive to the growth of bacteria. Persistent spasm of arterioles in Raynaud's disease may eventually give rise to dry gangrene.

The condition of thrombo-angiitis-obliterans, in which gradual obliteration of the lumen of vessels causes a decreasing supply of blood to the lower extremities, tends to result in gangrene. Severe inflammation resulting in thrombosis of vessels may lead to necrosis and gangrene. Bedsores are areas of gangrene and are the result of continual pressure, causing diminution of blood to the skin and superficial tissues.

REACTIVE OR REPARATIVE CHANGES

These occur as a series of changes which take place in order to remove a harmful agent and prepare the way for repair. The whole process is called inflammation and is the reaction of the tissues to irritation. The severity of the reaction will depend upon the amount of irritation, and therefore it is common to classify inflammation into acute and chronic types.

ACUTE INFLAMMATION

The irritation which provokes an acute reaction may be traumatic, such as a fall, a cut, a sprain or dislocation; it may be due to physical agents, heat, cold, or high-voltage electrical currents; it may be the result of the invasion of the part by bacteria either from elsewhere in the body or from the surface through a puncture wound. Whether the irritant be mild or severe, the inflammatory action will differ only in degree. Changes will occur both in blood vessels and in the tissues.

Vascular Changes

The immediate response of the blood vessels to irritation is dilatation. This is partly due to a reflex, set in action by the irritation of sensory nerve endings, and partly due to the paralysing effect on the involuntary muscle tissue in the walls of capillaries of chemical substances produced by bacteria and liberated by damaged cells. Not only do vessels already carrying blood dilate, but many capillaries which previously were closed now become patent and help in increasing the local blood supply. At the same time as the vaso-dilatation, changes take place in the endothelium of the blood vessels. The cells swell, lose their clear contour and their cohesiveness and project into the lumen of the vessels. In addition they become more permeable, so that substances in solution pass more readily through the cytoplasm. The result of these changes is far-reaching. As the vessels dilate and more capillaries open up, an increased flow of blood into the area takes place, bringing more cells and plasma. This is quickly followed by a slowing of flow, partly due to the diminished lumen of the vessels resulting from the swelling of the endothelium and partly to the increased viscosity of the blood, since much plasma has passed into the tissues, leaving the blood more concentrated. Sometimes the slowing becomes so marked that the blood clots in the vessels.

The slowing of blood flow gives time for further changes. Normally the red and white cells flow along together at the centre of the stream, but now the leucocytes begin to fall out and travel far more slowly along the vessel walls, till eventually the wall is lined by a continuous layer of white blood cells. These cells then work their way through the walls of the vessels till they lie free in the tissue spaces. This process by means of which the leucocytes emigrate into the tissues is known as diapedesis. It is made easy by the changes in the endothelium. The cell is actually attracted into the tissues, the attractive force being the substances liberated from the breakdown of the proteins of damaged cells, and the toxins produced by bacteria. These chemical substances pass into the capillaries and attract the leucocytes to the walls, then, travelling in the blood stream, they reach the bone marrow and attract the stored white cells into the blood. Thus as long as the attractive substances are being produced leucocytes will crowd into the area. The function of the leucocytes is to destroy the bacteria. Those which are damaged in the process liberate an enzyme which digests the damaged tissue and the fibrin.

Sometimes red cells escape through the vessel walls after the white, the tiny gap through which they pass quickly closing. No useful purpose appears to be served by this migration.

During the time in which all these changes are taking place, fluid from the blood is seeping out into the tissues, greatly increasing the flow of lymph from the damaged area. This increased tissue fluid formation is partly due to the fact that the capillary walls are more permeable, and partly to the fact that increased metabolism results in a rise in the osmotic pressure of the tissue spaces, and fluid is therefore withdrawn from the vessels. The exudation of fluid may become too great for the lymphatic vessels to deal with. It then collects in the tissue spaces and clots, so that the exudate becomes fibrinous. A useful purpose is served by the inflammatory exudate, since the toxins are diluted and the debris carried away. It also brings more nutrition to the tissues, and in addition, by clotting, forms a scaffolding along which the leucocytes crawl to reach the site of damage. This fibrinous exudate also acts as a basis for repair. Much of it is eventually removed by leucocytes, but unfortunately some becomes converted into scar tissue.

Tissue Changes

Some degeneration of cells and necrosis at the site of damage must occur. In the area surrounding this region, where the irritation is less severe, marked activity will immediately commence. Cells of various types, in addition to the leucocytes, crowd into the area. Large mononuclear cells, often known as macrophages, collect and multiply, their function being to absorb non-bacterial debris. Fibroblasts multiply and free themselves from their fibres, later throwing out fibrous threads. This process is probably the result of stimulation by chemical substances liberated by damaged cells.

Signs and Symptoms

The changes taking place give rise to certain clinical features easy to recognise. Active arterial hyperaemia and increased metabolism cause a rise of temperature of the part. Heat will therefore be a prominent sign. The area will be red, due to the engorgement, and if the inflammation is superficial or spreads to the skin, change in colour can be seen. Swelling will occur, partly due to the dilatation of vessels, and partly to the accumulated tissue fluid. The fluid will distend the tissues and give rise to pain because stretching and pressure on nerve endings will be the result of distension. If the tissues in the area are lax, less pressure will occur and so less pain, but if there is little room for accumulation of fluid, pressure will be severe and pain considerable. Partly owing to actual damage and degeneration of cells, and partly to pain, movement of the part will be limited and will evoke a protective muscle spasm.

TERMINATION OF ACUTE INFLAMMATION

When the changes of inflammation have occurred, various factors may influence the subsequent events. The severity of the damage, the cause of inflammation, the treatment given, the condition of the patient's general health and defensive mechanism will all affect the result. If the inflammation subsides and the area returns to normal, resolution is then said to have occurred. On the other hand, it may fail to clear, and the condition may then become chronic. If the irritation results in necrosis, then suppuration is likely to occur.

Resolution

When the irritant has been removed and damaged cells no longer liberate chemical substances, the blood vessels return to their normal size and the endothelium to its original state. The blood flow gradually recovers its accustomed speed. Excessive exudation of plasma and emigration of white cells therefore ceases. The fluid present in the tissue spaces can then be dealt with by the lymphatic vessels. Healthy leucocytes find their way back into the capillaries, while those which have been damaged are absorbed and digested by the macrophages. Fibrin, formed by the coagulation of exudate, is removed by the action of leucocytes. In this way the area returns to normal.

Suppuration

This is the formation of pus, and will only occur if necrosis has taken place. In fairly mild degrees of inflammation necrosis will not occur and suppuration should not be seen, but in severe cases some cells will die. Not only must necrosis take place but sufficient polymorphonuclear leucocytes must be present. The suppuration occurs in the following way. The cells degenerate and die, and protein-splitting enzymes, liberated by leucocytes and bacteria, break down and liquefy the necrosed tissue. The liquid material thus formed, together with the inflammatory exudate, leucocytes and dead and living bacteria, is known as pus. Bacteria are not essential for the process of suppuration, but are nearly always present. A necrosed area forms a very suitable medium for the growth of bacteria, and it is therefore quickly invaded by these micro-organisms from the blood stream, if they are not already present. Once in the area, they liberate the toxins which damage and destroy still more tissue cells.

The quantity of pus formed and the ultimate outcome depends on the severity of necrosis and, if bacteria are present, on their type. In addition, it depends on the defence which the tissues can put up against the micro-organisms. In mild cases only a small quantity of pus is formed, and this is absorbed by the lymph stream, and so the area returns to normal. In more severe cases, where pyogenic organisms are present, destruction of tissues continues, and more and more pus collects. Around the area the irritation is less intense. The tissues react by proliferation, and a fibrous capsule is formed. The result is an abscess. As more pus is formed, pressure within the abscess cavity rises, the wall tends to break down at its weakest point and the abscess spreads until it reaches a surface. The abscess track is known as a sinus.

It is apparent that for sinus and abscess formation, bacteria must be present, and these micro-organisms must be pyogenic (pus forming). Not all bacteria are pyogenic. The tubercle bacillus, for example, does not cause abscess formation. Its toxins destroy the protein-splitting enzyme of the polymorphonuclear leucocytes and the bacillus fails to act as an attractive force, so that leucocytes do not invade the area. If, however, a tuberculous area is invaded by other bacteria, pus may then be formed. Much pus formation means considerable destruction of tissue and return to normal cannot take place. The place of the destroyed tissue is eventually taken by fibrous tissue and, as will be seen later, scarring and contracture are likely to occur.

CHRONIC INFLAMMATION

This type of inflammation is characterised by the formation of fibrous tissue which tends to contract, often resulting in reduction in size of the area affected and loss of elasticity and pliability of the tissues.

Chronic inflammation is either the direct continuation of the acute form in which the irritant has grown milder, or it may be the result of some mild irritant which is not severe enough to evoke an acute reaction. Examples of mild irritants are repeated minor traumata such as frequent twisting of an ankle resulting in a chronic thickening of the joint structures; the constant inhalation of dust particles acting as a mild irritation and setting up a fibrosis of lung tissue in the condition of pneumokoniosis; the effect of mild poisons such as lead; or the action of tubercle bacilli or spirochaetes and other bacteria whose toxins are slow in their effects.

Changes

If acute inflammation passes into the chronic stage, it is because the former has failed to remove the irritant. The inflammatory exudate is therefore not absorbed and cell proliferation continues. The persistent irritant acts as a stimulus both to blood vessels and connective tissue cells and production of new cells occurs. Capillary buds grow into the exudate from the surrounding blood vessels, and where they meet new blood vessels are formed. At the same time the fibroblasts multiply and the inflammatory exudate gradually becomes converted into granulation tissue. In the course of time the new cells lay down fibres and eventually vascular fibrous tissue is formed. A chronic inflammation which has not followed an acute is due to an irritant which is insufficient to provoke marked degeneration of cells, vascular changes and inflammatory exudate. In this case the chief change is a thickening of the fibres of the connective tissue so that a non-cellular avascular fibrous tissue is the result.

The final result in either case is contraction, since fibrous tissue has a marked tendency to shrink. Should chronic inflammation occur in the walls of tubes, their lumen tends to be diminished; if it occurs in organs they decrease in size and their function is impaired. If it occurs in capsules or ligaments contraction results in limited movement.

Not only does the fibrous tissue cause contracture with all its ill effects, but while it is still vascular, if stretched, it gives rise to pain. When it is no longer vascular it ceases to be tender and painful, but its presence mats together the other tissues, reducing their pliability, and by dragging on delicate structures during movement gives rise to pain. In addition excessive fibrous tissue may well render the part anaemic because of the pressure it exerts on neighbouring blood vessels. Adhesions are the result of organised inflammatory exudate and blood clot and differ only from the fibrous formation described above in that they are usually in the form of bands which are sometimes covered with epithelium. Their effect is identical, they bind tissues together so reducing pliability and movement, and they cause pain and discomfort so that function is impaired.

VARIETIES OF INFLAMMATION

Many different names have been given to inflammation. In principle, all varieties of inflammation are the same, the changes are alike but the actual exudate varies with the nature of the tissue and the cause of the inflammation.

Thus the inflammation of serous membranes such as the pleura or peritoneum is characterised by a sero-fibrinous exudate, since special serous secreting cells form part of the tissue. As the exudate is sero-fibrinous in character and contains excessive plasma, fibrin tends to be deposited on the membrane, and the growth of new blood vessels results in organisation and the formation of new fibrous tissue. The result of inflammation of serous membranes is therefore likely to be adhesion formation.

Catarrhal inflammation is inflammation of a mucous membrane, in this case the special cells are mucus secreting and irritation of such a membrane results in increased mucus formation. In a chronic catarrhal inflammation, degeneration and fibrous tissue formation occur in the membrane, therefore the orifices of the glands are blocked and decreased secretion occurs.

Suppurative inflammation is an inflammation accompanied by necrosis and pus formation.

REPAIR

Repair is an important item in the restoration of damaged cells and the replacement of lost tissue. Its fundamental process is the formation of granulation tissue and this occurs in any area no matter what are its special characteristics. Thus granulation tissue will be found as the initial process in the healing of wounds, the repair of ruptured tendons, the union of broken bones, and in the organisation of inflammatory exudate and blood clot. A little difference may be found in the tissue eventually produced depending on the type of cells forming the damaged tissue. Bone is rich in bone-forming cells and repair is therefore characterised by the gradual development of osteoid tissue. Liver cells, endothelial cells and connective tissue cells have remarkable powers of regeneration and will form new cells of the same type as those which were damaged, but nerve cells have not this power and can only be replaced by fibrous tissue. In each and every case, however, the process of repair is by the formation of granulation tissue.

The stimulus. Much discussion exists as to the nature of the stimulus for repair. Two factors are probably present. The first is the break in continuity of the tissues. This is invariably followed by immediate activity of the edges. The second is the chemical substances liberated by damaged cells acting as stimuli to the surrounding tissues.

THE HEALING OF WOUNDS

Wounds may be roughly classified into those which are clean, with no loss of tissue and with the edges in apposition, and those which are open and have some tissue loss.

Clean incised wounds. In this case the sharp instrument causing the break in continuity acts as an irritant, and the immediate result is a vaso-dilatation at the edges. The tiny gap is filled by a small number of leucocytes and by tissue fluid. This exudate clots so that the edges of the gap become stuck together with fibrinous material. In the neighbouring tissue, the connective tissue cells multiply and grow out straight across the fibrin to make connection with others from the opposite side. This is immediately followed by a laying down of fibres by the fibroblasts, through a process not yet fully understood. These fibres bind the edges of the wound together. At the same time changes are occurring in the endothelium. Tiny capillary buds are thrown out, these join others and once joined they hollow out to form a lumen through which blood flows from the parent vessels. This tiny quantity of cells and blood vessels closing the gap is known as granulation tissue and may develop within twelve hours of the injury. During the subsequent few days the fibres contract and pull the edges of the wound firmly together. By means of a multiplication of epithelial cells the epithelium grows over the surface. The wound is thus usually completely healed in three or four days, leaving little obvious evidence of recent injury.

Open wounds with tissue loss. As there is loss of substance simple pulling together of the edges by fibres will be insufficient and more tissue must be formed. At first the gap is filled by inflammatory exudate and blood clot. Into this, new capillary loops and fibroblasts grow up from the base of the wound forming a layer of raised red dots known as granulations. Among these granulations will be a considerable number of leucocytes from the new blood vessels and macrophages from the surrounding tissues, their purpose being to resist the invasion of the open surface by micro-organisms. Gradually the wound is filled by granulations from below upwards and the new cells filling up the gap lay down fibres. In time these fibres contract. Eventually, provided the surface remains free from bacteria, epithelium will grow over it from the edges. This epithelium differs from the normal skin because at first it only consists of a layer or two of cells so that it is thin and transparent. It thickens quickly but never quite returns to normal because the special appendages of the skin do not regenerate and the skin covering the surface will have no hairs, sweat or sebaceous glands. As the gap is wider than in the case of clean incised wounds more cells are present, more fibres are formed and more contraction therefore takes place. As contraction continues the cells are flattened and the blood vessels gradually obliterated; thus in the course of three or four weeks the granulation tissue changes to vascular fibrous tissue and from vascular tissue to avascular scar tissue. It is evident that the more destruction and loss of tissue there is, the more scar tissue will eventually be formed. This may then be a serious disadvantage because contracture of the scar may lead to loss of pliability of the tissues and even to deformity. Should a wound become infected and considerable suppuration occur, much destruction of tissue results, and thus considerable quantities of scar tissue will eventuate.

HEALING OF OTHER SOFT TISSUES

Tendons consist of bundles of white fibres with rows of elongated tendon cells between. Healing of damaged tendons takes place in an identical way to that of wounds except that in some cases tendon cells take the place of the more usual fibroblasts. Partial rupture of a tendon leaving only a small gap is followed by the filling of the interval between the torn fibres by blood and inflammatory exudate. This clots, and the clot is then rapidly invaded by new capillary loops and young tendon cells. Thus is a new tendon formed. Complete rupture tends to leave a wider gap which cannot be completely filled by tendon cells, therefore the gap is closed by scar tissue as in the case of the healing of open wounds. In the case of a tendon this is not always a very satisfactory result because, though if left alone scar tissue tends to contract, if constantly subjected to movement it tends to stretch, thus lengthening the tendon and reducing the power of the muscle. Such a result may be prevented by bringing the two ends of the torn tendon together and holding them in a position until union has occurred by the formation of new tendon.

In a minor injury of muscle regeneration of actual muscle cells may take place but in a more severe injury the formation of scar tissue leads to loss of numbers of muscle cells with consequent detriment to its function. Cardiac muscle cells have no power of regeneration and damage must be repaired by fibrous tissue formation. Destroyed nerve tissue within the brain and spinal cord can only be replaced by connective tissue because highly specialised nerve cells have lost their power of regeneration.

REPAIR OF BONE

Here the process of repair is the same but two factors have to be taken into consideration. First, that an injury severe enough to break a bone must inevitably tear the periosteum and damage the soft tissue in the neighbourhood. Second, that the bone and periosteum are richly equipped with special bone-forming cells and many blood vessels. Beneath the torn periosteum the extravasated blood clots and this clot is rapidly invaded by new blood vessels and by fibroblasts from the damaged tissue. Thus in the usual way granulation tissue is formed, building up a soft splint on the external aspect of the damaged bone. The formation of this tissue is stimulated by the irritation of movement at a site where movement does not normally occur. The difference from normal repair by granulation tissue is that this tissue is rapidly invaded by osteoblasts which form bony trabeculae in the granulation tissue, so that scar tissue does not result.

When movement ceases, because the soft callus acts as a splint, the irritation lessens, blood flow returns to normal and under the influence of the osteoblasts, lime and calcium salts are laid down, hardening the callus.

A similar process occurs between the bone ends, but more slowly because less osteoblasts are available and blood vessels have been damaged. At first a mass consisting of spicules of dead bone, cartilage cells and fibrous tissue fills the gap, but gradually this is absorbed by bone-destroying cells and leucocytes, and its place is taken by true granulation tissue growing out from either bone end, eventually to meet and join. In time this too will be infiltrated by bony trabeculae and impregnated with lime and calcium salts.

Identical changes are seen in the surrounding tissues, not always with happy results. Healing of damaged tissue is necessary but much blood and exudate is likely to extravasate into undamaged soft tissue and if not rapidly absorbed will organise into granulation tissue.

RATE OF REPAIR

The rate of repair in the various tissues varies with many different factors. The vascularity of the affected area is an important consideration because a good blood supply is clearly necessary for growth of new tissue. For this reason bone, skin and muscle are usually quick to heal, while cartilage and tendon are comparatively slow. For the same reason the same tissue even may vary in its rate of repair. Thus some part of a bone may have a better blood supply than another part, while in some cases the arterial supply may be damaged at the moment of injury. Measures which aid the blood supply must inevitably aid repair.

Protection of young granulation tissue is another important point. Such tissue is easily damaged and each time its capillaries are ruptured delay in healing occurs. Rupture may easily be the result of excessive movement or, in the case of open wounds, of careless removal of dressings. These are points of which every physiotherapist should be aware. When the granulation tissue growing from either end of fractured bones is likely to meet, avoidance of movement which might rupture the fusing blood vessels is essential.

A third point to consider is the presence or absence of sepsis. Skin will not grow over infected surfaces and delay in healing therefore results from sepsis. Much longer time must elapse in the healing of infected wounds than in the repair of clean surfaces. Age and condition of general health are also factors to be borne in mind.

Chapter II

LOCAL DISTURBANCES OF THE CIRCULATION

DISTURBANCE OF THE FORMATION AND DRAINAGE OF TISSUE FLUID

Many of the degenerative and reactive changes previously described are the result of disturbances occurring in the local circulation. These disturbances will be either deficiency of blood in the area or a local excess. To the first, the term anaemia is applied, and to the second hyperaemia. It will be obvious that the health and function of the tissues will depend on an adequate and an adjustable blood supply, hence local alterations may profoundly affect the well-being of these tissues.

ANAEMIA

Local anaemia may result from many factors. A spasm of arteries, such as might occur if the vasomotor nerves are irritated, will result in a temporary reduction in the blood supply. Disease of the vessel walls bringing about a diminution in the lumen will inevitably cut down the amount of blood. An obstruction within the vessel will have the same effect. This obstruction may be caused by a thrombus within an artery, or by the impaction within it of an embolus. Pressure on the vessels may act as an occluding agent. A slowly growing neoplasm or scar tissue may, for example, exert a constricting force. The actual effect on the tissues depends upon the duration of the anaemia and this in its turn will depend upon the degree of spasm and the ability to establish a good collateral circulation in the area affected. If all the arteries of the area are not affected, then a certain sequence of events takes place. First, a sudden drop in blood pressure occurs in the vessels distal to the block and arterial flow slows, the part affected becoming cold and white. The arteries next constrict in order to raise the pressure and maintain the flow of blood. Metabolites accumulate in the tissues and as these act as vaso-dilators, collateral vessels now dilate so that blood enters them and the area begins to become warmer. In time the dilated vessel walls hypertrophy, showing an increase

c   33

in their muscular and elastic tissue to meet the new circulatory requirements. Little permanent change thus occurs in the affected tissues.

If, on the other hand, a good collateral circulation cannot be established, then the cutting down of arterial blood must of necessity result in degeneration and necrosis. Sometimes the cutting down of the blood supply takes place gradually, possibly as a result of a gradual diminution of the lumen of the vessels, or of arterial spasm or due to the slowly increasing pressure of a tumour, or excessive tissue fluid. Less and less oxygen and nutrient products are delivered to the tissues so that they shrink in size and atrophy occurs. The more highly specialised the cell, the more quickly it is affected by lack of oxygen and food supply, with the result that the highly specialised tissues gradually degenerate, leaving a larger supply of nutrition for the less highly specialised cells and fibres, with consequent increase in their quantity.

HYPERAEMIA

An increased amount of blood in some part of the circulatory system may be passive or active. An active hyperaemia means an increased flow of arterial blood into an area, while a passive hyperaemia supposes a part congested with blood because venous return is in some way obstructed.

Active hyperaemia may be a normal physiological process and is in reality the response of the blood vessels to a local need for extra blood. Every time muscles contract, such a condition occurs. Release of metabolites causes dilatation of arterioles and capillaries, including capillaries not previously patent. The result is a drop in peripheral resistance of the area, and blood pours into the dilated vessels. The ultimate result of such a process is increased oxygen and nutrition.

On the other hand, arterial hyperaemia may be the result of a pathological process. Vessels may dilate as a result of the release of chemical substances by damaged cells and by bacteria, or due to irritation of sensory nerve endings. Such a hyperaemia is seen in all inflammatory conditions and should result in removal of the irritant and repair of damage.

Passive hyperaemia means a condition of venous congestion, and it may be general or local. Since all the blood in the body must pass through the heart and lungs, general venous congestion is met with in some diseases of these organs. A stenosis of the mitral valve, giving rise to difficulty in the passage of blood from auricle to ventricle, results in congestion in the pulmonary and, later, in the systemic circulation. A fibrosis of an area of one or both lungs reduces the capillary bed and so makes it difficult for the right ventricle to pump blood through the pulmonary circulation, resulting in congestion in the systemic veins. Anoxaemia, cyanosis, oedema and structural changes in the tissues are likely to result from such general venous congestion.

Anoxaemia is the result of insufficient aeration of the blood during its passage through the congested or deficient pulmonary capillary bed. All cells and fibres of the body will suffer from an oxygen shortage and their metabolism and function will be impaired.

Cyanosis results from the slowing of the circulation. The slower the blood travels through the capillaries, the more oxygen will be given up to the tissues and the more reduced haemoglobin will be present in the blood. Cyanosis is particularly seen in the more distal parts of the circulation where flow is slowest.

Oedema is the result of a double change. Congestion in the veins brings about a passive dilatation of the capillaries and the blood pressure within them rises; hence greater filtration occurs. At the same time the low oxygen tension results in an increased permeability of the capillary endothelium with the result that plasma proteins and other substances pass through more readily. The osmotic pressure of the tissue fluid rises and fluid is not withdrawn into the capillaries.

Changes in the structure of the tissues inevitably follows decreased oxygenation, fatty and fibrous degeneration being characteristic features.

A local venous congestion is the result of some obstruction and may be sudden or insidious. A sudden obstruction is often the result of a thrombus. Pressure rapidly rises in the veins behind the obstruction with consequent excessive tissue fluid formation. A more gradual obstruction may have comparatively little effect because other vessels returning blood from the same area will dilate and in time a collateral circulation becomes established.

THROMBOSIS

Thrombosis may give rise to anaemia or to local passive hyperaemia and for these reasons it is considered separately.

A thrombus is a solid body formed within the cardiovascular system from the constituents of the blood. It is not entirely dissimilar from a blood clot, differing mainly in that it is formed while the blood is circulating, whereas a clot usually forms when the blood is stationary.

There is still much discussion as to the exact process of coagulation but it is accepted that thrombin, not normally present in the blood stream, acts on one of the plasma proteins, fibrinogen, in such a way as to form a soluble substance fibrin. This forms a meshwork in which the cells of the blood are entangled. The production of thrombin in the normal heart or blood vessels can only occur in the presence of an enzyme thromboplastin. This enzyme causes a reaction between the calcium salts and an inactive precursor of thrombin, thrombogen, both present in normal blood, whereby thrombin is formed. This essential enzyme is liberated from disintegrating blood platelets and tissue cells.

It would appear that three main factors are essential if clotting is to occur in the closed vascular system. These factors are: an alteration in the physical state of the endothelium; a slowing in the blood flow; an increase in the coagulability of the blood.

Physical state of the endothelium. One of the properties of the endothelium is to keep blood unclotted. When the tissue is injured, so that it is no longer smooth, thromboplastin is liberated and platelets, which have a natural tendency to adhere to any rough surface, become adherent. Thrombus formation is then liable to develop. Such changes in the endothelium may be brought about by toxins, by trauma, or by chemical irritants, or may be the result of degenerative changes of known or unknown origin. Whether or not thrombosis actually commences depends very largely on the rate of blood flow. A quick flow, such as occurs in arteries, will rapidly carry away the enzyme and lessen the chance of platelets becoming adherent. If the flow is slow, thrombosis is much more likely to occur.

Slowing of blood flow. This bears a very close relationship to the previous factor. A slow flow gives rises to the possibility of blood platelets and leucocytes falling out of the blood stream and adhering to the vessel wall. If the flow is unduly slow the oxygen tension of the blood will be low and the metabolism of the endothelial cells impaired, consequently it is not unlikely that a slow flow will mean an alteration in the physical state of the lining of the vessels.

The rate of blood flow is most likely to be altered in the veins, in which flow is already slower than in the arteries. Venous flow is markedly inpaired in congestive cardiac failure. It is also affected if the patient is confined to bed as may happen in long medical illnesses or after childbirth or operations. An additional factor may operate in cases of inactivity following operations. Thrombosis is known to develop particularly frequently following abdominal surgery. In these cases there is reflex and voluntary inhibition of the diaphragm, as a result of pain and fear. The diaphragm has a very great effect on venous return and this will, therefore, be markedly reduced in these cases.

Increase in the coagulability of the blood. A sudden rise in the number of blood platelets will markedly increase the tendency to clot. Such a rise is found post-operatively, the number steadily increasing from the second to the tenth day. Diseases of the spleen may have the same effect since one of the functions of this organ is believed to be the control of the number of platelets.

Increase in the viscosity of the blood predisposes towards clotting. This is particularly a danger in congenital cyanotic disease of the heart in which there is a marked rise in the number of erythrocytes.

The presence of thromboplastin in the blood stream will predispose towards clotting if any other factor is also present. After much handling of the tissues as may be necessary in difficult surgical procedures, such a condition will arise.

The actual process of thrombus formation. The first step is the deposit of platelets on the endothelium. These then gradually disintegrate and, in the process, thromboplastin is liberated. Fibrin is therefore formed from the moving blood, provided its flow is not too rapid. A small mass of platelets and fibrin develops. As the fibrin shrinks it squeezes out the serum rich in the enzyme and so more fibrin is formed. Since the natural tendency of platelets is to adhere to any rough surface more platelets are deposited. The white blood cells have a similar tendency and consequently a large mass may be formed, consisting of platelets, white cells and fibrin. A few red cells may find their way into the fibrous network, but these do not have the tendency to adhere and most of them, therefore, are carried on in the blood stream. A thrombus is therefore paler in colour than a true blood clot. Actually a thrombus in the vessels may be complicated by clotting because the thrombus, as it grows in size, will begin to occlude the vessel and relative stagnation of a long column of blood distal to the thrombus will occur. This will then clot in the normal way. A pale thrombosis may then have a red clot as a 'tail'. The final picture is that of a pale thrombus firmly adherent to the endothelium and, extending back from this, a long red blood clot not adherent, except to the thrombus, and moving freely in such circulation as is still present.

The site of thrombus formation. Thrombosis is not a frequent event in the heart or arteries because the flow of blood through them is rapid. Small thrombi do sometimes form on degenerative patches in the endothelium in arterio-sclerosis, and in congestive cardiac failure blood tends to stagnate in the atria and there may, therefore, be almost complete stasis in the appendages in which clotting may occur. A special form of thrombosis is seen in endocarditis, mainly confined to the cusps of the valves. These cusps are inflamed as a result of the action of toxins, considerable roughening develops at the line of apposition of the cusps and platelets tend to become adherent. Since the blood flow is rapid little fibrin is formed and, therefore, small hard masses, firmly adherent and mainly consisting of platelets, gradually form. These are the warty vegetations so often spoken of. Should the condition be a bacterial endocarditis there are many bacteria in the vegetations which are, therefore, softer and more easily broken off.

The commonest site of thrombi is the veins, since here the circulation is slower. Any vein may be involved but those of the legs are most frequently affected. Thrombi which develop in post-operative states, in long illness, and in chronic cardiac failure nearly always develop in either the deep veins of the calves, the femoral vein, just proximal to the entry of the long saphenous, or in the long saphenous vein. Occasionally thrombosis of the subclavian or axillary veins develops following strenuous use of the arm.

Fate of the thrombus. Organisation usually occurs if a thrombus is not infected. Cells and blood vessels grow into it from the vessel wall until eventually it becomes converted into fibrous tissue. Canalisation of the fibrous mass then follows. New blood vessels are formed within it and, as these meet and join, blood flows through them. There is also a tendency for the mass to contract and a larger channel between the thrombus and one wall of the vessel is therefore formed.

If the thrombus is infected by pyogenic organisms it is much softer and more friable. It usually eventually disintegrates and its septic fragments are swept away in the blood stream to set up septic processes elsewhere.

In either case, though it is obviously more common in the latter, the whole or a fragment of the thrombus may become detached forming an embolus and may enter the blood stream. Eventually this will become impacted in a vessel too small to allow it to pass. In this event the effect on the patient depends on the importance and the size of the vessel. Sometimes a long column of blood, which has clotted behind a thrombus, becomes detached, passes in the venous circulation to the right side of the heart and so on into the pulmonary artery, to become impacted at the point of division of the artery with immediate fatal results. Smaller detached fragments may block much smaller vessels with less serious results.

Effects of thrombosis. A small thrombus may have little effect on the circulation while a larger one may partly occlude the vessel. With larger thrombi the result depends very largely on how quickly a satisfactory collateral circulation can be established. In a case of insidious onset of thrombosis of the deep veins of the calf, slight oedema sufficient to mask the extensor tendons on the dorsum of the foot, slight fullness of the superficial veins, tenderness along the course of the vein and pain on stretching the vein may indicate the onset of the lesion. Sudden onset of thrombosis of the femoral vein would cause a rapid oedema extending up to the groin. Such an oedema usually produces arterial spasm and the limb would feel numb and cold. Tenderness would be present over the vein and pain felt in the groin. In axillary thrombosis of insidious onset, oedema gradually develops in the fingers and hand, spreading slowly up the limbs, and the superficial veins of the chest wall and medial side of the arm become distended. The severity of constitutional signs varies. In some cases the temperature and pulse rates are considerably raised, in others they are only slightly elevated. If the thrombus is the result of inflammation or a septic process, the constitutional signs will be more marked.

EMBOLISM

An embolus is a foreign body circulating in the blood stream. When it enters a vessel too small to allow it to pass, it becomes impacted and completely blocks the vessel producing a state of anaemia. Though the embolus is nearly always part or the whole of a detached thrombus, it can be a globule of fat derived from ruptured fat cells or it can be air. In the former case it is a complication of fractures in which the fat, in a liquid form, is released from the ruptured fat cells of the bone marrow and passes into the veins of the cancellous spaces. In the latter case air may enter the blood stream and so reach the heart where it becomes churned up with the blood, forming a frothy mass which interferes with the passage of blood through the heart. Emboli derived from a thrombus most often enter the venous circulation and so reach the right side of the heart to become impacted in the pulmonary circulation. Emboli formed in the left side of the heart may block the coronary or cerebral vessels.

Effect of embolism. Both thrombi and emboli block the vessels but the former usually produce a gradual blocking with a state of chronic anaemia. The effect of the latter is sudden, no time having been allowed for the dilatation of collateral vessels supplying the same area. In this case the result depends upon the presence of collateral vessels and the speed with which they open up. If the embolus impacts in a small vessel with many anastomosing branches, no ill effect may occur. If it obstructs a large vessel, such as the axillary artery, the limb would rapidly become cold, pulseless, cyanotic and oedematous. But warmth and colour would gradually return since blood can reach the limb through the branches of the subclavian artery, and provided these are healthy they will rapidly dilate. There may be some residual effects, but the health of the limb will be maintained. Should the obstruction occur in one of the main cerebral or coronary arteries which are entirely responsible for the nutrition of one area of the brain or heart, that area of tissue must inevitably undergo necrosis and infarction occurs.

INFARCTION

This results from complete obstruction of an artery which forms the sole supply of blood to an area of tissue. Such arteries are known as end arteries and are met with in the cerebral circulation. The cutting off of blood results in rapid death of the tissues. This mass of dead tissue acts as a foreign body and an inflammatory reaction, therefore, occurs around it. In the course of time the dead tissue shrinks and is absorbed and its place is taken by scar tissue.

DISTURBANCE OF THE FORMATION AND DRAINAGE OF TISSUE FLUID

OEDEMA

Oedema is the accumulation of fluid in the cells and fibres of the tissues and in the spaces between them. Its absorption into the cells and fibres renders the part firmer and heavier. Its presence in the tissue spaces gives rise to 'pitting on pressure'. If the area is firmly pressed on by the fingers or thumb, a pit or hollow is left when the fingers are removed; gradually the pit will fill again giving evidence that the swelling is a fluid one and that the fluid is under slight pressure.

NORMAL FORMATION OF TISSUE FLUID

Tissue fluid is formed under the influence of three main factors: hydrostatic pressure, osmotic pressure and the permeability of the capillary walls (see Fig. 1).

Hydrostatic pressure. The blood pressure in the capillaries is higher than the pressure of the tissue fluid, consequently blood plasma filters through the capillary wall into the tissues. At the venous end of the capillary, blood pressure is lower and less filtration therefore occurs.

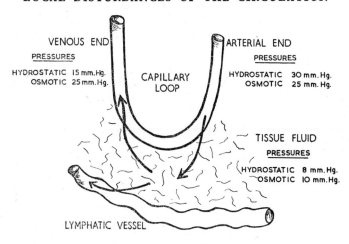

FIG. I. Diagram to illustrate tissue fluid formation and drainage

Osmotic pressure. The osmotic pressure of the blood is largely dependent upon the plasma proteins, particularly upon the serum albumen. The capillary wall is, under normal circumstances, not permeable to these proteins, consequently the osmotic pressure of the capillary blood is greater than that of the tissue fluid. An attractive force is therefore exerted to withdraw the fluid from the tissue space into the venous end of the capillary. At this end of the capillary there is a greater concentration of proteins because fluid has been lost at the arterial end.

Permeability of the capillary wall. The capillary endothelium is permeable to certain substances and not to others. Water, glucose and salts may all pass through, provided they are in greater concentration on one side of the membrane than the other. Plasma proteins cannot normally diffuse through the endothelial cells. This fact tends to keep the osmotic pressure of the blood high and that of the tissue fluid lower. This permeability can be altered. Any factor which brings about dilatation of the capillary will also increase the permeability of its cells, and it is then that plasma proteins may enter the tissue fluid.

Under normal circumstances a balance is kept between the fluid which is formed and that which is absorbed. Fluid passes into the tissues under the influence of the hydrostatic pressure at the arterial end of the capillary and is attracted back under the influence of the osmotic pressure at the venous end of the capillary. The fluid which does not return to the blood filters through into the lymph capillaries under pressure from the tissue fluid. The quantity of fluid varies with rest and exercise. Activity of the muscles brings about vaso-dilatation and increased formation of meta-bolites. Vaso-dilatation results in increased formation of tissue fluid, while increased metabolites may raise the osmotic pressure of the tissue fluid so that the attractive force of the capillary blood is lessened. The stiffness which follows strenuous exercise is the result of increased fluid in the tissue space.

FACTORS RESPONSIBLE FOR OEDEMA

Alteration in any or all of the three factors will result in excessive tissue fluid formation. As the lymph vessels also help to carry away tissue fluid, any obstruction in the lymphatic drainage will have the same effect.

Increase in hydrostatic pressure. This will, if it is sufficiently prolonged, cause oedema. It is usually not the only cause, since a rise in hydrostatic pressure in the capillaries means a disturbance of the circulation with change in the endothelium and increased permeability. A rise in hydrostatic pressure may be the result of general or local factors. If the heart fails to maintain a normal circulation there will be congestion in the veins and hydrostatic pressure will rise in the capillaries. Increased filtration will, therefore, occur. An obstruction in a large vein will have exactly the same effect though it will be localised to the area which is drained by that vein.

Fall in osmotic pressure. This will lessen the attractive force exerted by the blood and fluid will tend to accumulate in the tissues. A fall in the osmotic pressure may be the result of one type of kidney disease which results in a greater quantity of plasma proteins being lost through the kidney, or it may arise because the permeability of the capillary wall is increased and proteins are permitted to pass into the tissue spaces. This may arise in kidney disease; it will also occur in cardiac disease and in conditions in which the capillary endothelium is damaged.

The plasma proteins may also be deficient, as a result of starvation, and a nutritional oedema may develop.

Increased capillary permeability. Trauma or nutritional disturbances may alter the permeability of the endothelium. A capillary reacts to irritation not only by dilating but also by changes in the endothelial lining. A great quantity of fluid may enter the tissues as a result of this factor both in severe lacerations and in burns. Any factor which disturbs the nutrition of the cells will also increase their permeability. If the blood is circulating unduly slowly, it loses oxygen and gains more than the normal carbon dioxide. This disturbs the physical state of the endothelium and tissue

42

fluid increases. Oedema will therefore occur, not only following trauma but also in all cases of venous congestion.

Lymphatic obstruction. Tissue fluid may be formed normally but its drainage may be impaired, either because it is not adequately absorbed into the venous end of the capillary because hydrostatic pressure is too high or osmotic pressure too low, or because the lymph channels are blocked. Lymph vessels may be blocked by the action of parasites, as a result of inflammation, by pressure of tumours or scar tissue, or as a result of surgical stripping. Lymphatic glands into which the lymph vessels drain may themselves be involved, either as a result of disease processes such as carcinoma or because their removal is a surgical necessity.

EFFECTS OF OEDEMA

Oedema is closely related to general or local disturbance in the circulation, since it is either caused by circulatory disturbance or it brings it about.

The presence of extensive oedema is liable to set up an arterial spasm and so cause an anaemic condition of the area. If it fails to do this, it causes anaemia because, as the hydrostatic pressure of the tissue fluid rises, pressure is exerted on the capillaries and arterial inflow is retarded.

Persistent fluid in the tissue spaces interferes with the nutrition of the cells since fresh nutrient substances and gases are not available and waste products are not removed; metabolism is, therefore, seriously impaired.

Atrophy, loss of tone and elasticity, and defective resistance and healing properties must all inevitably result. The function of the area is therefore impaired.

In the course of time, the fluid will tend to organise into fibrous tissue and the area becomes indurated and hardened. The speed with which this occurs depends upon the characteristics of the oedema fluid. If it contains a high percentage of protein it will clot readily. This condition exists when the fluid is largely the result of increased capillary permeability and is less likely when the major factor in its formation is either raised hydrostatic pressure or low osmotic pressure. Should the fluid clot, it forms a mass foreign to the tissues and they will react by proliferation. Cells and blood vessels invade the clotted fluid and it gradually becomes converted into fibrous tissue. This may have serious results because the fibrous tissue tends to shrink. As it shrinks it may obliterate blood vessels, so causing anaemia and gross disturbance in local nutrition. It may, if it has occurred in the periarticular structures, cause gross limitation of movement in joints. Should the fluid have invaded muscles, pliability and extensibility will be impaired. Muscular contraction may be seriously hampered by the presence of scar tissue. Should oedema occur in serous membranes, adhesions may form resulting in interference with the movements of the underlying organs.

In addition to all these ill-effects, the presence of fluid distending the tissue spaces is a source of permanent discomfort and annoyance to the patient.

TYPES OF OEDEMA

Oedema occurs in many different conditions; often, therefore, a special name is used to indicate the type. Cardiac, renal and starvation oedema are examples of a generalised oedema. Local oedema is probably more common, and traumatic, obstructive, paralytic, and oedema due to poor muscle tone and laxity of fascia are illustrations of this type. In each, one or other of the factors previously discussed are responsible.

Cardiac oedema. While largely due to the rise in hydrostatic pressure in the capillaries, following failure of the heart to maintain a normal circulation, it may also be due to the low oxygen tension in the blood causing increased permeability of the capillary walls. The fluid formed has, therefore, a high protein content and will clot and organise. Until it clots it will pit on pressure.

The oedema of this type is found first in the periphery where circulation is the slowest, and it tends to gather in the most dependent areas. If the patient is up it will be seen therefore in the feet and around the ankles, gradually spreading up the legs. If the patient is in bed it will be seen also in the abdomen and sacral region. The quantity of fluid is always greatest at night, when the heart is tired, and least in the morning.

Renal oedema. This is the result of either a drop in osmotic pressure or a decrease in capillary permeability according to the disease affecting the kidney. In the first case the fluid will have a low specific gravity since its protein content is small; in the second case the protein content and, therefore, the specific gravity will be high. Since this oedema does not depend on venous congestion and slowing of the circulation it will not collect in the periphery nor will it be worse at night. It is often noticeable in the face, particularly in the lax tissue around the eyes, and is worse in the morning; it tends to be dispersed during the day by muscular action.

Starvation oedema. This is probably partly the result of a drop in the osmotic pressure of the blood as a result of a deficiency of proteins, partly due to nutritional disturbances of the endothelium resulting in increasing permeability, and partly to decreased heart action and slowing of the circulation.

Traumatic oedema. One of the most serious results of extensive burns is the great loss of fluid into the tissues. In a lesser degree this is also seen in injuries such as extensive lacerations, fractures and dislocations. Various factors enter into this type of oedema. Local hydrostatic pressure rises because the irritation of the sensory nerve endings and the release of a histamine-like substance brings about extensive vaso-dilatation and hyper-aemia. The injury also causes great increase in the permeability of the dilated capillaries. Lymphatic vessels and veins are also injured and possibly thrombosed with interference with the drainage of tissue fluid. Drainage is also impaired because damage usually implies diminished function, and the pumping effect on these soft-walled vessels of the muscular contractions and joint movements is either reduced or lost.

The fluid formed has a very high protein content and clots and organises readily. For this reason the final effects on the area may be serious if care is not taken.

Obstructive oedema. This develops if either venous or lymphatic obstruction occurs. This may be the result of deep venous thrombosis, lymphangitis, pressure of scars or tumours or removal of lymph glands and vessel. In a condition such as phlegmasia alba dolens (white leg) femoral thrombosis and chronic inflammation of the lymph vessels are probably both responsible. The oedema following radical mastectomy is an illustration of obstructive oedema which may be due to removal of lymph glands or to pressure by axillary scar tissue. The presence of fluid is mainly due to a rise in hydrostatic pressure and the fluid will have a low protein content and will clot only slowly. Nevertheless in the course of time it will organise.

Paralytic oedema. Oedema tends to result from muscular paralysis provided the vaso-dilators are not paralysed. In the latter case the vaso-constrictors are overactive and a cold limb results rather than oedema. When oedema occurs it is the result of either paralysis of the vaso-constrictors causing wide-spread vaso-dilatation, congestion and increased filtration, or it may be the result of decreased function and loss of the pumping effect normally exerted on the veins and lymphatics. If the circulation is slowed as a result of either or both of these factors, the oxygen tension of the blood will fall and the capillaries will therefore become more permeable. The fluid is likely to have a high protein content and will readily organise.

Oedema due to poor muscle tone and laxity of fascia. In the erect position, venous blood from the legs and abdomen has to return to the heart against the force of gravity. It would therefore have a tendency to stagnate in these regions if it were not for certain factors. In the first place, the deep fascia of the lower extremity is particularly strong and extensive and acts as a kind of elastic stocking to support the veins. Many of the muscles either insert directly into this fascia or send expansions to reinforce it. The fascia is, therefore, affected either by prolonged recumbency or by immobilisation of the limb in a rigid support since the muscles inserting into it will become weaker and hypotonic and the fascia will become less tense.

In the second place the tone of the muscles of the legs and abdominal wall plays a very important part in the prevention of 'pooling' of blood, thus any factor which causes decrease in tone may lead to venous congestion. Thirdly, the vaso-motor mechanism causes an increase in the tone of the veins when the posture is changed from lying to standing, but if this mechanism has not been fully in use for a period of time, then, when it is required, it does not act as effectively as it should. Oedema, therefore, tends to occur when a patient first gets up after a long period in bed, particularly if the illness has been one, such as rheumatoid arthritis, in which the muscles have been directly affected and their strength and tone reduced. It will also develop when a plaster splint has been removed after a prolonged period of immobilisation. In each case the inadequately constricted or supported vessels tend to dilate, venous congestion develops and excess tissue fluid is formed, partly under the influence of a raised hydrostatic pressure and partly as a result of increased capillary permeability. The fluid will have a relatively high protein content and will clot readily.

Idiopathic oedema. There are a few people in whom oedema tends to develop without known cause. This is an hereditary oedema which has certain peculiar features. It affects women mainly and may involve one or both legs. No treatment appears to be effective. It causes no outstanding symptoms but it brings about an unsightly thickening of the legs.

Chapter III

ATROPHY AND HYPERTROPHY.
HYPOPLASIA AND HYPERPLASIA

Alteration in the size of individual cells and fibres or of an organ as a whole is not uncommonly seen. Such alteration in size is invariably accompanied by alterations in function and in many cases, though not in all, is the result of disturbance of nutrition. For any cell or fibre to maintain its normal size once it reaches full development, it must carry out its normal function, its metabolism must continue undisturbed and its nervous connections must remain intact. It follows that disturbance of any one of these factors may cause increase or decrease in size. In addition such factors as the influence of toxins, the effect of the secretion of ductless glands and interference with the blood supply must all be considered.

ATROPHY

This is diminution in size of tissues. If the term is applied to muscles or organs it refers to the specialised elements and not to the supporting framework, although in certain cases the connective tissue may increase at the same rate or even faster than the atrophy of the histological cells. This increase of interstitial structures may be explained by the fact that the atrophied cells and fibres are probably receiving and using less nutrient products and oxygen and more are therefore available for the less specialised tissue.

Probably one of the commonest causes of atrophy is diminished function. It is often seen in limbs which have been immobilised for a period of time. This atrophy is due to impaired katabolism since it is a well-known fact that decreased katabolic processes mean decreased anabolism and therefore decrease in size. Disuse atrophy, as this type is usually called, is seen not only in muscles but also in other tissues which have lost their function, such as the ovaries after the menopause. Injuries and disease of joints are almost invariably accompanied by rapid and severe atrophy of the muscles acting on the affected joint. Such atrophy is usually much more profound

47

than could possibly be accounted for by disuse. The probable explanation is that either sympathetic fibres are disturbed and nutrition consequently impaired, or that reflex atrophy is the result of irritation of sensory nerve endings and so messages pass to the spinal cord and thus to the lateral and anterior horns of grey matter resulting in inhibition of activity of the cells. Atrophy is also seen in circulatory disturbances. A slow progressive diminution in the lumen of the main vessels of a limb means gradual cutting down of the nutrition to all the tissues of that part and all specialised cells and fibres consequently shrink in size. Involvement of skin, muscles, joint structures and bone is seen in advanced arterio-sclerosis and Buerger's disease. Continuous pressure is responsible for atrophy, partly because it reduces the blood supply to the part and partly because it impairs function and so katabolism. The presence of a tumour is liable to lead to atrophy of the tissue on which it grows.

In disease of the lower motor neurone atrophy will be present in all structures supplied either by the damaged neurones or by any other nerve fibres running with them. Several explanations arise for this: in the first place since no nerve impulses can reach the motor-end plate there can be no muscle tone or power of contraction and the result is abolition of katabolic processes with consequent atrophy of muscle fibres. In the second place, the vaso-constrictor fibres running with the motor fibres are also liable to be involved and if this occurs paralytic vaso-dilatation results in circulatory stasis and impairment of nutrition to all the structures in the region. Such atrophy is serious because it is likely to continue over a long period and will therefore be followed by degeneration of the tissues and permanent impairment of function.

Most cases of atrophy are local but a generalised atrophy is seen in chronic starvation and in fevers. In the latter case the toxins stimulate protein metabolism and a rapid wasting takes place particularly in the muscles. It is probably also partly the result of impaired digestion and absorption.

Effects of Atrophy. The primary effect of atrophy is decreased function. In the case of muscular tissue power depends on number and size of fibres. While atrophy does not normally affect the number it does affect size and therefore muscle power is markedly reduced as a result of atrophy. In addition atrophy may mean loss of elasticity which is particularly seen in the skin and may lead to limitation of function.

HYPERTROPHY

This is the increase in size of the specialised elements of a tissue. Increase in the quantity of the connective tissue such as is seen in some types of muscular dystrophy is not true hypertrophy. This change in size is always the result of increased functional demands except in those cases which are the result of overactivity of the ductless glands. An increased functional demand means increased katabolism, consequently increased building up and so increase in the size of fibres. It may be physiological or pathological. Physiological hypertrophy is not associated with disease, it is well illustrated in the case of the pregnant uterus or in the muscles of the athlete. The muscular tissue in either case is called upon to do extra work and hypertrophy results. Pathological hypertrophy, as its name implies, is associated with disease. An example of such an occurrence is seen in hypertrophy of the heart. Stenosis of the mitral valve hinders the flow of blood from the left auricle and the result is an increase in the breadth and length of its fibres. A similar hypertrophy may be seen in the involuntary muscular coat of the stomach in stenosis of the pyloric sphincter. It is well to realise that there is a limit to the amount to which any cell can hypertrophy and when this point is reached either hyperplasia results or the functional demand fails to be met. Pathological hypertrophy is sometimes compensatory. One group of cells and fibres enlarges to take over the work which should be done by damaged or lost tissue. This may be seen in one lobe of a lung when the other lobes have been removed or in one kidney when the other becomes diseased and fails to function.

A different illustration of hypertrophy is seen in diseases of the pituitary gland in the adult when hyperfunction results in enlargement of the girth of the bone and in thickening of the connective tissues throughout the body.

Effects of Hypertrophy. With the exception of the last type of hypertrophy increased size means increased function. Hypertrophied muscles have always greater power than normal muscles, provided that it is the whole muscle which is hypertrophied and not only a few groups of its fibres.

HYPOPLASIA AND HYPERPLASIA

These should not be confused with atrophy and hypertrophy. The latter terms invariably refer to size, the former to number or quantity. Hypoplasia and hyperplasia most commonly occur before the tissues have reached maturity and are then developmental defects often of unknown origin. Hypoplasia means a decreased number of cells or fibres and may be the result of disturbance of the ductless glands controlling growth and development, such as is seen in the pituitary dwarf. Hyperplasia is an increase in the number of cells and fibres either the result of increased activity of ductless glands during the period of growth, or the result of increased functional demands which cannot be entirely met by hypertrophy. Hyperplasia of bone marrow very readily occurs on a demand for increased blood; division of liver cells results in hyperplasia of the liver if a section of that organ is surgically removed. It is possible that some hyperplasia of cardiac muscle tissue may take place but it is not a feature of voluntary muscle cells.

Chapter IV

PRINCIPLES OF TREATMENT BY PHYSIOTHERAPY OF INFLAMMATION AND OEDEMA

INFLAMMATION

A very great proportion of conditions treated by the physiotherapist are inflammatory in origin and a clear understanding of the principles of treatment is therefore essential.

ACUTE INFLAMMATION

The changes of acute inflammation occur for a very definite purpose and should not be impeded. The first great principle of treatment therefore *is rest*. If the affected area is allowed to rest, nature will perform her function. Movement and handling at this stage simply increase the irritation so that the various changes are exaggerated and cannot fulfil their purpose. Rest may be gained in various ways according to the site of the lesion. The patient may be confined to bed, the limb may be splinted or the upper extremity may be supported in a sling. The main requirement is support so that movement does not occur and muscle spasm is avoided.

On the other hand absolute rest must not be maintained for too long because, if the circulation is slowed by diminished movement, absorption of exudate is reduced and organisation into fibrous tissue is then likely. The second principle of treatment is therefore *maintenance of normal circulation in the part affected*. This principle should be considered as soon as the height of inflammation is reached. At this stage, the purpose of the inflammatory change having been gained, resolution can be aided by promoting rapid absorption and preventing organisation. Circulation, and, therefore, absorption, can be aided by many different measures, but the simplest and most effective are the application of the constant current, electrical stimulation, and active exercise. No great range of movement is necessary to obtain these objects. If, for example, tearing of muscle fibres precludes early movement of the joint on which the muscle works, rhythmic contractions of the muscle in whatever support is being used, together with vigorous movements of other joints, will stimulate the circulation and prevent the sticky exudate from turning into fibrous tissue. In the case of an inflamed joint where movements might still be contra-indicated, tendons may be kept moving in their sheaths and the circulation be kept free in the joint structures by minimal faradic contractions using just sufficient current to produce movement of the muscle fibres, and pressure and relaxation on the blood and lymph vessels without producing movement at the joint.

In very severe trauma excessive changes tend to occur and blood from ruptured vessels may be added to the inflammatory exudate. In this excessive exudate and haemorrhage lies a danger—the blood and lymph vessels may be quite incapable of removing the extravasated fluid. If seen at once, steps may be taken to prevent this state of affairs, and *a third principle is the prevention of excessive exudate and bleeding.* Putting the part at rest immediately partly fulfils this principle; some measure to stop haemorrhage and constrict vessels may also help. Cold compresses, pressure bandages or evaporating lotions are suitable means.

In acute inflammation, particularly affecting joint structures, atrophy of muscle occurs very rapidly. *It is essential to keep the atrophy as slight as possible* because the first line of defence of the joint will be impaired if muscles are weak and atrophied. Because of its origin it is impossible to prevent all atrophy, yet muscles may be maintained in a reasonable condition by massage and active exercises. Both measures are used with care, and massage is omitted and exercises are rapidly increased as inflammation subsides.

From the physiotherapist's point of view, four main principles therefore stand out in the treatment of any acute inflammatory condition. They are: rest, prevention of excessive exudate, promotion of rapid absorption and prevention of organisation of exudate, and maintenance of muscle bulk and tone. It is immaterial whether the inflammation is that of a joint, as in rheumatoid arthritis, or an inflammation of fibrous tissue as in acute fibrositis, or of an organ as in pneumonia, the same principles apply, difference existing only in their method of application.

CHRONIC INFLAMMATION

As in the acute case, the physiotherapist must consider the changes which have occurred. The capsule or synovial membrane or other tissues may be thickened by the formation of new fibrous tissue; there may be anaemia, as permanently dilated vessels become thickened and blood-flow stagnates; part of the tissue may be adherent. As a result of these changes, movement is probably limited and muscles in the region grossly atrophied. The main objects of treatment can be clearly gathered from these facts. It is necessary to soften the indurated area and separate out the adherent tissues, to stretch the contracting fibrous tissues and to stretch or break down fibrous bands where they exist. In addition muscles must be brought back to their normal strength. The *first principle is to revascularize the area.* If a really acute hyperaemia can be produced some absorption of exudate not yet fully organised may occur. The tissues will be softened and relaxed and stretching made much easier. Revascularization of a localised area may be produced in many ways. Sometimes an injection of a local anaesthetic may be used; this will overcome vaso-spasm by paralysis of vaso-constrictor fibres and so will promote a hyperaemia. An even greater effect may be obtained by following the injection by the application of really deep frictions. Deep massage alone will prove effective.

These measures are most successful in such conditions as chronic bursitis or chronic non-tubercular teno-synovitis, and fibrositis. Stable galvanism, histamine or renotin ionisation or a strong dose of ultra-violet light can also be used to produce local hyperaemia, and are particularly effective if the thickened area is superficial, and a counter-irritant effect is desired.

Alternatively, some form of deep heating, such as long, or short-wave diathermy will be useful to increase the deep circulation.

The second principle is to follow the revascularisation by a deliberate attempt *to separate out, stretch and even break up the fibrous strands.* The best possible means of doing this is to apply deep transverse frictions and follow by passive manipulations, or, where suitable, strong faradism and vigorous active exercises.

If the chronic inflammation has resulted in muscle atrophy it is *essential to improve the condition of the muscle.* If muscles are in a very poor condition, faradism may be used to show the patient how to use his muscles, active contractions may then be combined with the faradism and very soon active work will replace electrical stimulation. Exercise may be quickly progressed and continued until the muscle condition equals that of the same group of the opposite limb.

SUPPURATIVE INFLAMMATION

It is well to remember that pus formation means destruction of tissue, and destroyed tissue must eventually be replaced, to a great extent at least, by scar tissue, with resultant alteration in function of the part. The great essential, therefore, where suppuration has occurred, is to limit as far as possible the production of pus and destruction of tissue, so that less fibrous tissue formation takes place.

The first principle of treatment, once the condition is established, is *to destroy micro-organisms and prevent their multiplication.* Destruction may be attempted by means of chemotherapy (that is the use of substances such as penicillin which destroy bacteria without devitalizing body tissues), by keeping septic surfaces clean; and by promoting free drainage of pus. If pus is allowed to escape easily, less pressure in abscess cavities will occur, less toxic absorption will take place and less destruction of tissue will eventuate. Destruction of bacteria and cleansing of surfaces may be aided by the use of short-wave therapy, ultra-violet rays and zinc ionisation. Once this principle has been fulfilled and free drainage is established, the next step is *to encourage rapid healing and to prevent contracture of fibrous tissue.* The promotion of a good blood supply will do much to promote rapid healing, and this can be aided by the use of infra-red or ultra-violet rays. Provided free drainage is present, circulation will be aided and fibrous contractures prevented by the use of small range, gentle, active movements, taking aseptic precautions in any necessary handling of the area.

Stiff joints are one of the complications of suppurative inflammation because circulation is impaired by the necessity for resting the part, and by the action of the toxins on the vessel walls. Oedema is also not an uncommon feature. A further principle of treatment is therefore *to prevent limited movement in joints.* Elevation of the part, and early active movements will relieve oedema and prevent joint stiffness. They can be commenced as soon as drainage is established. If the patient is being treated by saline baths the movements may well be carried out in the bath.

As in chronic inflammation, muscle atrophy is likely to be severe, and should be lessened by the measures taken to promote circulation and prevent stiff joints.

Later, when suppuration ceases, wounds are healed, and destroyed tissue has been replaced, massage may be used to soften and stretch fibrous tissue and loosen scars and keep them supple and free.

One principle applies to all types of inflammation—*the restoration of normal function.* Tissues may be pliable and elastic, joints may possess a full range of movement, perfect healing of ulcers and sinuses may have occurred and muscle tone and bulk may be normal, and yet the patient is unable to use his limb correctly. The lack may be partly mental, in that the patient is unable to realise that the part of the body is now organically sound. It is often due to a lack of co-ordination, the damaged structure not having learnt to fit in with healthy structures. This must be put right before the rehabilitation of the patient is considered complete.

OEDEMA

The treatment of oedema depends upon the type. General oedema is rarely treated by physical measures. In these cases the treatment is medical, and if the heart lesion or the kidney disease can be alleviated oedema is likely to disappear. Occasionally a case of cardiac oedema is met with by the physiotherapist, when the main object is to hasten the absorption of fluid by the lymphatic vessels and so give the patient temporary relief from discomfort until such time as the production of excessive fluid ceases. This oedema will be treated on the same lines as obstructive oedema but with particular precautions owing to the cardiac condition.

Local oedema more commonly presents itself for physical treatment and a careful consideration of the type must first be made.

TRAUMATIC OEDEMA

If the trauma is extensive some oedema is almost inevitable. The main principle of treatment is, therefore, the prevention of organisation into fibrous tissue. Efforts must be made to decrease the formation of the tissue fluid, to speed its absorption and to keep it moving so that it cannot clot. Less fluid will be formed if rest and firm support are given. To increase the speed with which the fluid is absorbed it is necessary to encourage its movement into areas in which the veins and lymphatics have not been damaged and to speed the flow of venous blood and lymph in these regions. Such measures such as superficial heat and massage to the region proximal to the injury will assist. Elevation of the limb is essential and, in this position rhythmic muscular contractions will press the fluid out of the tissue spaces. Provided the skin is intact and there is no fear of haemorrhage the depletive effect of anodal galvanism will help to move the fluid. In order to prevent clotting of the exudate it must be kept moving and rhythmic contractions are of the utmost importance. If these are difficult to obtain, minimal faradic contractions may be used temporarily. In nearly every case, functional use of the limb can be encouraged early, so stimulating the tissue drainage and preventing organisation.

OBSTRUCTIVE OEDEMA

The excess fluid in this case is the result of obstruction in the venous or lymphatic vessels, or in both. Whether or not the oedema will subside, depends upon how well the unobstructed vessels will dilate to do the work of the obstructed ones. The principle underlying the use of physical means is, therefore, the attempt to encourage the development of a good collateral circulation. Any measures which press the fluid out of the tissue spaces and force it proximally are likely to assist. Faradism under pressure, strong muscle contractions followed by relaxation, and kneadings given with deep pressure and relaxation are all effective. With the limb elevated, the fluid will be mechanically pushed on by slow, deep effleurage and vigorous active movements which press the fluid on in the veins and lymphatics. Regurgitation is prevented by the presence of valves.

In these cases of obstructive oedema the condition is sometimes a long-standing one and some of the tissue fluid may have organised into firm fibrous tissue which by pressure has further impeded the circulation. Special measures are then needed to soften this tissue. Any physical means which floods the tissue with blood and stretches it will be valuable; thus histamine or renotin ionisation and really deep massage may be used.

PARALYTIC OEDEMA

Since the excess fluid is the result of vaso-dilatation and lack of use, it is difficult to prevent its formation. Its continual dispersion and movement to prevent clotting are, therefore, essential. Unlike traumatic oedema this cannot be carried out by the use of rhythmic contractions and active movements. Passive means are therefore necessary. Elevation of the part is helpful. Artificial exercise of the paralysed muscles by means of the interrupted galvanic current will exert a pumping effect on the veins and lymphatics and will keep the tissue fluid moving. Passive movements of joints will have the same effect. Light massage is sometimes effective in dispersing the fluid into regions not affected by the paralysis, but care must be used not to increase the paralytic vaso-dilatation nor to bruise nor stretch the atonic muscle fibres.

OEDEMA DUE TO POOR MUSCLE TONE AND LAXITY OF THE FASCIA

Since the oedema is the result of lack of muscle tone and poor condition of fascia, the principle of treatment by physiotherapy is to bring back to normal the strength and tone of the musculature. This can be carried out by the use of maximal resisted exercises. During the time taken to bring the muscles and fascia back to normal, constant seeping of fluid into the tissues should be lessened by repeated elevation of the limb and by firm pressure in the form of Viscopaste or elastic bandages. Such fluid as does form must not be allowed to organise and measures such as those used in obstructive oedema are of value.

In all cases of oedema it is worth noting that the vessels in the region of the oedema should not be encouraged to dilate since this results in increased filtration. However, dilatation of vessels which are not always patent is desirable in areas proximal to the oedema. For this reason it is wiser to avoid the use of heat directly over the area. The immersion of an oedematous hand or foot in hot paraffin wax usually increases the tension in the tissues. Similarly the use of hot baths is unwise. If these are used for the legs they also mean that the treatment is being carried out in the dependent position. If, as a result of oedema and arterial spasm, the limb is cold and blue, heat can be given to the trunk; the limb is then indirectly warmed without increasing the oedema.

PART TWO

RHEUMATIC AFFECTIONS

Chapter I

CLASSIFICATION. RHEUMATOID TYPE OF ARTHRITIS

EXAMINATION OF THE PATIENT

CLASSIFICATION

From time to time many different classifications of rheumatic diseases have been drawn up, their very number indicating the difficulty which exists in arriving at a satisfactory grouping. Classification is not uncommonly undertaken according to the cause of the local signs and symptoms. Occasional cases of arthritis are due to infection by micro-organisms. Tuberculous joints, streptococcal, pneumococcal, gonococcal and dysenteric arthritis, as well as the arthritis seen in abortus fever, fall into this category. In the common forms of arthritis such as rheumatoid arthritis, ankylosing spondylitis and Still's disease, however, the cause is still quite unknown.

In the other common form of arthritis—osteo-arthritis—age, trauma, obesity and skeletal deformity play their part, but not all the causal factors are known, while in gout we see an arthritis which is the product of a general disturbance of purine metabolism in which heredity is the most important factor, though dietary and alcoholic excesses also play a part.

The method of classification given below is that proposed by the committee on nomenclature appointed by the Royal College of Physicians in 1936. (See Copeman, *Textbook of the Rheumatic Diseases*, page 11, Livingstone, 1955.)

1. ACUTE RHEUMATISM (Synonym: rheumatic fever) and *Subacute rheumatism.*

2. NON-ARTICULAR RHEUMATISM (Synonyms: fibrositis, myalgia). This group includes bursitis, panniculitis and, possibly, neuritis; also regional terms, such as lumbago, sciatica and pleurodynia.

3. GOUT, acute and chronic.

4. CHRONIC ARTHRITIS.

    (a) RHEUMATOID TYPE (Synonym: 'atrophic'). In its classical form it affects mostly women, often of the asthenic type. A polyarthritis, generally starting in the smaller joints of the extremities and travelling centripetally. General health is profoundly affected. The pathology is of an inflammatory nature and ankylosis common.

        i. *Unknown etiology.* This includes the classical type of rheumatoid arthritis of young women, and also Still's disease in children.

        ii. *Known etiology.* This includes all forms of infective arthritis, e.g. gonococcal, dysenteric; also sometimes cases of metabolic origin.

    (b) OSTEO-ARTHRITIC TYPE (Synonym: 'hypertrophic' and degenerative). Common in men. Generally monarticular, affecting larger weight-bearing joints. General health, blood tests, etc., unaffected. Pathology principally of degenerative nature—osteophyte formation, never ankylosis.

        i. *Unknown etiology.* This includes the so-called senile variety, e.g. malum coxae senilis.

        ii. *Known etiology.* This includes trauma; may be secondary to congenital joint deformity or other joint disease; central nervous disease—arthropathy.

    c) *Spondylitis* is also divisible into these two main types, the rheumatoid type being termed ankylosing spondylitis, and the osteo-arthritic type being termed spondylitis osteo-arthritica.

    '*Villus arthritis*', by which is meant a proliferation of the synovium and villi of the knee joints, in women at or around the climacteric, may ultimately either develop into rheumatoid or the osteo-arthritis type of arthritis—in most cases the latter.

No attempt will be made in this brief section to describe in detail all the conditions set out in this classification. Acute rheumatism is rarely treated by physical means. Many years after the attack, the physiotherapist may be asked to treat a patient suffering from congestive cardiac failure, the late result of the effect of acute rheumatism on the valves of the heart; this will, therefore, be dealt with in Part V. The conditions most often reaching the physiotherapy department—rheumatoid arthritis, osteo-arthritis, ankylosing spondylitis, and non-articular rheumatism—will be discussed here and a few of the main points in relation to some of the other conditions mentioned.

RHEUMATOID ARTHRITIS

The onset of rheumatoid arthritis is most common between the ages of forty and sixty, and it attacks women more often than men. The actual mode of onset varies from patient to patient. In a small percentage the disease comes on suddenly with an acute febrile illness and pain flitting from joint to joint. In the great majority of cases the onset is insidious. The symptoms are those of pain and stiffness. Often at this stage there may be no objective evidence of the disease process. Gradually swelling, deformity and restriction of movement develop. The small joints of the body are most commonly involved at first. Often the proximal interphalangeal joints of the fingers are first attacked. Gradually the disease involves the metacarpo-phalangeal, intercarpal and wrist joints and later the joints of the forearm, elbow and shoulder. Similarly the joints of the lower extremity may be involved. The temporo-mandibular joints and joints of the cervical spine are sometimes also affected. The hip joints, sacro-iliac joints and joints of the thoracic and lumbar spine are rarely attacked. The condition is almost always bilateral, though occasionally symmetrical.

There is no known cause for this disease.

CHANGES IN JOINTS

Changes in the joint structures often, though not always, progress through three stages.

Stage I. The synovial membrane becomes inflamed and is, therefore, hyperaemic and infiltrated by inflammatory cells. The secreting cells become more active and the result is an oedematous membrane and effusion into the joint cavity. Inflammation tends to spread to involve the periarticular soft tissues, the capsule, ligaments, tendon sheaths and bursae. These changes are reversible and if the disease is arrested at this stage it is possible for the joint to return to normal. This does often occur, though it is no criterion that the inflammation will not flare up again at a later date.

Stage II. If the disease progresses, granulation tissue is formed within the synovial membrane and periarticular structures. It tends to spread from the membrane over the periphery of the articular cartilage. The cartilage, now covered by this tissue, gradually thins and disintegrates, leaving areas of bone covered only by granulations. Sometimes granulation tissue invades the bone ends from the remains of the perichondrium and from the tissue growing in over the cartilage. Much decalcification of bone occurs, probably due to the hyperaemic condition around the bone ends.

With the destruction of articular cartilage and filling of the joint with granulation tissue, irreversible changes have occurred, but good function can still be obtained unless further progression develops.

Stage III. The granulation tissue gradually becomes organised into fibrous tissue and thus the soft tissues are matted together, with adhesions forming between the tendons and the capsule and between the articular surfaces. Contractures develop and deformity and gross limitation of movement result. In such joints the articular surfaces may be partly covered with cartilage and partly with fibrous tissue, giving rise to much irregularity, or they may be completely joined by fibrous tissue or even by bone. Where such changes have occurred, little improvement in function can be expected.

ARTICULAR SIGNS AND SYMPTOMS

Joints in which some or all of these changes have developed will show certain characteristic features. Pain and tenderness, swelling, limitation of movement, muscle atrophy and deformity are all to be expected, though they will occur in differing degrees according to the severity of the changes.

Pain is present in all three stages. In the first stage it is often continuous, and since several joints may be affected the patient's life may be a misery unless the pain is medically controlled. Movement increases the pain, hence joints tend to be held rigid. In the second stage, pain is often less noticeable at rest but is marked on movement or weight-bearing, so that if the knees or ankles are involved walking is a real difficulty. In the third stage, when inflammation has subsided and fibrous tissue has formed, there is usually no pain at rest and only on movement when the fibrous tissue is stretched and a pull is, therefore, exerted on sensitive tissues.

Tenderness will always be present when there is any active inflammation in the joint. It can be elicited by gentle pressure of the joint and by palpation along the joint line. The degree of the tenderness is a good indication of the activity of the arthritis. When the inflammation has subsided there may still be tenderness but this is localised and not on pressure of the joint. It is felt over structures which are being persistently irritated

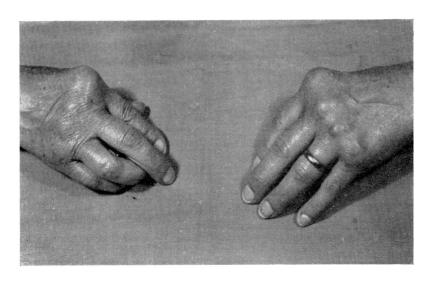

PLATE I. RHEUMATOID ARTHRITIS
(a) Showing deformity of hands

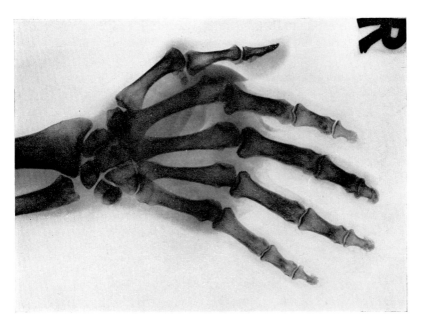

(b) X-ray photograph of same patient

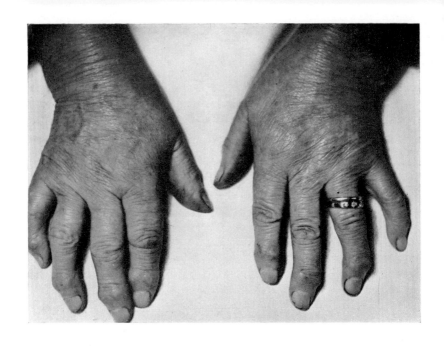

PLATE II. (a) and (b) Heberden's nodes

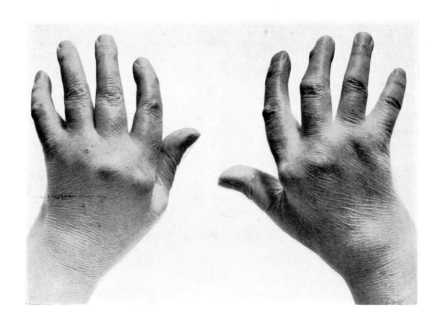

by stretch, the result of abnormal postures. For example at the knee there is often localised tenderness over the ligamentum patellae, the tibial attachment of the medial ligament, and the insertion of the hamstrings. In the latter case, the tenderness may be explained by the fact that the hamstrings are often contracted and then pull on the periosteum at their insertions.

Swelling is usually present at all stages of the disease. In the stage of early inflammation the swelling is soft and often fluctuating owing to the presence of effusion. Sometimes there is oedema not limited to the joint only; for example, the whole finger or fingers and hand may be puffy, while if the joints of the lower extremity are affected there is often oedema of the feet and legs. Later, as granulation tissue forms, the swelling feels firmer and more spongy. It is often at this stage more noticeable owing to muscle atrophy proximal and distal to the joint giving rise to the spindle-shaped or fusiform swelling so often described in textbooks.

Muscle spasm is a common feature. In the first stage the spasm is protective, its object being to prevent movement of a painful joint. It tends to become a habit and is, therefore, often prolonged into subsequent stages.

Muscle atrophy is an outstanding feature and is largely the result of disuse. If movement causes pain then the patient moves the joint as little as possible. In some patients atrophy exceeds that which could be explained by disuse alone. In these patients there is probably also reflex inhibition of muscles. Atrophy is a serious feature because it means less protection of the already damaged joint and more likelihood of the development of fixed deformity.

Deformity is one of the greatest dangers to fight against in rheumatoid arthritis. Each damaged joint has a characteristic 'deformity' pattern. There is some position in which the capsule and ligaments are most relaxed and there is, therefore, most room for swelling with minimal pressure on nerve endings. In addition, at each joint some muscle groups are more powerful than others. In many cases gravity has a powerful influence over the direction of deformity. Thus we find a flexed knee, a dorsiflexed everted ankle, clawed toes, adducted and medially rotated shoulder, flexed elbow, pronated forearm and flexed wrist. At the hand the deformity is difficult to explain, but usually it consists of ulnar deviation of the fingers, flexion of the metacarpo-phalangeal joints, hyperextension of the proximal interphalangeal joints, and adduction of the thumb (see Plate 1).

At first the deformities are held by muscle spasm, but later they become more fixed due to contracture of the muscle framework, permanent shortening of the muscle fibres and shortening of the fascia and ligaments. Eventually fibrous or bony ankylosis may develop in the deformed position.

Limited movement is another serious feature of the disease. In cases of gradual onset there is often at first a history of stiffness first thing in the morning which wears off during the day but reoccurs after exercise and at night. If an acute attack develops the joint movement becomes grossly limited by muscle spasm. Later, movement is restricted in all directions as a result of muscle weakness and contractures, and, sometimes, because of gross destruction of the articular surfaces. Eventually, in some cases, movement is completely lost, due to fibrous or bony ankylosis.

It will be realised that no two cases are exactly alike, and that each case varies from time to time. Thus there may be one joint in Stage I, another in Stage II, and several in the third stage, all at the same time. A joint in Stage II or III may suddenly flare up and show all the features of acute inflammation. The disease is in fact unpredictable.

CHANGES IN OTHER TISSUES

Skin. A common feature is the formation of subcutaneous nodules around bony points, particularly around the elbow and along the posterior border of the ulna. These nodules have been found to consist of a central area of necrotic tissue, a zone of phagocytic cells and an outer ring of proliferating connective tissue.

Muscles. Similar nodules form in the connective tissue framework of the muscles, and there is usually atrophy of the muscle fibres. Thus there is a generalised reduction in muscle bulk throughout the body predisposing to faulty posture and defective function.

Lymphatic glands. These often show enlargement. The spleen is occasionally enlarged and a gland which can be readily palpated is the epitrochlear at the elbow.

In general, during a fairly active phase of the disease the patient presents, in addition to the joint troubles, a picture of ill health. Continuous pain leads to a sense of frustration, marked depression develops as the patient finds she cannot play her proper part in the family life. There is a raised sedimentation rate, anaemia, loss of appetite, a feeling of lassitude and often loss of weight.

PROGNOSIS

There is no known cure for this disease, but it is known that it usually eventually burns itself out. It is impossible to make a definite prognosis in the early stages of any case. In about twenty-five per cent of patients the disease burns itself out within a year or two, leaving no crippling or deformity. In ten per cent the disease progresses inexorably in spite of all treatment, eventually leaving the patient a bed-ridden cripple. In the remaining sixty-five per cent of cases the disease follows a course of exacerbations and remissions until it finally burns itself out after perhaps ten or twenty years. There is hope for this large group because, with proper care and their own co-operation, they can usually be kept ambulant and able to lead useful lives.

PRINCIPLES OF TREATMENT

In spite of continuous research, no cure has yet been found for the disease; treatment therefore has three main objects: improvement of health and so of the ability of the patient to fight the disease; relief of symptoms; and maintenance of the function of the joints.

Improvement of health. The first principle is *rest*. During an active phase of the disease when one or more joints are acutely inflamed and the general health is particularly poor, rest can only be obtained by spending a good deal of the day in bed. The patient is often given this rest in hospital because in this way she is relieved from household tasks, is able to make social contacts which may have been impossible for some time and may be helped by seeing others who are bearing and coping with disabilities greater than her own. Unless weight-bearing joints are acutely affected, the patient is usually allowed to get up for toilet purposes and often for longer periods during the day, but this type of rest can never be satis- factory if the patient is tense because of social or financial worries, and here the help of the almoner may be necessary. Some relief from tension can be gained by training in relaxation and by the practice of breathing exercises. Good food, easily digested and containing adequate first-class protein and vitamins, is helpful. The anaemic condition, if present, is treated by iron preparations. Ability to fight the disease appears to be increased by the use of gold therapy, though it is still uncertain how this is so effective.

Relief of symptoms. The symptom which worries the patient above all is persistent pain, hampering activities, reducing sleep and so lowering general health and morale. Relief of pain is, therefore, an important principle. This may be carried out by the use of analgesic drugs. Aspirin, phenacetin and codeine, either separately or combined are still most widely used. Barbiturates are used to help sleep.

Some use has been made in recent years of cortisone, hydro-cortisone and A.C.T.H. Briefly it may be said that the object is to raise the circulating level of hydrocortisone above that which is normal in the ordinary individual. It has been found that this results in a suppression of many of the changes of inflammation. It reduces malaise, temperature and the sedimentation rate. Consequently it usually results in a rapid improvement in the state of the joints and general health of the patient. Within a few days the pain and stiffness may have subsided, the patient feels better, swelling goes down, and, within a week, in these cases, joints in Stage I may be completely normal, while those in State II may be less swollen and free from pain.

The picture is not, however, as bright as it looks, since none of these substances touches the actual disease. The relief of pain, swelling and stiffness may be dangerous since it gives the patient a false idea of his state, and this, together with the analgesic effects of the drugs, may lead him to overuse and damage the affected joints. In addition there are certain harmful side effects of the drugs which may preclude their use. Excessive gain in weight, psychological changes, oedema eventually leading to heart failure, and gastro-intestinal disturbances are some of the possible and more serious side effects. Because of these dangers, together with the fact that if these drugs are withdrawn the arthritis often flares up again, salicylates in the form of aspirin are still the most valuable drug available.

Pain, swelling and muscle spasm may also be relieved by the use of splints, heat, and in some cases suitable movements; these will be discussed later.

Maintenance of the function of the joints. During the long course of the disease it is clearly essential to limit the crippling which will tend to result from the progressive changes. While it is not possible to prevent changes, it is possible to limit them. The main principles are, therefore, to reduce swelling and lessen organisation, to limit muscle atrophy, to retain movement and to prevent deformity. These principles are fulfilled by the application of splints and by means of physiotherapy. In addition, the patient can do a very great deal to help himself if he has patience, courage and perseverance.

THE PART PLAYED BY PHYSIOTHERAPY

The physiotherapist can play some part in the fulfilment of all three main objects.

The general health. As has already been seen, partial bed rest is, in many cases, necessary. This has certain disadvantages. Circulation is slowed, general muscle atrophy develops, breathing is restricted and joints tend to become stiff. Good posture is difficult to maintain. Often the mattress sags, the pillows are unsuitably arranged, and the bedclothes are heavy on the feet. The result is that the head is pressed forward, the shoulders rounded, the chest narrowed and the lumbar curve obliterated. The knees may be flexed and the feet dorsiflexed and everted. The patient, un-checked, tends to hold the arms in to the side, with the forearms resting across the abdomen, and, consequently, the wrists and fingers are flexed. All these disadvantages can be, at least, reduced by the use of physical measures. Slowing of the circulation and generalised muscle atrophy due to disuse may be dealt with by the use of easy movements. Each muscle group and each joint, excluding those which are acute or subacute, should be given free, simple movements. If the patient is fit enough, this is best carried out in a small class.

Posture requires special attention. In order to gain the patient's co-operation the value of good, and the dangers of faulty, posture should be explained. The ideal position for the greater part of the day is lying on a firm mattress placed over fracture boards, with a single pillow under the head and a board at the feet projecting up vertically above the level of the toes. There should be no pillow under the knees, and the arms should rest on pillows with some degree of abduction of the shoulders, and the wrist supported in a few degrees of extension. At least once daily, the patient should turn into prone lying to ensure maintenance of the lumbar curve and extension in the hips. When the patient sits up in bed it is necessary to see that there is a firm back rest with the pillows arranged vertically and not in the 'arm-chair' position. If the patient is allowed to get up for periods during the day, careful attention should be paid to her posture, both in sitting and when she is walking.

When the position has been corrected the patient is shown this position, if possible using a mirror, and she is taught to feel and sense it as well as to see it. Rhythmic contractions of the main muscle groups are added. As soon as the patient is allowed to begin active movements, progression is made to simple exercises to strengthen the transverse and longitudinal back muscles, the extensors of the cervical spine, hips and knees and the abdominal muscles.

Breathing exercises are most important to aid the posture of the chest as well as to stimulate the circulation. General and local chest expansion should both be taught.

Training in relaxation is essential if full rest is to be obtained. Nearly all patients are tense, partly due to worry and partly due to continuous pain. The first step is to explain what is meant by relaxation and its value, and this is followed by an attempt to find a position in which the patient is really comfortable and can relax. Usually the best method to follow is to teach the patient the difference between the 'feel' of contracted and relaxed muscles by starting on muscles and joints not as yet affected. Gradually progression can be made to painful joints. It will take patience and considerable time before any degree of relaxation can be obtained, but eventually it is possible for the patient to relax completely.

Relief of symptoms and maintenance of the function of the joint. These are so closely related that the physical measures to fulfil these objects will be discussed together. They depend upon the condition of the individual joints. For the purpose of selecting suitable treatment, joints may be classified into four main groups, provided it is realised that there is no clear line of distinction between each group, and that a joint may be in one group at one time and in another later.

The acute joint. Joints in this group usually present with continuous pain and extreme tenderness, so that the patient can hardly bear to have the joint touched, muscle spasm resulting in complete absence of movement, swelling, heat and a tendency to hold the joint in the position of ease. The first principle of treatment for such a joint is rest and this is usually obtained by splintage. Often, at this stage, a complete plaster is used. The physiotherapist is not usually asked to apply this but when dealing with the bed exercises she will note that it is comfortable, not too tight and fulfilling its purpose. After a few days it is usual to bivalve the plaster, and if there is improvement attention may then be paid to the relief of residual pain, stimulation of absorption of inflammatory exudate, prevention of muscle atrophy and of deformity and the regaining of movement. Infra red or radiant heat will have a sedative effect on nerve endings and, by producing superficial vaso-dilation, may relieve deep-seated congestion.

In the case of puffy fingers and hand, citrate ionisation has recently been found to be of considerable value, and with the physician's permission it should be tried. It is thought that the citrate ions, driven in by the constant current, check the tendency to thrombus formation in the digital capillaries.

Rhythmic muscle contractions should be taught; this is difficult if there is a bilateral condition, but if one joint is not acute the patient can get the idea and feel of the movement on the less acute joint. As soon as the physician permits, the splint is removed for very gentle assisted active movements carried out within the limit of real pain. Gradually, as the inflammation subsides, the splint can be discarded until it is worn only at night. Heat can be omitted and the range of movements increased.

The active but non-acute joint. Probably the greater number of joints are found in this stage. The characteristics are ı) pain is not continuous but it tends to be troublesome in the morning and at night and on movement; 2) tenderness is still present but it is not elicited so easily, the patient is able to tolerate light handling of the joint; the range of movement is greater but is not by any means full, and often muscle spasm will be precipitated when a certain point in the movement is reached; the muscles usually show considerable atrophy; swelling is marked and feels soft and spongy since it is usually rather the result of granulation tissue growth than of effusion; deformity is often present, though it is not yet a fixed deformity. More vigorous treatment is now necessary, but it must be carried out with care, avoiding anything which might stimulate the inflammatory process. The main objects now are to prevent organisation of the granulation tissue, to build up the muscles and prevent the deformities becoming permanent. To carry out the first object, stimulation of the deep circulation is necessary and short-wave therapy is probably the method of choice. Carefully chosen active movements are essential to fulfil the second and third aims. Positions are selected to help the patient to get the maximum possible range, for example, shoulder movements are more easily carried out in lying position. Any measures which aid movement should be used, where they are suitable. Suspension and pool therapy are most valuable. Active movements are assisted and skill is required to encourage relaxation of antagonistic muscles.

In addition to assisted active movements, some movements against maximal resistance should be included in order to build up the muscle power. The resistance may in fact be only very slight and it should not cause pain. Often there is a small part of the range in which resistance can be given without causing pain.

Particular attention is necessary to the incipient deformities. Thus it is particularly important to exercise the lumbricales to prevent toe clawing, and if necessary surged faradism may be used to start the retraining of these muscles. Similarly, special work is usually needed for the plantar flexors of the ankles, and for the quadriceps. Night splints are valuable to prevent the development of these deformities, and it is usually the duty of the physiotherapist to make and supervise these splints. The most usual are back splints to prevent flexion deformities of the knees, and hand splints to correct the tendency to flexion of the wrists and ulnar deviation of the fingers. Sometimes day splints are helpful; thus, for example, short cock-up splints to support painful wrists are invaluable and they allow comfortable use of the fingers. Metatarsal pads or bars are useful for painful metatarso-phalangeal joints. A back splint is necessary for the knee when weight-bearing if the quadriceps is not strong enough to straighten the knee against the force of gravity. It will be remembered that deformity will develop as a result of pain, muscle spasm and muscle weakness.

The chronic joint, when the actual disease is still active. This joint is usually no longer painful at rest because the inflammatory process has, for the time being at least, subsided. It may, however, be painful on movement as a result of fibrous tissue contracture and irregularity of joint surfaces. Tenderness on pressure and along the joint line is, for the same reason, no longer likely to be present but there is often localised tenderness over tight tendon or ligamentous attachments. The joint is still swollen but the swelling is firmer since it is caused by fibrous thickenings. Movement is usually limited as a result of contractures and habit spasm of muscles; occasionally ankylosis may have occurred. Deformity and gross muscle atrophy are most commonly present.

The chief objects of treatment are very similar to the previous group, but as the inflammation is no longer present they can be pressed rather further.

Localised tender areas, often causing considerable discomfort, can quite often be cleared by a few treatments using counter-irritant measures such as histamine or renotin ionisation, strong doses of ultra-violet rays or deep kneadings and friction.

The position of the joints can in many cases be improved, though not fully corrected, in the following way. The soft tissues are first warmed, softened and relaxed by the use of heat, inductothermy often proving most successful. Stretching is then attempted by means of deep massage. Gentle passive stretching may also be used if the physician permits. The patient is then encouraged to use the muscles which would correct the deformity, against resistance, the object being twofold: first to relax any habit spasm in the muscles holding the deformed position, and secondly to strengthen the weak group. Then follows an effort to use the group action of joints, the patient being encouraged to stretch the whole limb out against resistance.

Muscles are strengthened by resisted exercises again, provided resistance does not cause pain. It is important to remember that so long as the disease is active it is possible by faulty treatment to re-start an inflammation in the joint. For this reason forced movements are not permitted and any movement causing real pain is avoided.

The chronic joint when the disease has burnt itself out. The real point at issue in this stage is whether any improvement of the joint condition is possible. In some cases it is a matter of training the patient to make the best use of what function, if any, remains. In others, some useful improvement can be obtained. In the first case, the patient can often be helped to lead an independent existence by the provision of suitable equipment. Such 'gadgets' as special tap turners, bottle openers, long-handled combs, potato peelers, may make all the difference.

In the second case, treatment will follow the lines of the previous group, but there is no fear of lighting the condition up. At this stage the patient's health is improving and he is often able to tolerate more vigorous treatment.

Throughout all stages of treatment the stress must be laid on function. The practice of functional activities is essential and the physiotherapist constantly asks herself if there is any particular thing the patient is unable to do in the way of dressing, feeding, getting about and doing the household tasks. The next question is what stands in the way of her doing these things, and can this be overcome?

It is, of course, equally important to realise that inflamed joints need rest, and, during a period of return of pain and swelling, rest must be given, but, even during this period, gentle active movements are soon restarted provided they do not involve weight-bearing or resistance. The patient does require instruction to the effect that he cannot 'work off' the active conditions.

EXAMINATION OF THE PATIENT

Before the physiotherapist can treat the patient a careful examination is necessary. This examination fulfils a special purpose and is only partly similar to that carried out by the physician.

THE PURPOSE OF THE EXAMINATION

This is three-fold. First, its purpose is to find out something of the patient's background, without which an assessment of suitable treatment cannot be made. Secondly, it is essential to know the state of the general health, how much work the patient is capable of, and what medical treatment she is having. Thirdly, it is necessary to have a knowledge of the present state of each affected joint. This changes so frequently that it is possible that the joint may not be in the same state when the patient reaches the department as it was when the patient was seen by the physician. The actual physical examination is always preceded by a thoughtful reading of the patient's notes. These will nearly always give the facts about the patient's general health, the level of the erythrocyte sedimentation rate, the condition of the blood. Also in the notes will usually be found the social history of the patient, including such points as the number and age of the family, the type of house, and the amount of help in the home. A detailed account of the state of the joints at the time of examination will also be included. It might well be asked what more do we need to know. The answer is not, in fact, difficult to seek. We must add, in order to carry out adequate and safe treatment, the state of the skin which tells us whether certain physical measures are suitable; the power of the muscle groups which guides us as to the most suitable type of exercise; the presence of pain, including how and when the pain is produced; the degree of tenderness and its site, both of which help us in the placing of pads and electrodes and in the use or omission of massage and exercises. It is also necessary to know the degree of deformity and, if movement is limited, the reason for this limitation in terms of spasm, contracture or ankylosis. Perhaps, most important of all, we have to ask: is the patient independent, what can he not do for himself?

No assessment of the needs of the patient from the point of view of physiotherapy can be made without first carrying out such an examination. Especially is this so when the physician, having gained confidence in the physiotherapist, orders physiotherapy.

METHOD OF EXAMINATION

The first step in any examination is the study of the notes written by the physician. In most hospitals these are readily available. In some cases the X-ray photographs and report will also give useful information.

The second step is the observation and questioning of the patient. To classify it as a step in an examination is actually erroneous, because the powers of observation will be used throughout the whole procedure, but it is useful to find out as much as possible by using the sense of sight before proceeding to confirm or supplement by palpation and the use of various tests.

The patient should, as far as is possible, be left to undress, get on the bed and settle down by herself, careful watch being kept to note her particular difficulties. When she is comfortably settled, warm, and in a good light, her co-operation is obtained by an explanation of the purpose and method of the examination. While talking to her, her general appearance will be noted. It is possible to begin to assess how depressed, how tense, how ill she may be. A slight idea of the general muscular condition and posture and what joints are affected may also be obtained. It is suitable at this point to question her as to what she has found difficult in the way of dressing, feeding, toilet arrangements, and household work, explaining that it may be possible to find ways of helping her if she would like help. It is helpful to enquire about her aches and pains, when pain is felt, whether it interferes with sleep, what movement she can do.

Often the patient, once started, talks far too much, but it has to be remembered that a great deal can be learnt by what the patient says and how she says it; and though patience is needed, it is well rewarded in the knowledge gained by the physiotherapist and in the greater confidence obtained by the patient.

The third step is the careful examination of each individual joint. To make this clear the knee joints will be taken as an illustration, but the same procedure may be used for any joint. The patient should be in the lying position with the head and shoulders comfortably raised, and no pillow should be used beneath the legs.

Observation. The physiotherapist stands at the foot of the bed so that the two legs can be viewed together and equally. A careful check of the bulk of the quadriceps muscle, the position of the knee, the contour of the joint, the presence of swelling should be made. The two knees are compared since there is rarely symmetry in this disease. Note may also be made of any movements the patient makes, because if the knees are painful she often cannot keep them still for long.

Palpation. The swollen area should be gently palpated with the finger-tips to ascertain whether it feels soft or spongy or firm. If fluid is suspected, the flat hand may be gently placed above the suprapatellar pouch and pressure exerted towards the toes. If there is effusion the fluid will move and the patella will be floated off the lower end of the femur. Gentle pressure by the fingers of the free hand will cause the patella to tap against the femur. This tap can be felt and heard.

Palpation is then carried out to note the presence or absence of tenderness and whether the tenderness is the result of 'activity' within the joint or a localised tenderness of ligament or tendons. The joint is gently grasped between the hands and they are then gradually approximated, careful note being made of how much depth of pressure is required before pain is experienced. The patient is watched during this procedure because, in spite of explanation, some patients will not readily admit to pain. Note is, therefore, made of muscle contraction, wincing, and facial expression. With the finger-tips, palpation is carried out along the joint line, over the medial ligament, the ligamentum patellae and the insertions of the hamstrings.

Some knowledge of the state of the muscles may be gained by palpation. Tone can be tested by touch; the muscles vary in softness or firmness according to their state of tone.

Measurements are useful if there is any doubt as to difference in size, and for record purposes to check progress of the joint. The bulk of both thighs, the circumference of the joint and the degrees of flexion and extension should all be measured and charted. Actual graphs are probably better than a list of figures as progress can be more readily seen at a glance. Copies of the records should be available for the physician, and, in most cases, should be given to the patient provided she has been warned as to the likelihood of exacerbations and remissions in the disease.

Movements are next carried out. A careful explanation of what is required is given. The hip is gently flexed and the patient then asked to bend the knee while the thigh is supported. Note is made of the range actively obtained and the speed and smoothness of movement. Extension of the knee joint follows, the same points being noticed. If the movement is not full an attempt is made to perform passive movement in order to ascertain whether the passive movement is greater, the same, or less than the active. While performing these movements a careful look-out is kept for the onset of pain and muscle spasm. One of the objects of these tests is to find out what particular change is leading to limited movement. If there should be no movement at all, it is likely to be either because there is bony ankylosis or because there is severe muscle spasm; the latter could be both seen and felt and can usually be confirmed because other signs of an 'acute' joint will be present. Very slight movement is often the result of complete loss of cartilage and fibrous ankylosis; the former can be confirmed by a glance at the X-ray photographs. Some limitation is often present either due to habit spasm or contractures. To test this, resistance, if it is not too painful, should be given to the movement. For example, if extension is limited and it is doubtful whether this is due to hamstring spasm or capsular contracture, resistance is given to attempted knee extension and if spasm is present this should be felt and seen to relax.

Power of muscle must be estimated. It is necessary to know if the patient is able to contract the quadriceps, or if she can extend the knee against gravity. If the patient is unable to extend the knee actively against gravity but it can be fully extended passively, then the quadriceps is not strong enough for her to be walking without some form of knee support. It is obvious, therefore, that a careful check of this point should be made.

An estimate of the power of muscles at any joint is important because the muscles protect the damaged joint structures. Testing of power is carried out very carefully because pain should not be precipitated. Assisted and free movement are tested first and then gradually increasing resistance is given, but this is kept within the limit of pain.

Gait and stance should be observed as part of the examination of any lower extremity joint. It is valuable to note the position of the hip, knee and foot in standing, also how the line of weight is falling. The method of walking gives helpful information, and if the patient walks reasonably well an attempt may be made to climb stairs. If the patient is walking and standing badly, it is useful to observe whether sticks or crutches help.

Summary

At the end of such an examination, which, incidentally, is rarely completed in one session, it should be possible to make a tentative assessment of what the patient can do and what can be done for the patient, and on this a scheme of treatment is planned. It is important to realise that the scheme has frequently to be modified and changed as the general and joint condition changes with the exacerbations and remissions. Thus repeated examinations and close observations are necessary throughout the whole course of treatment.

ADDITIONAL NOTES

THE RELATIONSHIP OF PHYSIOTHERAPY TO THE VARIOUS DRUGS USED

Aspirin, phenacetin, codeine group. The patient will sometimes tell the physiotherapist that she is not taking the number of aspirins ordered by the physician because she is afraid she may become addicted or that they may lose their effectiveness. The physiotherapist should report this to the physician, because it is widely held that, since this disease is incurable and often does not burn itself out for many years, the patient should not suffer unnecessary pain. Pain, if persistent, lowers the morale and this in its turn lowers the pain threshold. The aspirin group of drugs is usually harmless, has few side effects and the drugs are not drugs of addiction, consequently it is important that the patient should take as many as the physician allows.

Cortisone, A.C.T.H., Butazolidine. It has already been seen that in many cases these drugs have spectacular effects, but that they also can have harmful side effects. Since the physiotherapist is often seeing the patient daily or at least more frequently than the physician, she should be on the look-out for these and be ready to report them at once. The physician is always anxious to know whether the drugs are resulting in improvement of the condition of the joint and the physiotherapist should keep a chart showing the weekly measurements of the size, and of the range of movement of the affected joints. If the joint rapidly improves advantage is taken of this in the treatment, but care must be taken not to 'overdo' the use of the joint, because the actual disease process is not cured, the drugs are analgesic, and the patient feels so much better that he is anxious to get on and in the process may damage the joint further.

Gold therapy. The patient may be treated as usual during a course of gold therapy. Sometimes the patient feels rather more stiff after the early injections and a little less treatment may then be indicated. Signs of side effects in the form, for example, of skin rashes should be watched for and reported. If ultra-violet light is being given it will be remembered that gold is a sensitizer and doses should be reduced.

LENGTH OF COURSE OF PHYSIOTHERAPY

It is not possible to say exactly for how long a patient should be treated. Each case varies. In general it may be said that the object is to teach the patient how best to help herself so that she can carry on at home. One of the most important points is to teach her the relationship of rest and exercise. It is clearly stressed that when a joint is really painful at rest it needs rest and the splints provided for this purpose should be worn and the joint should be saved as much as possible. As the pain subsides, exercise should be restarted, at first without weight.

In selecting exercises during a course of treatment stress is laid on those which can be done at home without apparatus. The patient can often be taught to use heat lamps and wax at home. As long as the patient needs a form of treatment which cannot be done safely at home and as long as her full co-operation and understanding have not been obtained, she needs to attend the department. Thus, one patient may require only a few weeks of treatment; another, months. Usually it is found that a course of about three months may be followed by return to work, but with assiduous practise of home exercises. Often the patient returns for another course of treatment during periods of exacerbations.

THE ATTITUDE OF THE RELATIVES

In the early stages of the illness the relatives are usually kind, helpful and considerate. Often, in fact, too much is done for the patient and, in an effort to make her comfortable, wrong treatment is given. Quite often the patient is carefully nursed, for example, with a pillow under the knees producing a flexion deformity. Later, the relatives may get rather tired of a depressed, frustrated sufferer and sympathy and tact are not conspicuous. It is not usually the physiotherapist's place to deal with the relatives, but occasionally a word of advice is asked for and should be given. It is necessary, therefore, to have an understanding of the difficulties and of the way in which the relatives can help.

USE OF GADGETS, SPLINTS AND APPLIANCES

If it is suggested to a patient that she should use splints or gadgets, she often objects that this will result in her joints becoming stiff and in an inability to do the things which she still can do. This is, of course, not true, provided the appliances are suitably used. Splints are necessary at certain times and for certain purposes. They are needed when joints are in an acute stage in order to give rest and gain resolution of inflammation. For this purpose they are most often complete or bivalved plaster splints and are applied by the physician and worn until the inflammation begins to subside. After this they are gradually discarded. There will be a time when they can be taken off for treatment and the physiotherapist has to re-apply them carefully and see that they are still suitable. Again, they are worn, often as night splints, to check the tendency to increasing deformity. The physiotherapist may be asked to make and supervise these. They are applied in the best possible position which can be obtained and re-made as, and when, the position improves. The patient has to be taught their purpose and how to apply them. Splints are often needed to support joints whose muscles are not as yet strong enough to perform this function. Thus metatarsal pads or bars may be worn while the lumbricales are being re-educated and back splints to control flexion of the knees during a period of quadriceps insufficiency. Short cock-up splints are particularly valuable for the wrists when dorsiflexion is becoming increasingly limited and when their condition is painful, making use of the fingers difficult.

These are best made of material which will not be destroyed by water so that the work of the housewife is not interfered with.

If the physiotherapist is called upon to make splints, there are certain points she should consider. They must be light, as it is not desirable to add weight to an already weakened limb; they must fit well for obvious reasons; the patient must know how to apply them and how to take care of them. They should be renewed whenever necessary and they should not immobilise more joints than is essential.

Gadgets may be considered as equipment which enables a patient to do things he could not do before. They may make a very great difference to the patient's independence and happiness. After examination it may be realised that for a considerable period the patient may not be able to wash the back of her neck or do the back of her hair. Twisted combs and long-handled brushes may make all the difference. The fingers may be so crippled that she cannot turn on taps or unscrew jars; gadgets are available to make these possible. It is essential that the physiotherapist should find out what the patient cannot do and then try to see if there is any equipment which will help. Another problem is that of sticks or crutches. Patients do not usually like these because they feel that if they once start using them they will not walk without their aid again. Often it is necessary to explain that sticks or crutches will help by sharing the weight between the arms and legs and so taking some of the strain from the affected leg joints. Sometimes the hands are unsuitable for sticks and elbow crutches are more useful. Whatever is ordered, it is essential to see that they are of the right length and are being properly used.

SURGERY IN RHEUMATOID ARTHRITIS

There is but little scope for surgery in rheumatoid arthritis. In cases which are virtually monoarticular and severely disabling, arthrodesis is sometimes carried out, as it is in cases where one knee becomes the seat of a flexion contracture which cannot be rectified by non-operative measures. In such cases the physiotherapist gives invaluable service in restoring maximal function in the limb in which arthrodesis has been done.

Chapter II

STILL'S DISEASE. INFECTIVE ARTHRITIS

STILL'S DISEASE *~ mainly children up to 5 years.*

This is a widespread arthritis of the rheumatoid type occurring in children. It is very similar to the adult type of rheumatoid arthritis but differs in that it is much more severe. More joints are involved, the lymphoid tissue throughout the body is inflamed, the constitutional reaction is much greater. There is nearly always fever and severe malaise. The muscles are usually very tender and this, together with the fact that so many joints are in an acute condition, makes the child very unwilling to be handled. As a rule the young patient lies in bed, tense and frightened, a picture of misery. Often the small joints of the neck are affected so that there is considerable danger of a flexion deformity of the head.

The condition usually persists for several years and when it burns itself out it leaves the child with much crippling and deformity. The treatment follows very closely that used for the adult form of rheumatoid arthritis. As there is even more danger of fibrous ankylosis of joints, it is most important that they should be splinted in the position for optimum function. Thus it is essential that the wrist should be fixed in slight extension.

Particular care should be taken of the posture in bed and the child should be encouraged to lie on the face for a brief period each day in order to avoid flexion contractures of the hip.

Heat seems to give considerable relief in these cases and hot-water baths are often valuable. A full length bath encourages relaxation and permits of easier movement.

During the acute phase the main objects of physiotherapy are to relieve pain, prevent deformities and maintain the function of the joints.

INFECTIVE ARTHRITIS

The gonococcus, pneumococcus and streptococcus are the organisms commonly responsible for infective arthritis. Streptococcal arthritis may follow streptococcal tonsillitis, while pneumococcal arthritis arises as a rule in association with pneumonia. In both streptococcal and pneumococcal arthritis the exudate is usually purulent, while in gonococcal arthritis, which tends to follow in the wake of an attack of acute gonorrhoea, the effusion in the joint is sero-fibrinous. Whatever the causal organism, the arthritis may be monoarticular or multiple joints may be involved. The knee is very commonly affected, particularly by gonorrhoea. Antibiotic therapy with penicillin or sulphanilamide drugs, usually bring about a speedy resolution of the arthritis but the joints have a strong tendency to be left stiff and virtually immobile, and in the prevention of this unfortunate legacy the physiotherapist is often of great value. Abortus fever and bacillary dysentery sometimes produce a variety of infective arthritis which is very similar to rheumatoid arthritis.

Apart from antibiotic therapy, rest is the main principle of the treatment of the joint or joints involved. Often a plaster splint is necessary, though it is sometimes bi-valved so that the condition of the joint can be watched. As soon as the acute symptoms have subsided it is essential to prevent further muscle atrophy and to try to prevent organisation and adhesion formation within the joint and between the periarticular structures. For this reason, assisted active movements within the limit of pain are essential, and rhythmic muscle contractions should be given repeatedly. The administration of deep heating is not wise while the condition is active since the metabolism and activity of the micro-organisms might be increased. Superficial heating for the relief of pain and relaxation of muscle spasm is safe and useful. Massage may help the condition of the muscle groups but should not be used over the joint.

Main treatment — Hydrotheraphy

Chapter III

OSTEO-ARTHRITIC TYPE

OSTEO-ARTHRITIS Degeneration

This type of chronic articular rheumatism shows less well-marked constitutional changes than the preceding varieties. In addition, it differs in that the joint structures primarily involved are the articular ones, bone and cartilage; periarticular soft structures are only secondarily affected. In the majority of cases osteo-arthritis develops in the middle-aged and elderly, and appears in those joints which are most subjected to strain: either the weight-bearing joints, such as the hip and knee, or those which, according to the particular occupation are most used, such as the spinal articulations of the agricultural and manual worker, or the terminal interphalangeal joints of the hands of the gardener and cleaner.

Though much discussion exists as to the exact cause of the development of this type of arthritis, it is likely that the resistance of the joint structures is reduced by the 'wear and tear' of life. Minor traumata, sufficient to damage delicate joint structures, though insufficient to produce joint symptoms, may be responsible for the insidious onset of changes in cartilage and bone. Such strains and stresses may be seen in the arthritis of certain definite occupations, as in the vertebral column of the miner and the elbow of the blacksmith.

Direct trauma, such as a fracture involving the articular surfaces and damaging the cartilage, is often followed by osteo-arthritis. Faulty posture is a possible cause of degenerative changes because it upsets the mechanics of the joint, and abnormal strain is, therefore, brought to bear on cartilage and bone, as well as on joint capsules. For example, osteo-arthritis of the spine is often a secondary condition to structural kyphosis and scoliosis. Congenital abnormalities are liable to produce trouble in the same way. In many cases, early senile changes are probably the beginning of a chronic arthritis.

Obesity may be a contributory factor in osteo-arthritis of the hip and knee, while varus or valgus deformity and repeated damage of the menisci are often followed by this type of arthritis of the knee joint.

Some authorities now believe that in certain cases the cause of the degenerative changes is a thrombosis of the vessels supplying one or more bone ends. This would result in the cutting off of blood and in necrosis of the bone.

PATHOLOGICAL CHANGES

These probably vary with the cause but the eventual condition of the joint is likely to be similar, whatever the cause.

Should thrombosis of the vessels supplying one of the articular surfaces occur, necrosis of bone will result, and since the central part of the articular cartilage obtains its nutrition from the bone, this will degenerate, and eventually disappear. Meanwhile, in order to try to bring more blood to the bone, the vessels of the synovial membrane and capsule will dilate and a state of engorgement and congestion results. It has been found that in this attempt to introduce more blood vessels, the capsule becomes adherent to the bone. On each movement of the joint, therefore, it pulls on the bone and little masses of bone, osteophytes, develop.

If the changes are the result of wear and tear, they usually begin in the articular cartilage at the point at which the trauma is applied. Degenerative changes resulting in a gradual break-up of the cartilage develop and the underlying bone, no longer protected by the 'shock-absorber' action of the cartilage, undergoes sclerosis, becoming hard, white and smooth like ivory (the process of eburation). At the points at which trauma is not experienced and pressure is lessened, chondro-osseous proliferation occurs. It is thought that this may be the result of increased activity of the remnants of perichondrium at the point where the articular cartilage and synovial membrane blend. Little masses of cartilage, which later ossify, therefore develop; these lead to an irregular widening of the articular surfaces. The loss of part of the articular cartilage and the development of osteophytes result in loss of joint space and a rough irregular articular surface causing much difficulty in movement.

Whatever the cause, the periarticular structures are eventually affected. Congestion or abnormal use will result in a hypertrophy of the synovial membrane with diminished secretion of synovial fluid. Fringes and folds become enlarged and liable to be trapped on movement. The fibrosis of the capsule and ligaments resulting from continuous minor strain is followed by contracture which, in its turn, will lead to limited movement and deformity.

SIGNS AND SYMPTOMS

In the early stage of the condition, there is usually hypotonia of the muscles acting on the affected joint, laxity of ligaments and a tendency for the joint to 'give way'. The range of movement is usually full, but the patient complains of pain at the extremes of each movement. There is also a feeling of stiffness on using the joint after a period of rest, and pain on weight-bearing or after prolonged exercise. As the degenerative changes progress and fibrous thickening in the soft tissues develops, signs and symptoms become more pronounced. Pain and tenderness, enlargement of the joint, muscle atrophy, limitation of movement, deformity and crepitus are all common features.

Pain and tenderness. Pain is a very variable feature and does not necessarily bear any relationship to the degree of cartilaginous or bony change, since the cartilage is devoid of nerve endings. According to its cause, it may be present at rest, particularly in bed when the limb becomes warm, or only on movement, or it may be persistent. It is most often felt after prolonged exercise or after a period of rest. It is usually experienced in the joint but may be referred. Referred pain occurs most often in osteo-arthritis affecting the joints of the spine since, as a result of changes in the joints between the articular processes, the intervertebral foramina may be narrowed and the spinal nerve roots compressed.

Pain may be the results of many different factors. Nipping of the hypertrophied synovial membrane, thrombosis of the blood vessels of the joint, fibrosis of the capsule or accessory ligaments, weakness and fatigue of muscles, rubbing of 'young' osteophytes over one another, may all be causes.

Nipping of the hypertrophied synovial membrane gives rise to sharp pain and muscle spasm at one point of one particular movement. It ceases as soon as the fringe is released, leaving soreness and tenderness due to the inflammation which follows the trauma.

Thrombosis of the blood vessels results in ischaemia, and this causes pain as metabolites accumulate. This pain is, therefore, present early, is persistent and is not usually accompanied by limitation of joint movement. It tends to pass off as necrosis develops.

Fibrosis tends to cause trapping of nerve endings, so that when the contracting tissue is stretched, pain is felt. This pain is appreciated at that point in the range of movement which begins to stretch the contracted capsule or ligaments. As the disease progresses and contractures increase, pain is produced earlier in the movement. This may account for the onset of pain when the limb begins to get warm at night.

The pain which is felt after prolonged exertion usually arises as a result of stimulation of sensory nerve endings by the presence of accumulated fatigue products.

Tenderness is due either to the inflammation of the synovial membrane which follows nipping, or to pressure on young osteophytes.

Joint enlargement. The swelling of an osteo-arthritic joint is usually a hard swelling. It is the result of an increase in the size of the bone ends by excessive throwing out of bone, though it may also be partly due to fibrous thickening of the synovial membrane and capsule. Occasionally there will be an effusion into the joint. This will develop following trapping of the synovial membrane or minor strain of the joint.

Muscle weakness and atrophy. In the early stage, muscles are hypotonic and their endurance rather than their power is decreased. Later, as pain and contractures develop, limited use and reflex inhibition lead to atrophy and weakness. The atrophy is rarely as obvious as it is in rheumatoid arthritis because the condition is not a constitutional one. In addition it is confined to the muscles acting on the joint.

Limited movement. At first movement is usually limited only slightly when the shortening tissues are stretched. At this stage the movement can often be completed passively if the patient will tolerate the discomfort. Later muscle weakness, spasm, and contractures will limit both active and passive movements in all directions. When the joint space is lost and the cartilage is denuded, movement becomes mechanically difficult and is still further hampered by the absence of synovial fluid and therefore of lubrication.

Deformity. This is a characteristic feature of the advanced condition. It may be the result of alteration of the alignment of the articular surfaces when part of the cartilage has been completely worn away. In the knee joint, for example, it may be only one condylar articulation which is affected and knock-knee may then develop.

Deformity is also the result of thickening and contractures of the soft tissues, the direction depending upon which part of the capsule is most fibrosed. Thus at the hip joint the antero-lateral part of the capsule is usually eventually grossly thickened, and flexion and lateral rotation at the joint gradually develop.

Muscle imbalance will also predispose towards deformity, quadriceps weakness leading to flexion deformity at the knee and abductor weakness to adduction deformity at the hip. Spasm of a powerful muscle group will have a similar effect.

Often one deformity leads to another compensatory one; at the hip, for example, a flexion deformity, with increased pelvic tilt due to tight hip flexors, will result in a lordosis, and an adduction deformity will lead to a scoliosis.

86

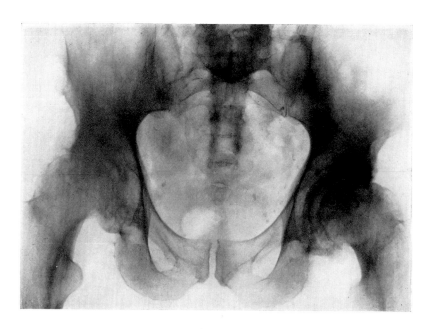

PLATE III. OSTEO-ARTHRITIS OF BOTH HIPS

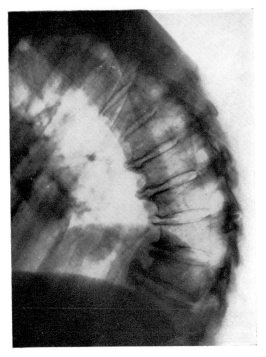

(b) Osteo-arthritis of the spine. Note the spurs of bone

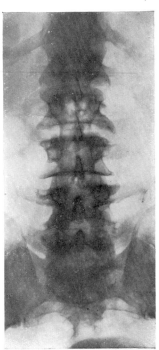

A characteristic deformity of osteo-arthritis results from the development of Heberden's nodes. These may be either bony outgrowths, usually on the lateral side of the distal inter-phalangeal joints of the fingers, or small red cystic nodules containing gelatinous material. The former are often painless but unsightly, while the latter tend to develop suddenly and are then very painful (see Plate II (a) and (b)).

Crepitus. In most osteo-arthritic joints, crepitus can be felt on movement. It usually occurs in joints in which there is irregular loss of cartilage and some bony outgrowths. Grating sound

X-ray evidence. Changes can be seen in the X-ray photographs in advanced cases. The joint space is reduced and may be irregular in size. Sclerosis of the thin layer of compact tissue is appreciable. Bony outgrowths and cystic cavities are readily detectable (see Plate III). Too much emphasis should not, however, be laid on these findings since the actual bony changes do not necessarily tally with the degree of pain and loss of function.

Acute attacks. Occasionally osteo-arthritis of a joint suddenly becomes acute. There is then swelling, intense pain, muscle spasm and very limited movement. This may follow minor strain, to which such joints are prone, or may be the result of trapping of some part of the hypertrophied synovial membrane.

PRINCIPLES OF TREATMENT BY PHYSIOTHERAPY

There are four fundamental objects of treatment in these cases; the first of these, and the most important to the patient, is the relief of pain; the next three of equal importance, are the strengthening of muscles, the prevention of deformity and the maintenance or improvement of the range of movement.

Relief of pain. There is no known cure for the osteo-arthritic joint, there can only be relief of symptoms. Of these, pain is the most outstanding and worries the patient most, in advanced cases seriously interfering with daily activities and with sleep. The relief of pain is, therefore, of the utmost importance. Measures taken to fulfil this object depend upon the cause of the pain.

If pain is the result of ischaemia following thrombosis the application of 'deep' heat may, by stimulating the collateral circulation, relieve pain. Should pain be due to fibrosis of the capsule and synovial membrane, deep heating may again be successful, but in this case indirectly only, by softening the tissue so that it can be more readily stretched. Then the pain

87

soothing

because cartilage is deep. Short wave.

also wax bath.

which occurs on movement, because soft tissue is being stretched, will occur less early. Deep heating should be followed by deep massage and passive stretching to the limit of discomfort but within the limit of pain. Occasionally, especially where there are cystic cavities in the bone, the application of heat increases the pain during its administration. In this case treatment should be changed to the use of the constant current. Softening will then be gained by the stimulation of the circulation through the interpolar effects of the current.

In many cases pain is the result of congestion of the blood vessels in the capsule and synovial membrane. Relief can very often be obtained if counter-irritant measures are adopted. Renotin ionisation or kathodal galvanism are most effective, while a more lasting effect is obtained by means of strong doses of ultra-violet rays, obtaining a third or fourth degree erythema. The first two measures should be followed by deep massage, provided the area is sufficiently superficial.

If nipping of a synovial fringe is causing pain, the avoiding of the particular movement will stop the irritation and the inflammation of the fringe may be relieved by the use of 'deep' heat or the constant current. Should pain occur in joints in which there is only a very small range of movement and this movement is painful, then it may be possible to relieve pain, either by a complete remodelling of the joint, that is by an arthroplasty or by preventing movement at the joint through the use of splints, or by means of surgical fixation, that is, by arthrodesis. These measures are not the province of the physiotherapist, but she will modify her treatment accordingly.

It is apparent that a careful examination of the patient to estimate the cause of pain is necessary before the choice of a suitable measure is made.

Strengthening of muscles. This is necessary in all cases of osteo-arthritis because the muscles are an essential support of the joint. Strong muscles will also be one factor in the prevention of deformity. All muscles acting on the joint should therefore be exercised in such a way as to increase their power and their endurance. Particular attention should be paid to those which will resist the tendency to the development of deformity. Thus at the hip, the extensors and abductors require special care. It will be borne in mind that three half-hour periods of exercise weekly will not achieve this object; it must be made certain that the patient practises repeatedly at home.

Prevention of deformity. The development of deformity at a joint will not only lead to increasing muscle weakness, to pain and to limited function, but also result in strain on other joints and compensatory deformities.

For this reason deformities should, if possible, be avoided. The first essential is an understanding of the mechanics involved. Deformities will develop in the direction encouraged by the pull of the stronger muscle groups and by contracture of the capsule, which will naturally thicken most at the point at which it is usually most well developed to take the normal strain. They will also develop in the position in which least strain is thrown on the capsule and ligaments, that is the so-called 'position of ease'. At the hip, therefore, the tendency is for a flexion, adduction, lateral rotation deformity; at the knee, flexion and valgus; at the elbow, flexion.

This tendency is more easily checked than it is corrected once developed. The three most important measures are passive movements and active assisted movements, active strengthening exercises and the use of night splints. Passive movements and active assisted movements are particularly valuable because in the early stages of the condition full range can be obtained, but often this is not done and consequently an insidious contracture develops. At this stage the joint should be gently and carefully carried through its full range, particularly in that direction which would correct the possible deformity. This should be followed by resisted exercise of the muscles. Should there be already any shortening when the patient first attends for treatment, passive stretching should be preceded by heat or by the use of the constant current.

If there is a tendency to contracture, night splints holding the joint in the best possible position are valuable.

Maintenance of full range of movement. As has already been seen, limitation of movement often develops insidiously as a result of muscle spasm, weakness and contractures. It is essential, therefore, that the joint should be carried through its full range, both actively and passively, daily. The correct range may be obtained by comparison with the opposite limb if this is unaffected.

For those cases in which range is already limited, steps should be taken to ascertain the cause of the limitation and measures chosen accordingly. If muscle spasm is the main factor, the patient is taught to relax the muscles, and it is usual to practise active movement within the limit of pain only. All measures possible should be taken to encourage the patient to carry out a wider range.

If contractures are responsible for limited movements, steps should be taken to stretch the soft tissue, followed by work to strengthen the muscles.

Occasionally a patient is seen in whom movement is so limited that there is little hope of increasing the range, in fact an arthrodesis is likely. These patients must be encouraged to develop compensatory mechanisms.

A stiff hip is not so detrimental if the lumbar spine is reasonably mobile, so that adequate flexion is possible, and if the knee is more than normally mobile so that good flexion will allow the patient to put on her own shoes and stockings working from behind instead of in front.

Again, a stiff knee will be helped by good range in the hip and, particularly, in the ankle.

EXAMINATION OF THE PATIENT

This will follow the same lines as that used for patients suffering from rheumatoid arthritis. Its purpose is to find out those things which make for suitable selection of treatment. Let us take for example the patient sent to the physiotherapy department ordered heat and exercises for an osteo-arthritic hip. It is essential to know whether there is pain and when it is felt, what is the state of the muscles, if there is any deformity and what is its cause if present, and how much limitation of movement there is. The first step, having read the notes and examined the X-rays, is to watch the patient as unobtrusively as possible as she walks into the department, noting how she walks, the presence of any limp and the facial expression. She is then observed as she undresses. Can she, for example, flex the hip to undo the shoes, and, if not, how does she manage?

Observation. Careful note is made of the position of the leg in lying. Are the hip and knee slightly flexed? If the pelvis is horizontal, what angle do the two legs make with the pelvis? Is the affected one adducted? Does one leg lie in greater lateral rotation than the other? The position of the lumbar spine is also noted. The gluteal muscles and the quadriceps are carefully observed, as these often show some atrophy. Comparison is made with the unaffected side.

Palpation. This is carried out to detect the presence of tenderness. Gentle pressure is given just below the middle of the inguinal ligament and around the great trochanter.

Measurements. The length of leg is measured, since real or apparent shortening may be present. The bulk of the thigh and the degree of movement of the hip should also be estimated.

Movements. Free active movements should be tested. Each movement is first carried out at the unaffected hip so that a careful comparison can be made. In the early stages the movement may be so little affected that, unless this is done, slight limitation is not detected. While the movements are being performed a close watch is kept for any movement of the pelvis and for the speed and smoothness of performance and signs of pain. Any movement which is even slightly limited is next tested passively and note is made as to what is the 'feel' of the limitation. Does it in fact feel like a bony block, or is there an elastic resistance, or is it muscle spasm due to pain?

If there appeared, during this observation, to be a flexion deformity, the opposite hip should be fully flexed and note made as to whether the affected leg increased in flexion during this test. Ability to correct this deformity may be tested by asking the patient to try to keep the affected leg on the bed while the unaffected hip is being flexed.

Slight limitation of adduction can best be checked by abducting both hips together. The mobility of the lumbar spine and knee should also be tested.

Power of muscles. Each group of muscles must be carefully checked by comparison with the unaffected hip using free and resisted movements, providing the latter are not painful. The abdominal muscles should be included in this test.

Posture. The patient is seen in the standing position and a careful note is made of the position of the legs, pelvis and spine. With a marked adduction deformity the patient will attempt to bring the two legs parallel with one another by lifting the pelvis on the affected side, then to bring the foot onto the ground; the knee on the unaffected side is flexed. If there is a hip flexion deformity, the pelvis will be tilted forward and there will be a marked lordosis and protuberant abdomen. If outward rotation of the hip has occurred, the patella will face laterally instead of directly forward, and the foot will be turned outwards.

Gait. This will next be examined and will be followed by a check on such functional activities as the ability to mount steps, to get up and sit down, and to put on the shoes and stockings.

This type of examination may be carried out for any affected joint. It allows an estimation of the most suitable form of heat and the right type of exercise. It gains the co-operation of the patient, who will realise that the exercises are chosen with a thorough understanding of the condition.

ADVICE TO THE PATIENT

It has already been pointed out that exercises three times weekly are of little value. Since exercises form, in most cases, the main part of the physical treatment, it is essential that they are practised daily and, if possible, several times daily. Each patient is given a written list of carefully chosen exercises with full instructions as to how, when, and how often they should be done. The value of each exercise is explained, together with a little information as to what is likely to develop if they are not practised.

Instruction is also needed in relation to the amount of activity which should be undertaken. Usually this is done by the physician, but sometimes it is left to the physiotherapist. Exercise is absolutely essential if stiffness and limitation of movement is to be prevented. The patient is, therefore, instructed that rest in bed is harmful and that the more the joint is moved the better. But on the other hand weight-bearing without movement is not good and the patient is, therefore, advised, if the joints of the lower extremity are affected, not to stand more than is essential. A stool of suitable height will make it possible to sit while washing dishes, peeling potatoes and even while ironing. But should an acute attack occur, then the joint should be rested. If this advice is followed the patient can do a very great deal to make himself more comfortable and slow the progress of the disease.

Chapter IV

SPONDYLITIS

There are two main types of rheumatic spondylitis, namely, spondylitis osteo-arthritica and ankylosing spondylitis.

SPONDYLITIS OSTEO-ARTHRITICA

The term osteo-arthritis is often used when there are spurs of bones and lipping of the margins of the vertebrae, but this is a normal age change, some degree of which is seen in all middle-aged and older subjects.

TRUE OSTEO-ARTHRITIS

This attacks the lateral intervertebral joints and is similar in pathology to osteo-arthritis of any other synovial joint. The joints of the cervical region are most often involved, as they lie almost horizontally and therefore take the weight. Cervical osteo-arthritis or, as it is frequently called, cervical spondylosis, is believed often to result from repeated disc prolapse. It is extremely common and may produce no symptoms.

One of the important points to be noted is that degeneration and bony proliferation are taking place in very close proximity to the intervertebral foramina, and a large osteophyte, or slight alteration in the alignment of the articular surfaces, may bring about narrowing of a foramen and, therefore, compression of a nerve root. If a foramen is narrowed it may still be large enough not to press on a nerve root at rest, but on certain movements pressure may readily be exerted. In this case nerve-root pain is intermittent. Thickening of the capsule and periarticular structures may also result in pressure on a nerve root.

In the cervical region osteophytes form bars on the posterior aspect of the intervertebral joints, and these may press on the spinal cord itself producing paraplegic manifestations.

Pain and limited movement are the chief features of true osteo-arthritis. Pain is present on movement, is relieved by rest, but is worse on moving after a period of rest. This pain is felt in the back or neck, but often root pains also occur and either radiate into the arm or leg in the distribution of the nerve roots involved, or are felt as girdle pains round the trunk if the intercostal nerves are affected. Both passive and active movement will be limited and they are guarded by muscle spasm.

Physical treatment should be carried out following the same principles as indicated for osteo-arthritis (see page 87), but the use of traction and support is often of value for osteo-arthritis of the cervical region in patients complaining of intermittent root pains. Pressure may be relieved if the vertebrae are separated, and surprising improvement sometimes follows traction applied to the head with the patient lying on an inclined plinth with the feet lower than the head. Traction will be used daily, progressing the length of time for which it is applied. Sometimes a plaster collar moulded over the shoulders and extending to the chin and external occipital protuberance is a great help. This can be removed for heat massage, exercises and traction.

LIPPING OF THE VERTEBRAE AND THINNING OF THE DISC

It is not uncommon to find that after a period of years degenerative changes develop in the intervertebral disc which becomes considerably thinned. The nucleus pulposus becomes smaller and easily herniates, probably into the body of the vertebra above or below. The buffering effect of the disc is then lost and pressure on movement is no longer distributed evenly over the surface of the vertebra. The front of the body is therefore subjected to greatest strain and it tends to respond by throwing out extra bone (see Plate IV (a) and (b)). Sometimes the annulus fibrosus may become so thin that the edges of the vertebrae actually come into contact on movement and irritation also results in bony proliferation. Bony spurs are formed and occasionally these may fuse, bridging across the gap between two vertebrae. There is sometimes an involvement of the articular joints, with the changes of a true osteo-arthritis, when the disc changes have developed, since the thinning of the disc may lead to altered alignment and persistent strain on these joints.

Quite often the patient is free from symptoms, but sometimes there is the gradual onset of stiffness and aching in the affected region of the back. Occasionally nerve roots may be involved, since much narrowing of the disc space will reduce the size of the intervertebral foramen.

The principles underlying the physical treatment of patients suffering from this condition are not clear. It is probable that physiotherapy can

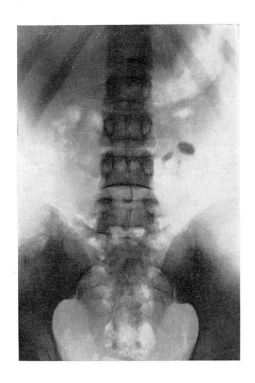

PLATE V

ANKYLOSING SPONDYLITIS

(a) Early case. Showing bilateral sacro-iliac arthritis. Note sclerosis and loss of joint space in right joint. No evidence of changes in spine

(b) Advanced case. Note continuous outline of right side of vertebral column showing calcification of ligaments

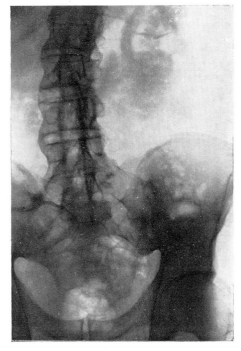

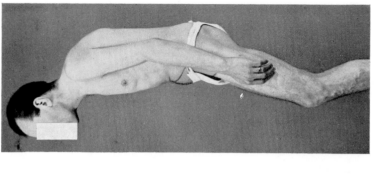

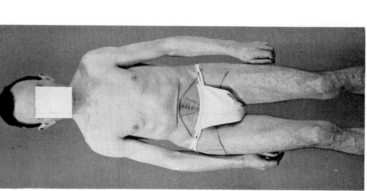

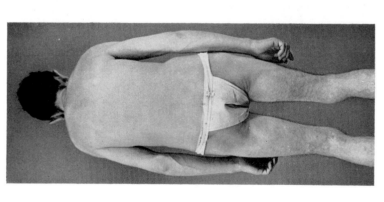

PLATE VI. ANKYLOSING SPONDYLITIS

Showing deformity in advanced case. Note emaciation, flexion deformity, position of head, scoliosis, flat lumbar spine, diminished costal angle

do little to help. If there are attacks of pain and stiffness with muscle spasm, relief may be obtained by the application of deep heat and massage.

Should narrowing of the disc space be the cause of root pain, help may be given by traction and by teaching the patient to keep the spine erect and to avoid the 'slump' which is such a characteristic of many middle-aged and elderly patients. Strengthening the abdominal and back muscles and training good posture will both be of value.

ANKYLOSING SPONDYLITIS

(Synonyms: Spondylitis Ankylopoetica; Spondylose Rhizomelique; Marie-Strumpell Disease).

Ankylosing spondylitis is a condition characterised by rigidity of the spinal column and thorax, often associated with considerable deformity. There has been much discussion as to whether it is simply a rheumatoid arthritis affecting the spine or whether it is a separate entity. In this country it is usually considered to be a separate disease. This opinion is based on the fact that the sex incidence, joints affected and main changes are dissimilar, though its inflammatory nature, the general ill health, the anaemia and raised sedimentation rate are all symptoms which are also present in rheumatoid arthritis. This condition, unlike rheumatoid arthritis, does not respond to gold therapy but does respond to X-ray therapy.

About ninety per cent of patients suffering from ankylosing spondylitis are men, the usual age of onset being between twenty and forty. Cases occurring later in life are reported, but it is probable that in these patients the condition has actually been present for some years before it was diagnosed.

The cause of the condition is unknown, though the onset of symptoms is often related, by the patient, to some slight injury such as a fall or a blow on the back. The proximal joints are affected first. Almost invariably it begins in the sacro-iliac joints and spreads up the spine. The atlanto-axial and atlanto-occipital joints often escape, but the thoracic joints are involved with those of the spine and spread also occurs to the joints of the shoulder girdle. The condition spreads downwards to the hip joints and occasionally to the knees. The small distal joints are rarely affected, although sometimes changes do occur similar to those seen in the rheumatoid type of arthritis.

CHANGES

There is uncertainty as to the exact series of changes which are taking place, but in advanced cases two definite changes can be seen in X-ray films, namely osteo-porosis and bony ankylosis (see Plate V (a) and (b)).

Osteo-porosis. Rarefaction is seen early in the pelvis, particularly near the sacro-iliac joints, and in the bodies of the lumbar vertebrae. When the condition is well advanced the vertebrae are so soft that the superincumbent weight causes them to be compressed.

Bony ankylosis. Lime and calcium salts, absorbed from the bone, are deposited in the capsule and ligaments and in the edges of the articular cartilage and intervertebral discs. Eventually the articular surfaces are often joined by soft spongy bone and the ligaments become completely ossified (see Plate V (b)). The lateral ligaments, the supra- and interspinous ligaments, the anterior longitudinal and ligamenta flava are particularly affected. The ligaments of the costo-vertebral and costotransverse joints are also attacked. At the hip calcification begins in the acetabular labrum and spreads to the capsule.

MODE OF ONSET AND PROGRESS

The onset of the disease is often insidious. Sometimes there is a pre-spondylitic phase, developing between the ages of about 14 and 20, in which there is a complaint of stiffness and vague pains in the legs and trunk. Sometimes there is general malaise and a slight pyrexia. Usually these symptoms disappear rapidly. If the patient is examined at this stage the sacro-iliac joints will probably show a bilateral arthritis. Some years later there may be aching and stiffness in the lumbar region. Usually this increases gradually until the lumbar region may have become completely ankylosed. Sometimes remissions occur and these may last years. It is not uncommon after a period of quiescence for the condition to reoccur in the thoracic or cervical regions. In some cases the disease progresses until the spine and chest and even the hips are completely rigid.

SIGNS AND SYMPTOMS

Pain is a fairly constant feature though it varies in the time of onset; some patients have almost complete rigidity of the lumbar spine before the onset of pain. Aching, discomfort and pain are usually first felt in the lumbar region, since the condition almost invariably commences in sacro-iliac and lumbar joints. Gradually, with the spread of the arthritis,

96

pain extends up the whole back. Many patients complain of pain round the chest and abdomen or pain extending into the limbs, and sciatica is an occasional complaint. These pains are the result of irritation of the spinal nerves, or are referred from spinal segments into the area of distribution of these segments. If limb joints are involved, pain is also felt in relation to these joints.

Tenderness can sometimes be elicited by gentle pressure over the spinous processes or adjacent muscles.

Muscle spasm is practically always to be seen in the spinal muscles or muscles of other affected joints. As the condition ceases to be active and pain is alleviated, spasm persists because it has become a habit. This spasm is responsible for a great deal of the limited movement and deformity.

Limited movement is an early feature in whatever joints are involved, due to the inflammatory changes and muscle spasm. In the limb joints the progress of the arthritis is extraordinarily rapid, and fibrous or bony ankylosis results in complete loss of movement. In the spine, rigidity of the affected area may be partly masked by movement in neighbouring regions, but if the patient is carefully watched, a flattening of the affected area on movement can be easily recognised. Joints between the ribs and vertebrae, early involved, quickly stiffen and a much-diminished thoracic mobility is soon apparent, progressing until respiration becomes entirely abdominal. *muscle atrophy of muscle of back muscles.*

Deformity in ankylosing spondylitis varies very much from case to case and no adequate explanation of this fact can be given. It seems that whatever treatment is undertaken, some patients will eventually develop a severe flexion deformity of the spine and hips, while others retain a remarkably good posture (see Plate VI).

All cases show loss of the lumbar concavity, and flattening of the lumbar spine may even amount to a lumbar kyphosis. If one hip joint is affected there is nearly always a scoliosis also. Practically every patient suffers from flattening of the chest, diminution of the costal angle and decreased width of the intercostal spaces, these thoracic changes hampering the action of lungs and heart and causing laxity of the abdominal wall. If the cervical spine is involved, the weight of the head on the softened cervical bodies causes an increase in the cervical concavity and the head is carried forward on the shoulder while the chin is thrust forward. The dorsal curve is usually increased.

The general health is poor. Nearly all patients are grossly underweight and look and feel ill during the long active stage. The blood sedimentation rate is high and, as long as it remains raised, the condition may be considered to be active. Owing to the impairment of the action of the lungs, chest complications are very likely and bronchitis is a common feature. Iritis is another fairly common complication of this disease.

EXAMINATION OF THE PATIENT

Before commencing physiotherapy a thorough examination of the patient must be carried out. This may be conducted on the lines discussed for cases of rheumatoid arthritis. It is essential to know the state of the patient's health, the blood sedimentation rate, the medical treatment being given, and what chest complications, if any, are present. Careful observation must be made of the condition of all muscle groups, particularly noting muscular spasm or atrophy. Deformity must be noted, as must also the range of movement in all affected joints. The mobility of the thorax should be tested and records of weight, chest expansion and vital capacity made. Where there is much deformity a spinal tracing should be taken. It is of value to see the X-ray photographs in order that the presence of bony ankylosis or calcification of ligaments may be noted.

TIME TO COMMENCE PHYSIOTHERAPY TREATMENT

If treatment is to be really effective it must begin as early as possible in the active stage, since once calcification has occurred, no further movement in that region can be obtained. The ideal is to commence before the spinal articulations have become involved, but unfortunately patients rarely present themselves for treatment at this stage.

X-RAY THERAPY

Once diagnosed, these patients are treated by a course of deep X-ray therapy. This is usually given daily over a period of a month and the whole course may be repeated later if necessary. During the course general and local reaction will be experienced and this must be borne in mind in planning a course of physiotherapy. Exactly how the treatment obtains its good effects is not fully understood, but it is followed by decrease of pain, and, therefore, increased range of movement. Sometimes when response to X-ray therapy is poor Corticoid therapy is given.

OUTLINE OF PHYSIOTHERAPY

The active stage. This may be considered to be the stage during which the erythrocyte sedimentation rate is raised. Often the severe symptoms

98

may subside and the general condition of the patient improves, but so long as the sedimentation rate is raised the condition has not completely died out and further exacerbations are possible.

Treatment is best commenced by *teaching relaxation*. Muscle spasm is so often responsible for much of the pain, limited movement, and deformity that great improvement can often be gained by a few sessions of relaxation exercises alone. One obvious difficulty experienced by these patients is that of getting into a comfortable position, and this is particularly so where much deformity of the spine exists. The first step in relaxation training is, therefore, to teach the patient how to obtain a comfortable, relaxed position. It is usually necessary to teach a relative how to help the patient to acquire such a position at home by the judicious use of pillows. Once the patient is adequately supported and really comfortable (usually in as near the lying position as possible) he may be taught relaxation of all unaffected muscle groups. When the ability to relax these groups is attained, special attention is paid to 'spastic' groups. The patient usually finds the most difficult groups to relax are the anterior neck and pectoral muscles. Assistance may be given by the use of massage. Once the patient thoroughly understands the purpose and method of gaining relaxation he is told to practise many times during the day and especially before going to sleep at night, and in this way he falls asleep much more quickly—one step in the improvement of his general health. As time goes on and the ability to relax improves, less pillows will be needed to make him comfortable. heat + massage.

Concurrently with training in relaxation, efforts are made to *improve thoracic mobility* and consequently to increase the chest expansion and vital capacity. With the patient in a relaxed position general and local breathing exercises are taught. Local breathing aims at increasing lateral and posterior costal, and apical expansion, and can best be taught by the use of manual pressures and later by strap exercises. When the breathing has improved, abdominal breathing may be controlled by the use of a tight abdominal binder or by teaching the patient to contract the abdominal muscles strongly at the end of inspiration.

Once breathing has improved and the ability to relax increases, the next step is *to strengthen the extensor muscles* of head, spine, hips and shoulders and the abdominal muscles, so that a better posture can be held and a tendency to a flexion deformity resisted. Isolated muscular contractions should be taught first: for example, with the anterior neck muscles relaxed the patient is encouraged to contract the posterior neck muscles. The same procedure is then carried out for the rhomboids, latissimus dorsi, sacrospinalis, the extensors of the hips and the abdominal muscles.

Progression may be made by adding manual resistance and later resistance in slings by springs. Exercises for trapezius, latissimus dorsi and gluteus maximus in modified lying or side lying positions are also useful. When the muscular strength has improved sufficiently, similar work may be carried out in sitting and standing. The same strengthening work is also necessary for any muscle groups which act on other affected joints.

The *maintenance and improvement of the range of movement* in affected joints must depend on the wishes of the physician. Usually, since deep X-ray therapy results in improvement of the condition, it is considered wise to encourage active movement at the affected joints, giving every assistance possible. It must, however, be borne in mind that an active inflammatory process is present and no forcing under any circumstances is permissible. For this reason it is wiser to omit mobilising movements in slings and to rely on free, active, unassisted movements choosing good starting positions and eliminating gravity and friction.

Those joints which are not as yet affected, but which are always liable to become so, should be given full range active movements at each treatment.

When the course of deep X-ray is completed, or before, if the physician wishes, the patient may join a class of patients suffering from the same condition. All the work can be given and progressed as group work, and in addition easy games and light activities can be added. These patients are young and nearly always most co-operative, consequently they enjoy working together.

Some physicians prefer to keep their patients in hospital during the first course of X-ray therapy, others allow them to attend daily for treatment. If the patient is in hospital the physiotherapist will find that close co-operation with the sister of the ward is essential. It is necessary, if the patient is being nursed on fracture boards or in a plaster shell (with the object of preventing or correcting deformity), that he should be comfortable and able to relax, otherwise correction of deformity will be resisted by muscle spasm. If the physician wishes the patient to remain in bed, the majority of the work advocated can be carried out in the lying position.

Home exercises are essential whether the patient is in hospital or is an outpatient. Very careful instruction and explanation of their purpose and value must be given, particularly stressing the importance of relaxation and breathing exercises.

Precaution. Heat and massage should not be given to the back during or for some months following the X-ray therapy since the condition of the skin following X-ray therapy is not suitable.

The chronic state. This is the stage at which the sedimentation rate is normal and the patient is no longer complaining of ill health. At this stage bony ankylosis is complete and there is, therefore, no hope of increasing the range of movement. It is, however, sometimes possible to relieve aching and fatigue, due to ligamentous and muscular strain, by the application of heat, massage and relaxation exercises. Some improvement in posture can often be obtained by strengthening the postural muscles. Breathing exercises must always be given because, though improvement in mobility may not be obtained, the lungs are exercised, their circulation stimulated, gaseous interchange is increased, and the resistance of the lung tissue is raised so that chest diseases are less likely to arise. Again, home exercises are of paramount importance.

Chapter V

MENOPAUSAL OR
CLIMACTERIC ARTHRITIS. GOUT

MENOPAUSAL ARTHRITIS

This condition appears to be primarily a chronic synovitis rather than a true arthritis, but if untreated it tends to develop into an osteo-arthritis. *Women. 45-55*

Usually a few months after the cessation of the menopause, or a year or so before or after, the patient begins to complain of pain, aching and stiffness in the knee joints. On examination it is found that there is hypothyroidism, the patient is overweight, the skin dry, the hair and eyebrows thin. Locally, the knees appear enlarged, due to synovial thickening, there are pads of fat on the medial side of the knee joints and often a tender spot over the medial ligament of the joint. The range of movement is usually full but the joints feel stiff, particularly on getting up from sitting and on kneeling or walking up and down stairs. Pain is sometimes quite severe. Though the knee joints are most commonly involved, the feet and hands may also be stiff and painful.

PATHOLOGICAL CHANGES

In the early stages the changes appear to be chiefly in the synovial membrane. The folds and fringes proliferate. Since the synovial membrane of the knee joint is outstanding in the number of its fat-filled folds, it is this joint which is nearly always the seat of trouble in a menopausal arthritis.

In addition to changes in the synovial membrane there is nearly always hypotonia of muscles and laxity of ligaments, particularly noticeable in the lower extremities; thus considerable strain is thrown on the joint structures, which, if untreated, leads to the development of degenerative changes in bone and cartilage. If muscles and ligaments are weak, flat foot is likely to occur, and this may result in further strain on the knee joints and may account for the tenderness over the medial ligament.

PROGNOSIS

If a menopausal arthritis is treated early there is considerable hope of improvement, because changes in bone and cartilage have not yet occurred. If untreated the condition invariably progresses to an osteo-arthritis with no hope of cure.

PRINCIPLES OF TREATMENT BY PHYSICAL MEANS

Since this condition is associated with overweight and glandular disturbance, treatment obviously implies an attempt to reduce weight, usually by restricted diet and use of thyroid extract, and the administration of oestrogen preparations. Physical treatment should be directed towards the local condition. Improvement of circulation to the synovial membrane may be obtained by the use of diathermy. Muscular tone and ligamentous strength may be increased by means of faradism and non-weight-bearing exercises. Posture may be improved, and particularly the posture of the feet in standing and walking. If flat foot is present, it is treated so that strain on the knees through faulty distribution of weight and inelastic gait is avoided.

Note. It may be noted that another type of arthritis, of the rheumatoid variety, sometimes commences during the time of the menopause. It attacks the small joints of the hands and feet and tends to spread to the larger joints. It is not nearly so amenable to treatment as the previous type. This type is dealt with on the same lines as rheumatoid arthritis.

GOUT

Gout is a metabolic disorder in which the metabolism of a purine is upset. The quantity of uric acid in the blood stream rises and from time to time there occurs a sudden precipitation of this substance into the tissues in the form of crystals of sodium biurate. These crystals are deposited in the cartilage, bone ends, synovial membrane and periarticular structures, and, in addition, in other poorly vascularised structures such as the cartilage of the ears. These form the chalk stones or 'tophi' characteristic of gout.

During an acute attack of gout the deposit of sodium biurate in joint structure sets up an acute inflammatory reaction and the joint affected, commonly the metatarso-phalangeal joint of the first toe, becomes red, hot, swollen and exquisitely painful and tender to touch, while over it the skin is stretched and shiny. Such an attack lasts with varying degrees of intensity of pain over several days and then, as the joint symptoms subside, the skin desquamates. Usually the joint condition clears completely. If repeated attacks take place, arthritic changes will eventually occur and the joint will become stiff and the range of movement limited.

For such cases the treatment is purely medical. Colchicine is the drug in common use for sufferers from acute gout.

Some patients suffer from a chronic form of gout in which acute attacks do not occur. For many weeks or months the patient complains of some pain, swelling, and stiffness, usually in the small joints of the hands or feet, particularly the metatarso-phalangeal joint of the great toe and similar joints in the fingers and thumb. Occasionally larger joints are also affected. Very often the joints fail to clear completely. In most cases tophi form, and, acting as irritants, result in degenerative osteo-arthritic changes. If the tophi form in superficial tissues the skin directly over them is so thin and shiny that they can be seen through it. Eventually, they tend to ulcerate through, leaving ulcers which rarely heal.

Again, for these cases treatment is mainly medical, Atophan and sodium salicylate being the most effective drugs. These cases do sometimes appear for physiotherapy because both general and local physical measures will help the patient. These patients benefit from any treatment which stimulates general metabolism or aids elimination by the skin. General breathing exercises, petrissage to all muscle groups of the body, and general muscular contractions are all of value.

Affected joints appear to benefit most from the application of salicylic ionisation followed by active movements.

Peri-arthritis. — Arthritis around joint

e.g. Slddda. ? no.

Chapter VI

NON-ARTICULAR RHEUMATISM — FIBROSITIS

It has been seen that a factor common to all rheumatic lesions is the involvement of fibrous structures. In articular rheumatism changes occur in the synovial membrane, cartilage and bone, while in non-articular rheumatism it is other fibrous structures of the body which are involved. In the latter condition the tissues particularly prone to be affected are the aponeuroses, origins, insertions and sheaths of muscles, the capsules and bursae of joints and the subcutaneous fatty tissue.

The term fibrositis implies an inflammatory condition of any of these structures, but in some cases inflammation is not present and pain and stiffness are due to other factors. The term is then incorrect. For want of a better word, however, it is still in constant use and is a satisfactory term provided that it is clearly understood that the term covers a wide range of lesions of fibrous tissues, many of which are not inflammatory. In many cases, no structural abnormality is present and the symptoms are wholly determined by psychological influences.

The main characteristics of the condition are pain, which is not relieved by rest, tenderness of muscles, stiffness and 'trigger' spots. These trigger spots are localised areas of tenderness from which pain is referred segmentally. Usually the cause of the symptoms is not obvious.

CLASSIFICATION

Many attempts at a classification of these lesions have been made. Grouping may be made according to the area involved, namely: lumbago, pleurodynia, torticollis; but it is now more usual to classify according to the exact tissue involved. Thus a reasonable grouping might be made as follows:

Intra-muscular rheumatism, in which the fibrous framework, tendons or aponeuroses are involved.

Periarticular fibrositis, in which the capsule and periarticular structures are attacked.

Panniculitis, an involvement of the subcutaneous tissue.

Bursitis, a lesion of bursae.

CAUSES *Etiology*

The cause of the soft tissue lesions is unknown but certain factors appear to be closely connected with the lesion. In many cases there appears to be a *psychogenic factor*. Some patients suffering from fibrositis, on examination are found to have some emotional disturbance, the patient being worried or upset. It appears that one of the manifestations of emotional disturbance is an increase in tension in the muscles which will be accompanied by tenderness and stiffness, caused by an accumulation of fatigue products in the muscle.

A second factor is probably *infection*. Painful nodules often appear in the soft tissues during an infectious illness, particularly influenza. These often disappear as the illness improves but in some cases they fail to do so.

Cold and damp play a considerable part. Some patients appear to be less able to adapt to changes in temperature, possibly because all rheumatic subjects show a poor peripheral circulation. In these people sudden chilling of the overheated skin will often provoke an attack of fibrositis.

Trauma may be responsible for fibrositis. There may be a definite injury, but more often it is the continuous strain of faulty posture. Faulty carriage of the head may well be responsible for a great many cases of fibrositis of the neck and shoulders; in the same way, an increased pelvic tilt will throw a continuous strain on the ligaments, muscles and fascia in the lumbar region and give rise to aching and fatigue in the back.

Fibrositis may sometimes be the result of *retention of fluid* within the tissues. The cause of this is not yet known, but it is possible that this retention may be one of the causes of the acute stiff neck of sudden onset.

Fibrositis is known to *accompany the articular rheumatic disorders*. It is, for example, often found in the medial ligament of the knee in rheumatoid and osteo-arthritis.

Stiff neck and lumbago, traditionally attributed to fibrositis, are usually caused by *minor degrees of disc prolapse*, and tearing of a few muscle fibres may account for so-called fibrositis in other areas.

Psychosomatic   The reaction in body of a mind disturbance

PATHOLOGY

Since in many cases the chief feature of the condition appears to be the presence of nodules which are the source of pain referred segmentally, the natural query arises as to what these nodules are. Much work has been done on this subject and it has been found that a variety of changes gives rise to them.

They may be literally the result of inflammation of fibrous tissue and they are then masses of fibrous tissue. In this case, if they are sufficiently superficial as to be palpable, the nodules are usually found to be small and firm and are most often found in the tendons and aponeuroses. They are probably the result of continuous strain or of trauma. Sometimes the nodule may be palpated in the muscle belly. It is then most likely to be caused by contraction of a group of muscle fibres due to irritation of a nerve. In these cases it may be very difficult to isolate the site of the real lesion.

Nodules are quite commonly found along the posterior extremity of the iliac crest, up to the lateral edge of the sacro-spinalis and over the whole of the area of trapezius. Copeman has pointed out that these nodules are, in fact, oedematous fat lobules. Since the fat lobules are enclosed in a firm fibrous membrane, any swelling will result in tension and pain. The reason for the oedema is as yet uncertain. Occasionally the fat lobules have been found to herniate through the membrane and their blood supply has then been impaired.

In some cases no nodules can be detected. In these cases the changes may be those of inflammation as in peri-articular fibrositis, or there may be accumulation of the products of metabolism in a muscle or group of muscles which is in a state of tension.

In many cases in which diffuse tenderness is present, no changes can be found.

SIGNS AND SYMPTOMS

Pain may be felt in one muscle group or in several. It may appear to start at one point in a muscle, tendon or ligament and to radiate from this point. Pain felt diffusely in a muscle group is usually made worse by movement but it is not actually relieved by rest. Pain starting from one definite spot can often be 'set off' by pressure on that point, and such a spot is known as a 'trigger point'. Thus from a trigger point in supraspinatus, pain may radiate to the skin over the insertion of deltoid since both structures are innervated by the fifth cervical segment. Pain arising in the capsule of the shoulder joint may be felt down the whole arm including the radial side of the forearm, to the thumb, index and middle fingers, since the capsule receives its innervation from the fifth, sixth, seventh and eighth cervical segments, while these dermatomes extend right to the hand (see Fig. 8).

Tenderness. The nodule itself, if it is the cause of the pain of which the patient is complaining, will be tender on pressure. Often, if there are fatigue products in the muscle, the whole muscle or group will be tender on palpation.

Stiffness. The patient complains of the area feeling stiff, particularly after severe exercise; for this reason there is an unwillingness to perform movements.

Atrophy and limitation of movement. Pain and stiffness may give rise to disuse and some generalised atrophy may be found. Thus a painful shoulder leads to fixation of the arm in the adducted and medially rotated position, and there may then be some atrophy of the abductors and lateral rotators and slight limitation in shoulder movement due to adaptive shortening.

EXAMINATION OF THE PATIENT

In the majority of cases the patient is sent to the physiotherapy department diagnosed as fibrositis, capsulitis or intra-muscular rheumatism. Further information is needed before correct physical treatment can be carried out. It is absolutely essential to try to find the exact site of the lesion so that treatment can be directed to this and not to the site of referred pain.

It is important to take a careful history, particularly noting where the pain was first felt, since this is usually a true guide to the site of the lesion.

Observation is important in order to note the general appearance and posture. The presence of spasm, of swelling and of changes in colour should all be noted. The way the patient holds the affected part is a useful sign.

Changes in muscle tone, swelling or atrophy can be particularly well detected by the sense of touch and generalised tenderness can also be appreciated at the same time. Palpation for trigger points should not be carried out until the movements have been tested. It is simpler to isolate the tissue at fault first and then palpate for the exact site of the nodule.

Test of movement is the most important part of the examination. Where pain is referred, each joint within the area supplied by the same segment of the spinal cord should be tested. If pain is felt in the arm, movement of fingers, wrist, forearm, elbow, neck, shoulder girdle and shoulder should all be examined. Each movement which can normally be carried out in the joint, should be tested passively and actively. The patient should then be asked to try to perform the movement against such resistance that it will ensure that no movement actually occurs in the joint. In this case, no structure is stretched but certain muscles contract strongly. While the movements are being tested note should be made of pain, limitation by muscle spasm, unusual sounds such as snapping, clicking and crepitus

The actual findings in the examination will enable the lesion to be isolated to a certain structure. First, if there is pain on passive and active movement in the same direction an inert structure such as the capsule is at fault. Secondly, if pain occurs on active movement in one direction and passive in the reverse, a muscle or tendon is probably concerned, and should pain arise when such resistance is given so that no movement occurs, the lesion is definitely in a contractile structure. The significance of these findings was first pointed out by Cyriax, and there are many other points which arise and which are of value in estimating the exact site of the lesion. For a full account of these, reference should be made to his book, *Rheumatism and Soft Tissue Injuries*.

When a lesion has been tracked to a definite structure, careful palpation should then be made to find a tender spot. If pressure on such a spot reproduces the patient's pain, then it is probably the real lesion.

Such an examination is not easy, it takes time and needs care and skill, but it does mean that in many cases the real lesion can be treated.

PRINCIPLES OF TREATMENT BY PHYSIOTHERAPY

Physical treatment depends on the site and nature of the lesion. *Prophylaxis — is to prevent fibrositis (occurrence)*

Acute diffuse tenderness and pain in a muscle group. Whether the cause of this state is inflammation or retention of fluid, there is pain and spasm and the most successful treatment is support. In the lumbar region, this can be given in the form of strapping; in the neck it is more difficult and rest in bed with the head properly supported on pillows is the method of choice. Superficial heat will relieve pain by its sedative effect on nerve endings. Whatever the nature of the condition, as soon as the acute pain begins to subside it is essential that the exudate or fluid should not be allowed to organise or scarring and impairment of movement will result. Measures which stimulate the venous and lymphatic drainage of the area and keep the fluid moving are valuable. Anodal galvanism, deep but not intensive heating, light massage, may all be used, adapted to the patient's tolerance.

As the condition improves and pain lessens, deeper massage should be given and exercise introduced. The chief purpose of the exercise is to prevent clotting of exudate and fluid and so to maintain a full range of movement. *They must not wear flannel*

Diffuse tenderness in many groups without obvious trigger points. In most patients suffering from this type of fibrositis the origin is due to stress and anxiety. The first principle of physical treatment is to teach the patient

change of occupation. Open air is good

to relax. The value of relaxation should be explained and any method which proves satisfactory may be used. Relaxation must then be practised regularly at home and particularly at night so that sleep is more easily achieved.

Palliative treatment may be given to carry away fatigue products in the muscles. Inductothermy and massage are suitable. It must be realised that relaxation is far more important. Heat and massage make the patient more comfortable but do not touch the cause of the condition.

Localised nodules in aponeuroses, tendons and deep fibro-fatty tissue. The object of physical treatment is to promote absorption of blood or retained fluid, to reduce fat herniation by stretching the fibrous envelope or to stretch and soften scar tissue. All these will be achieved if the area around the nodule is flooded with tissue fluid and the blood and lymph capillaries are dilated. One of the best methods of gaining this end is the use of counter-irritation if the nodule is superficial, and deep heating or constant-current applications if it is deep. This is followed by deep massage localised to the nodule. Vigorous kneading and finger kneading will help to produce vaso-dilation and circular or transverse frictions will stretch out fibrous tissue. Full range active movement will stimulate the circulation and aid stretching.

Localised nodules in the belly of the muscle. Since these are areas of reflex spasm, local treatment is of no avail. Spasm may be relieved by the measures previously discussed but the condition will return. A more careful search for the lesion is necessary. It is almost always neural in origin, and if it is found, treatment should be carried out on the lines indicated for neuritis (see Part IV, Chapter XI).

Pain arising in the arm or leg from soft tissue lesions will be discussed further when Brachial Neuritis and Sciatica are described (see Part IV, Chapter XI).

PERIARTICULAR FIBROSITIS (CAPSULITIS)

This discussion of fibrositis has mainly considered localised lesions in muscles, tendons and inert structures. Further attention must now be paid to a well-recognised fibrositic condition which occurs almost solely in the shoulder joint. This is an inflammation, of unknown origin, of the capsule and periarticular structures leading to pain, stiffness and severe limitation of movement.

Many cases of stiff and painful shoulders are traumatic in origin, as, for example, the stiff shoulder which occasionally follows fractures round the shoulder joint or a Colles fracture. Again, stiffness may occur when movement at the joint is difficult or impossible, such as is seen in some cases of hemiplegia. Stiffness in these cases probably results from circulatory stagnation, oedema of the periarticular structures and adhesion formation.

On the other hand a certain number will report for treatment complaining of discomfort in the shoulder and pain radiating into the arm, who can give no history of injury, and it is these cases which possibly may be classified with other non-articular rheumatic conditions. The cause of the onset of symptoms is unknown. Inflammation probably commences in the subacromial bursa, supraspinatus tendon and upper part of the capsule, and then spreads to the rest of the capsule. Acute or chronic inflammation results in thickening and contracture of the capsule, degeneration of bursae and tendons and extensive fibrous tissue formation.

The characteristic onset of the condition is aching and stiffness in one or both shoulders, worse at night or on movement. Pain is felt in the shoulder or may be referred to the lower third of deltoid. After perhaps some weeks, pain becomes much more severe and begins to radiate into the forearm, hand and fingers. It is now present even when the limb is at rest, and it interferes with sleep, the patient being unable to lie on the affected side. Slight swelling may be identified round the edge of the acromion and the whole region of the joint may now be tender. Movement is limited in all directions by muscle spasm, the patient holding the arm rigidly to the side. Some muscle atrophy takes place, most noticeably in the deltoid and supraspinatus and the lateral rotators, since these muscles tend to be inhibited during the period of severe pain.

Gradually pain subsides but often limitation of movement increases as adhesions form, and a long period of discomfort and stiffness ensues. All movements are limited, but the most limited are abduction and lateral rotation, since abduction causes friction between the inflamed structures and the acromion, while if the limb is adducted it is also medially rotated and tends to become fixed in this position.

OUTLINE OF TREATMENT BY PHYSIOTHERAPY

Treatment must depend on the stage of the condition.

During the acute phase, when pain is severe and felt in the whole arm and movement is guarded by muscle spasm, *rest* is indicated and physiotherapy contra-indicated. Complete rest in bed is by far the most effective measure. In bed the arm can be supported in as much abduction and lateral rotation as can be obtained, a much safer position than that obtained by the use of a large arm sling, since in the sling the arm is fixed in medial rotation and lateral rotation is liable to become limited. Without full lateral rotation abduction and full elevation cannot be obtained.

As pain subsides *active movements* may be instituted but these must be painless and will therefore not at first include abduction or lateral rotation. The best movements to use are either lying, fully supported and relaxed, arm elevation through flexion, or lax stoop sitting, with the sound arm supported on a plinth or table, and easy relaxed pendular swinging of the affected limb. In either case, gentle downward traction on the arm should be exerted because, as a result of muscle spasm, the head of the humerus is usually 'hitched up' in the glenoid cavity, with the result that on movement pressure by the acromion is brought to bear sooner on the inflamed structures. With the patient in the lying position the physiotherapist should place one hand gently but firmly in the axilla while the other grips and exerts a downward pull on the lower end of the humerus. This traction may be maintained during active movement. If pendular swinging is being used, traction is obtained partly by the weight of the limb and partly by the addition of a light weight in the hand.

As the condition improves other shoulder movements may be added —always within the limit of pain. Lateral rotation should be practised at first with the patient lying flat on the back, elbow flexed, fingers pointing vertically upwards, the patient attempting to press the posterior aspect of the forearm against the plinth while avoiding any abduction. Later this movement may be practised in standing back to a wall, and other lateral rotation exercises may be added. Abduction is first taught in lying and the assistance of the slings and pulleys may be added if desired. Gradually the active work is progressed, always within the limit of pain, keeping a careful watch for recurrence of acute symptoms.

In the chronic phase, either before or after the acute phase, when pain is felt only in the shoulder on movement and not at rest, when it does not radiate down the arm, when the patient is able to lie on that side at night, and when active movement is stationary, more drastic treatment is indicated. Circulation may be improved by the deep heating effect of the short-wave current and absorption of the fibrous thickening aided by the introduction of chlorine or iodine ions by the direct current.

With the tissues relaxed by the heating effect, the muscles acting on the joint should be thoroughly loosened and softened by kneading and picking-up manipulations; traction may then be applied to the capsule in the way previously described. This should be followed by free active exercises and assisted work, either by self-assistance with double-handed pulleys or by assistance with poles and springs. Care is needed in the supervision

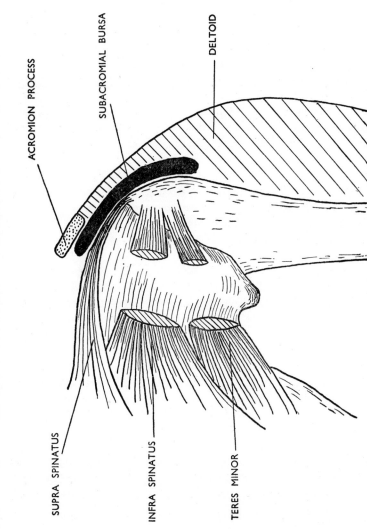

ACROMION PROCESS

SUBACROMIAL BURSA

DELTOID

SUPRA SPINATUS

INFRA SPINATUS

TERES MINOR

(AFTER STONE)

Fig. 2

of active work for a stiff or painful humero-scapular joint because so much 'cheating' often takes place through movement of the shoulder girdle or trunk. The patient should either be placed in lying for the movement so that the scapula is at least partly fixed, or the scapula and clavicle should be steadied by the physiotherapist, or, at least, the patient should be in such a position that the movement can be adequately watched. For this reason class-work is not always very satisfactory.

It is essential to teach the patient to use the correct humero-scapular rhythm. If possible, the patient should sit in front of a mirror with both shoulders and arms free from clothing. Abduction of the unaffected arm may then be carried out. This is followed by abduction of the affected arm. At the beginning of the movement the patient is taught to press the shoulder down and lift the elbow sideways, making the space between the elbow and the side of the trunk as wide as possible. She watches the movement in the mirror, noting and correcting any tendency to elevate the point of the shoulder. It is often valuable to move both arms at the same time in order to compare the performance.

Elevation of the arm is then practised in the same way and this is followed by rotation.

Resisted exercises must also be included to restore the power of the shoulder muscles, especially that of the abductors and lateral rotators. Even if the actual range obtained is small there is usually some part of the range in which resistance can be given without producing pain.

Rapid progress in these cases should not be expected. If a time is reached when increasing range is no longer being obtained by voluntary active movements, then the physician will probably consider the advisability of manipulation. If manipulation under anaesthesia is carried out, the physiotherapist should be in attendance to note what range is obtained, so that immediately the patient recovers from the anaesthetic physiotherapy may be employed to maintain and improve upon the range already obtained by the physician.

The constant daily practice of shoulder movement is absolutely essential, and it is necessary to explain this to the patient. Each patient should be given a list of exercises and instructed as to how these should be performed at home. Recovery should take place within a year.

SUBACROMIAL BURSITIS

Subacromial bursitis may be the result of trauma or may occur in rheumatoid arthritis, in which condition the bursae are peculiarly prone to be affected. On the other hand the condition may develop insidiously without obvious cause, and it is this condition which is considered here.

It will be remembered that the articular surfaces of the shoulder joint are surrounded by a loose capsule with which are blended the tendons of supraspinatus, infraspinatus, teres minor and subscapularis. These four tendons form a cuff round the joint and are often spoken of as the 'rotator cuff'. Covering the greater tuberosity and blending with the rotator cuff is the subacromial bursa separating these structures from the deltoid muscle (see Fig. 2). In addition, the bursa extends up beneath the acromion, protecting the supraspinatus tendon from constant friction. The floor of the bursa is adherent to the supraspinatus, coraco-humeral ligament and capsule, while the roof is adherent to the under surface of the coraco-acromial arch; thus as the humerous moves in the glenoid cavity the upper part of the joint moves in relation to the arch, and ease and freedom of movement are guaranteed. Should either wall of the bursa become inflamed and the floor and roof then become adherent, movement at the shoulder joint will be seriously impaired.

This type of subacromial bursitis is characterised by pain in the shoulder (sometimes referred to the insertion of deltoid), tenderness along the lateral edge of the acromion, reversed scapulo-humeral rhythm and a painful arc of movement occurring on both passive and active abduction between about 60° and 120°.

The condition usually yields to conservative treatment but occasionally excision of the bursa or of the acromion may be necessary. Conservative treatment is carried out on similar lines to that of capsulitis. Some physicians advocate the use of a large arm sling for a week or fortnight in order to limit the movements which cause pain. Short-wave therapy and movements should be started during this phase. The movements are commenced and progressed in the way already described (see page 111).

Causes of Peri-arthritic shoulder.
1) Acute o chronic infections eg Rheumatoid arthritis.
2) Trauma, e g) dislocated sholder Such has beentput back again 2) Strain
3) immobilisation - damaged caused due to immobilisation
4) Referred from other sources

PART THREE

DISEASES OF THE
RESPIRATORY SYSTEM

Chapter 1

INTRODUCTION. SIGNS AND SYMPTOMS. EXAMINATION OF THE PATIENT. PRINCIPLES OF TREATMENT

I t is not within the scope of a book of this nature to describe in detail the structure and function of the respiratory apparatus but certain points do deserve special consideration if the physiotherapist is to work intelligently in the chest unit.

The lungs are each covered by a completely closed pleural sac, one layer of which lines the chest wall and floor, the other covering the lung. The layers are normally in contact but move smoothly over one another owing to the small amount of serous fluid secreted by the epithelial cells of the membrane. A potential cavity does, however, exist. Pressure within each pleural cavity is less than that of atmosphere. It varies below this point, rhythmically with respiration, dropping during inspiration and rising with expiration.

The lungs are composed of a great number of lobules bound together by highly elastic connective tissue. Each lobule is a miniature lung since it consists of a terminal bronchiole, ending in vestibule, atria, infundibulae and alveolar sacs, blood and lymph vessels and nerves. The lobules are connected together to form lobes. Each lung is divided into two main lobes by an oblique fissure which, commencing above and behind the hilum, runs back and up to cross the posterior border a little below the apex of the lung, then sweeps down and forward to terminate at the lower border just behind its anterior extremity.

The upper lobe lying above this fissure includes the apex, anterior border, most of the medial surface and some part of the costal surface. The lower lobe consists of the base, nearly all the posterior border and some of the costal surface.

In the case of the right lung there is an additional transverse fissure dividing the upper lobe into an upper part and a lower part known as the middle lobe.

Each lobe consists of a number of segments, each with its own bronchus (see Fig. 3A, I, II, B, C, D). Each segment is quite distinct from its fellow and occasionally this may be apparent on the surface of the lung by means of slight visible indentations. A knowledge of these segments is essential in both medical and surgical cases if postural drainage is to be carried out effectively.

The right lung shows ten segments, the left nine. From the right upper lobe bronchus three bronchi are given off to the three segments; an apical passes up to supply an apical area forming the dome of the lung and projecting above the clavicle; a posterior bronchus passes backwards into a posterior segment; and an anterior bronchus passing antero-laterally to the anterior segment.

The middle lobe bronchus divides into two to supply the superior and inferior segments of the middle lobe. The right lower lobe bronchus gives off a bronchus which passes, exactly opposite the origin of the middle lobe, directly backwards into the apical segment of the right lower lobe. The bronchus then divides into four to supply the remaining four segments of the lower lobe, that is the cardiac segment, anterior-basal, lateral-basal and posterior-basal segments.

The ten segments of the right lobe are therefore anterior, apical and posterior of the upper lobe, superior and inferior of the middle lobe, and apical and anterior, posterior and lateral basal of the lower.

The left lung differs hardly at all except that it has no cardiac lobe, and that, because its main bronchus is more oblique, the apical bronchus of its upper lobe is more vertical.

The upper lobe bronchus gives off four main bronchi to five segments. An apical to the apical segment, an anterior to an anterior and a posterior to a posterior segment. The fourth is the lingular bronchus which divides into two for the superior and inferior segments of the lingular area of the upper lobe. The lower lobe bronchus is similar to that of the right lower lobe with the exception that it has three divisions instead of four because there is no cardiac lobe in the left lung.

The nine segments of the left lung are, therefore, apical, anterior, posterior, superior and inferior lingular of the upper lobe and apical, anterior basal, lateral basal and posterior basal of the lower lobe.

In structure the bronchi consist of an outer coat of fibrous tissue and cartilage, a middle coat of smooth muscular tissue and an inner mucous coat which has a lining of ciliated columnar epithelium on a basement membrane. This inner coat contains a considerable quantity of elastic fibres and lymphoid tissue. As the tubes narrow and become smaller their structure gradually changes.

INTRODUCTION

No cartilage is found in the walls of bronchioles of less than one millimetre in diameter, while in these the muscle tissue is conspicuous and
forms sphincters at the end of the alveolar ducts. The lining of the alveoli
is probably incomplete and capillaries may push their way between the
cells, consequently the blood is in almost direct contact with the alveolar
air.

Mechanism of Respiration

Inspiration occurs as a result of the contraction of certain muscles, particularly the diaphragm and intercostals, whereby the size of the thoracic
cavity is increased and pressure within the pleural cavity is consequently
reduced. As pressure on the external surface of the lung drops while that

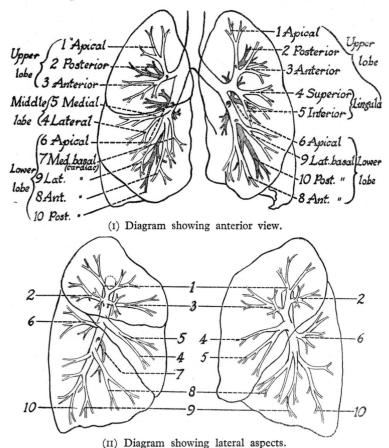

(I) Diagram showing anterior view.

(II) Diagram showing lateral aspects.

Fig. 3A. Diagrammatic representation of the bronchi.

on the internal surface remains the same, the lung expands, pressure within it drops and air is therefore drawn in. The stimulus which brings about the contraction of the muscles is an automatic rhythmical discharge of impulses from the cells of the respiratory centre which is influenced in its rate by nervous and chemical factors.

Expiration is not a muscular action but depends largely on the elastic nature of the chest wall and the lungs. When the impulses passing to the respiratory muscles are sufficiently diminished, the muscles relax and the

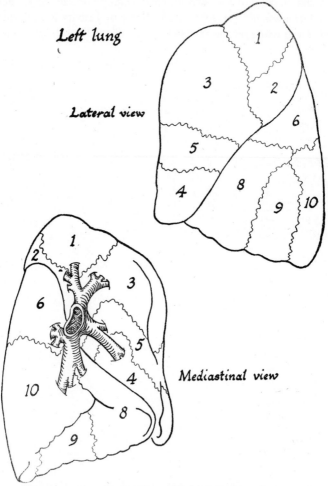

Fig. 3B. Diagrammatic representation of the left broncho-pulmonary segments.

chest wall therefore sinks back to its normal position, the diaphragm ascending, partly as a result of the recoil of the abdominal wall. As the thoracic cavity diminishes in size, intra-pleural pressure rises. The suction effect of low pressure on the external surface of the lung is diminished, and consequently the elastic lung tissue recoils with rise of intra-pulmonary pressure and outflow of air. It should be noted that the ability to breathe out fully depends on the elasticity of the lung. The low intra-pleural pressure is always tending to suck the lung out and this tendency is resisted by the elastic tissue. Should this elasticity be lost on expiration, though

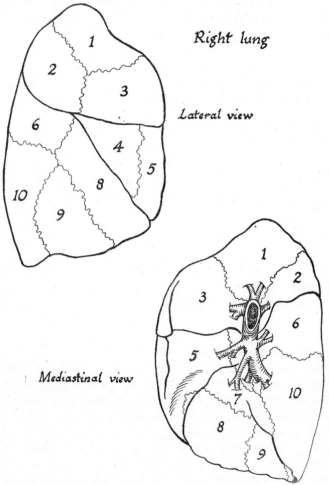

Fig. 3C. Diagrammatic representation of the right broncho-pulmonary segments.

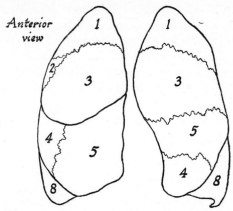

Fig. 3D. Diagrammatic representation of the segments.

intra-pleural pressure rises, it is still less than that within the lung and the lung will therefore tend to remain expanded.

The Removal of Secretions

The cells of the mucous membrane lining the air passages from nose to respiratory bronchioles secrete a tiny quantity of mucus which moistens the tubes and traps small foreign bodies in the inspired air. Any irritation of the mucous membrane results in a marked increase in the formation of mucus which may form a thick viscid layer over the surface or may collect in the smaller tubes acting as a mucus plug and preventing entry of air. If the excess mucus is allowed to remain in the bronchial tree certain dangers arise. It may result in collapse of the area of lung into which air cannot enter, the air distal to the block gradually being absorbed. It may undergo the process of decomposition as the stale mucus becomes invaded by micro-organisms and pus may be formed. In any case if decomposition occurs toxins will be liberated which, acting as irritants, will set up a chronic inflammation with weakening of the tubal walls and fibrosis of the mucous membrane and surrounding tissue.

Normally excessive mucus or foreign substances can be eliminated by coughing. The patient takes a deep breath to fill the lungs with air, closes the larynx, vigorously contracts the muscles of forced expiration in order to raise intrapulmonary pressure, then relaxes the glottis and a sudden outrush of air occurs, carrying with it the offending substance. The excessive secretion, however, may be so deeply placed in the small tubes or even in the alveoli that there is no current of air behind it, and consequently coughing is ineffective. Provided the secretion is in that part of the tube proximal to the respiratory bronchiole, its movement upward is aided by the action of the cilia which will bring the substance into a region where coughing is effective. Under certain circumstances, in spite of these means, secretions do tend to accumulate; coughing may be suppressed either because the cough reflex is inhibited as a result of the action of an anaesthetic or because the patient voluntarily inhibits coughing through fear of pain; the action of the cilia may cease because cold or an anaesthetic decreases their activity, or because as a result of a chronic inflammatory process, degeneration of the mucous membrane has occurred with loss of the ciliated epithelium. It is also possible that pus, mucus or inflammatory exudate is so viscid that it adheres to the walls of the tubes, or it may have collected in cavities and therefore is no longer capable of stimulating the cough reflex.

In these cases certain steps may be taken to aid its removal. Breathing exercises or percussion on the chest and agility exercises will help to loosen mucus while gravity may be used to drain cavities. Sometimes suction drainage may be necessary.

Postural Drainage

The principle of postural drainage of secretion lies in the above facts. If the secretions can be moved towards the extra pulmonary bronchi and trachea, then they can be eliminated without strain by coughing. The patient is therefore placed in the position in which gravity will cause fluid secretions to flow towards these areas of the bronchial tree. Two facts must be known if postural drainage is to be successful; first, where the material is accumulating; and secondly, the direction of the bronchus which will drain this area. Once these facts are known the arrangement of the patient's position presents no difficulty. The positions set out below form a basis but minor adjustments are often necessary according to the exact site of the cavities and it is of great advantage to have an X-ray of the chest handy for reference (see Plate 4(a), (b), (c), (d), (e), (f) and (g)).

UPPER LOBE

(a) *Apex* by apical bronchus—upright.

(b) *Anterior area* by antero-lateral bronchus—lying flat on the back.

(c) *Postero-lateral area*—lying on opposite side turned about 45° towards the face (in the case of the left lung the shoulders should be slightly raised as the bronchus is more vertical).

MIDDLE LOBE AND LINGULAR PROCESS—middle and lingular bronchus—lying on back but slightly turned to the opposite side, hips raised about 10 inches.

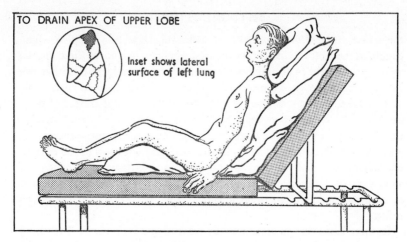

TO DRAIN APEX OF UPPER LOBE

Inset shows lateral
surface of left lung

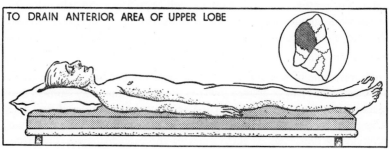

TO DRAIN ANTERIOR AREA OF UPPER LOBE

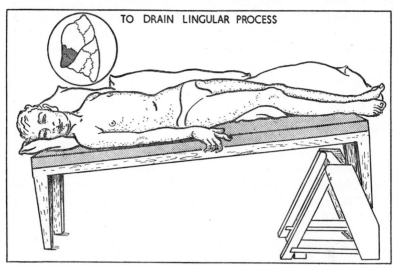

TO DRAIN LINGULAR PROCESS

Top, Fig. 4(a), Centre, Fig. 4(b), Bottom, Fig. 4(c).

LOWER LOBE

(a) *Apex* by dorsal bronchus, patient lying flat on face.

(b) *Anterior area* by anterior basic bronchus, patient lying on back, hips raised about 12 inches.

(c) *Lateral area* by lateral basic bronchus, patient lying on opposite side, hips raised about 12 inches.

(d) *Posterior area* by posterior basic bronchus, patient lying on face, hips raised about 14 inches.

'Tipping' may be gained by raising the foot of the bed or plinth by means of a bed elevator or bed blocks. Alternatively, pillows may be used

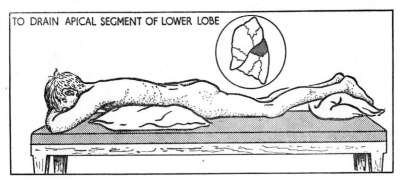

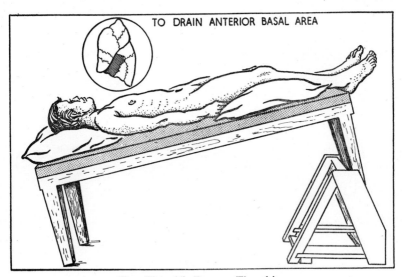

Top, Fig. 4(d), Bottom, Fig. 4(e).

beneath the hips. In cases where the deepest 'tip' is required the patient may lean over the side of the bed with the hands on a stool or the floor, according to the height of the bed, or a Nelson bed may be used. In choosing the method and height of 'tipping', attention must always be paid to

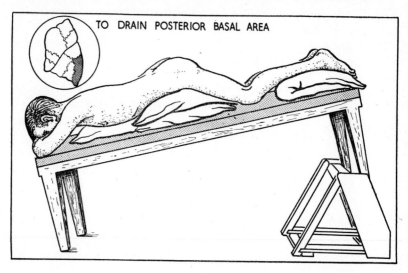

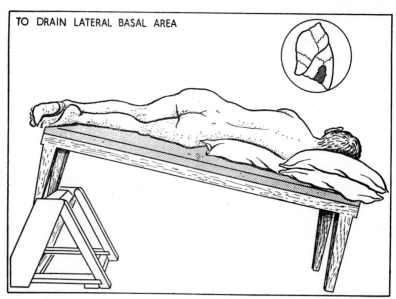

Top, Fig. 4(f), Bottom, Fig. 4(g).

the age and condition of the patient. Obviously a bronchiectatic child can stand a deeper and longer 'tip' than an elderly patient who has recently had a lobectomy.

Breathing Exercises, Percussion and Agility

In some cases postural drainage alone is insufficient to move thick secretions. Purulent material or viscid mucus may sometimes be loosened and dislodged, in suitable cases, by preceding 'tipping' by agility exercises. Any exercises which produce considerable movement in the trunk are useful, such as quick trunk forward and downward bending, brisk double arm circling, running and jumping. Obviously age and condition of patient have to be considered before agility work can be used. Material can often be loosened by percussion on the chest wall. The patient is then placed in the drainage position and vigorous shaking and clapping are given over the affected area of the lung, the strength of the percussion movements being modified according to the condition. Deep breathing exercises will, by the movement of the lung tissue, help to dislodge accumulated material; particular emphasis should be laid on expiration. These exercises can be combined with percussion and carried out in the same position.

SIGNS AND SYMPTOMS OF RESPIRATORY DISORDERS

There are certain outstanding signs and symptoms of disorders of the respiratory system which should be familiar to the physiotherapist. These are: cough, expectoration, dyspnoea, diminished thoracic movement and pain. In addition haemoptysis, loss of weight and deformity may also be present. These symptoms do not necessarily indicate a respiratory lesion, in fact they may well be evidence of other diseases particularly cardiac, but they are likely to be present if something goes wrong in the respiratory apparatus.

Cough may be simply a habit or it may be the result of a reflex irritation. Thus, for example, disorders of the stomach may result in irritation of the afferent fibres of the vagus nerve and so cause a 'stomach' cough. Usually, however, a cough is due to irritation of the nerve endings in the mucous lining of the trachea and bronchi, either by mechanical irritants such as dust, smoke, a foreign body or a growth, or as a result of the action of micro-organisms setting up an inflammatory reaction and increased secretion. In both cases the cough may be dry or it may be accompanied by expectoration. The cough may show other characteristic features. It may, for example, be seasonal such as the 'winter cough' of a chronic bronchitic. It may be worse on change of posture or at certain times during the day.

Expectoration. The sputum varies considerably both in quantity and appearance. It may be practically negligible or may be in excessive quantities as so often happens in lung abscess or bronchiectasis. If it appears clear but viscid, it is mucoid sputum characteristic of irritation of the mucous membrane of larynx, trachea and main bronchi by such factors as smoke or dust. A scanty but stringy type of sputum usually occurs at the beginning of an acute infection, due to a fibrinous exudate. Purulent sputum will appear in severe infections and is yellow or greenish in colour. If it is pink or reddish, this will be due to the presence of blood which may be fresh or altered according to the length of time between haemorrhage and expectoration. It is not necessarily a serious sign to find evidence of blood in the sputum.

The physiotherapist should know the amount of sputum and its type, and if the patient is being treated with postural drainage the amount expectorated during the treatment should be carefully measured. Care must be taken not to confuse sputum with saliva or with secretions from the nasopharynx.

Dyspnoea. Coope defines dyspnoea as the 'word used to cover difficult, painful or disordered breathing'. Another term, not quite so accurate, but in common use, is shortness of breath. It is not necessarily a sign of disease of the respiratory system. It may be, for example, a sign of cardiac or renal disease and it is, also, normally present in severe exercise. There are, however, many factors in respiratory disease which may be the cause of shortness of breath, these will include: loss of thoracic mobility; fibrosis or loss of elasticity of the lung tissue; narrowing of the bronchial tubes; thickening of the alveolar lining; low vital capacity; anxiety may also play a contributory part. Loss of thoracic mobility, fibrosis or loss of elasticity of lung tissue and narrowing of the bronchial tubes entail greater effort on the part of the respiratory muscles to move the chest wall or lung, or to widen and lengthen the tubes. A greater number of afferent stimuli, therefore, reach the respiratory centre. If the alveolar lining is thickened, there is a greater difficulty in absorbing oxygen, while if the vital capacity is very low there is little interchange of gases between the inspired and the dead space air. In both these cases the chemical factors influencing respiratory rate will be changed.

Anxiety may play its part because it produces tension and therefore increases afferent stimuli. Direct disturbance of the respiratory centre may also lead to dyspnoea.

Dyspnoea may be inspiratory, when it is due to obstruction to air entry or expiratory, where there is bronchial spasm or extensive loss of lung elasticity.

If dyspnoea is present when the patient is sitting up the term orthopnoea is used.

Pain. Pain in the thoracic region is again not necessarily proof of respiratory disease. The lung itself has no pain nerve endings and is therefore insensitive to pain. Either the pleura, the ribs and thoracic muscles, the heart or the intercostal nerves may be affected if the patient complains of pain. If the pleura is inflamed the pain is of the sharp lancinating type, worse on each inspiration, so that thoracic movement is restricted in that area. Pain, the result of muscular or bony lesion, may be very severe but all movements, not only respiratory, will increase it and there will be localised tenderness and evidence of muscle spasm. Pain due to involvement of the intercostal nerves will radiate along the course of the nerve. If pain is cardiac in origin it will usually be felt behind the sternum and may radiate up the left side of the neck and into the axilla and the medial side of one or both arms.

Limited respiratory movements. Limitation in chest movement may be the result of a loss of elasticity of the lung tissue resulting in fixation of the thorax in a position of inspiration. Again it may be the result of collapse or fibrosis of one or more lobes resulting in diminished movement on one side of the chest; pleural adhesions may have the same effect. Shallow breathing results in little movement at the sides, posterior aspect and lower part of the chest wall.

It is important to realise that limited respiratory movements may be the result of other factors such as ankylosing spondylitis and kyphosis or scoliosis.

Haemoptysis. This term means the spitting of blood from the larynx, trachea, bronchi or lungs. If it is expectorated at once it is unchanged and is therefore bright red and frothy in appearance; such a haemoptysis is usually the result of a sudden rupture of a fairly large vessel. This might be the result of trauma, or of destruction of a vessel in a tuberculous patch, or a bronchiectatic cavity. Blood coughed up may amount to several ounces. The sputum is usually streaked with blood for several successive days.

It is not uncommon to see minute quantities of blood in the sputum in acute inflammatory conditions of the lung due to excessively dilated or ruptured capillaries.

Sometimes the blood is not coughed up at once but is mixed with mucus or pus. It is then changed in colour and may have a brownish-red appearance or may colour the sputum faintly pink.

Loss of weight is a feature of many diseases and does not necessarily occur in all respiratory disorders. It is, however, a feature of infective or malignant chest conditions and weight should therefore be carefully watched. Active tuberculosis, bronchiectasis and carcinoma are the three conditions in which weight is most likely to be lost.

Deformities. Although deformity is not in any way a diagnostic sign of respiratory disorders, many chest diseases are complicated by alteration in the shape of the thorax, by curvature of the spine and by inequality in the shoulder girdle. Difficulty in expiration, over use of the accessory muscles of respiration, imbalance of the muscles on either side of the chest and spine, painful conditions affecting one side of the chest, general poor muscle tone resulting from imperfect oxygenation of the blood, all these will lead to thoracic and spinal deformity. Expiratory dyspnoea leads to the chest being held in the position of forced inspiration. In time the muscles and ligaments will adapt themselves to this new position and the chest will take on a barrel-shaped appearance, in which the shoulders are high, the antero-posterior diameter of the thorax is as wide as the lateral, the costal angle is wide and the ribs are more horizontally placed.

Accessory muscles of respiration lift the upper ribs and the neck appears unduly short and the shoulders high. These muscles are constantly in action if respiratory dyspnoea is present and gradually they become shorter.

Muscle imbalance is a natural result of lack of movement of one side of the chest or of chest surgery. Following a thoracoplasty, for example, extensive division of muscles is necessary and one obvious deformity is the lateral shift of the trunk towards the sound side.

Unilateral painful respiratory conditions lead to deformities because the patient tends to limit chest movement on the painful side and to lean to this side. In a pleurisy, therefore, a scoliosis is liable to develop its convexity towards the unaffected side.

In all respiratory conditions there is likely to be a decrease in gaseous interchange and oxygenation of the blood may be incomplete. The metabolism of all the muscles of the body will, therefore, be impaired and their tone and strength is likely to be decreased. General posture is, as a result, defective and a general 'slump' develops to which any special fault arising from the particular chest condition may be added. A child suffering from bronchiectasis, for example, will in all probability show poor general posture and in addition may show a thoracic scoliosis particularly if the bronchiectatic condition is unilateral. The usual position is one in which the head is carried forward. This means that the muscles attaching to the clavicle and first rib (the scalenes and sterno-mastoid) are relaxed and the chest sinks forward, the costal angle is reduced and the ribs are more vertical with narrowed intercostal spaces. Poor tone of the rhomboids allows the scapulae to glide forward and the chest is then narrowed in its lateral diameters. All these thoracic deformities though at first postural, become fixed as soft tissues adapt themselves to the new position. Respiration is, therefore, grossly affected.

EXAMINATION OF THE PATIENT PRIOR TO TREATMENT BY PHYSICAL MEASURES

A routine examination should be carried out in order to elicit certain essential facts. It is necessary before planning treatment to be aware of the state of general health, the vital capacity, the extent of thoracic expansion and whether this is equal on the two sides. A knowledge of the range of movement obtainable in the joints of the thorax, spine and shoulder girdle is valuable, while details of any thoracic deformity should be known. It is essential to know if there is any cough and if so whether it is productive, and the quantity and nature of the sputum.

Before proceeding to examination the case notes should be read and X-rays studied.

Interrogation

The patient is encouraged to recount the history of his illness and symptoms. This, together with his answers to questions, should elicit any important facts as regards the family history, his occupation, habits, home conditions, possible contact with infection, the presence of cough, sputum, pain and alterations in weight.

Observation

During the interrogation, certain points such as general appearance, colour, posture and health will have already been noted. A more detailed inspection is now carried out. The *shape of the chest* may first be considered. Normally the chest is wider from side to side than from back to front, and the diverging costal margins form about a right angle with one another. Various changes may occur, the antero-posterior diameter may be increased so that it equals the lateral and the chest assumes a barrel-shaped appearance. Alternatively, the antero-posterior diameter may be decreased and the anterior aspect of the chest becomes flat instead of slightly convex.

In this case the costal angle will be decreased and the inter-costal spaces diminished. Some thoracic asymmetry may be noticed—either a flattening or a 'bulging' in one area. A localised flattening nearly always indicates some underlying lung disease, though it can be the result of muscle atrophy in a lower motor neurone lesion. Abnormalities may also be present which are not the result of respiratory disease but which predispose towards infection. Such may be the pigeon breast in which the sternum is thrust forward and the sides of the chest flattened—a feature common in a case of rickets. A groove extending downwards from the sternum to axillary line, known as Harrison's sulcus may be produced by the pull of the diaphragm on softened bones in the same condition.

The *respiratory movements* should be carefully watched. Note should be made of the type of breathing, apical or diaphragmatic, the depth and rate and whether or not the accessory muscles of respiration are being used. A careful check should be made to see if any particular area of the chest is moving less freely than the rest. Any sign of cyanosis or dyspnoea will be easily detected during this examination.

It is well also to examine the fingers since in chronic infective conditions '*clubbing*' is often present.

Palpation

The physiotherapist should place her hands lightly on the chest, so checking any variations in thoracic movement on each side of the chest. Often slight differences in amount of expansion can be better detected through palpation than observation. Any tenderness originating from lesions of bone or muscle will then also be noticed.

Range of Movement

The range of movement of thoracic, vertebral and shoulder girdle joints should next be tested. If these joints have not been exercised to their full extent, owing to deformity or to diseases of the respiratory system, they will become permanently limited in range, so further reducing the possibility of good chest expansion and correct posture.

Measurements

The chest expansion should be measured. It is usual to take three measurements, apical expansion at the level of the angle of Louis, lateral costal at the level of the tip of the sternum and diaphragmatic at the level of the tip of the tenth rib. These measurements must be carefully recorded. The patient should be weighed and, if a spirometer is available, the vital capacity taken.

PRINCIPLES OF TREATMENT BY PHYSIOTHERAPY

Broadly speaking the chest diseases may be divided into acute conditions such as acute bronchitis, pleurisy and pneumonia, in which, at least during the acute phase, no physiotherapy is indicated, and chronic diseases such as chronic bronchitis, bronchiectasis, emphysema and asthma, where treatment by physical means can play an important part. A third group of cases are those which are going to have, or have had, some surgical treatment. As these are surgical cases they will not be dealt with here.

THE CHRONIC CHEST CONDITIONS

All chronic chest conditions show certain characteristic features, particularly tenseness of neck and thoracic muscles, limited chest expansion, and reduced vital capacity, faulty breathing, defective posture, poor general health, and in many cases cough with or without expectoration. The principles of treatment will therefore be similar but modified in their fulfilment according to the special features of each separate condition.

Relaxation

In most chest cases general and local tenseness is present. Difficult breathing engenders fear, and fear results in a condition of hypertonicity. This sets up a vicious circle because, as has already been seen, hypertonicity leads to an increased respiratory rate. Many patients with respiratory disorders are afraid, either that they may be suffering from conditions such as lung cancer, or tuberculosis, or that they may be unable to continue their work. An important step in treatment is, therefore, to find out what the patient is worrying about and if possible to relieve him of this worry. This is, of course, done by the physician, but the patient often talks to the physiotherapist more freely and any information in relation to such worries should be reported to the physician. The physiotherapist can also help by giving the patient very careful training in the art of relaxation. Both general and local relaxation require training because, in addition to general tenseness, if either inspiration or expiration require special effort the accessory muscles of respiration are liable to be brought into action, and all muscles round the shoulder girdle show increased tone in order to give these muscles a firmer origin; much unnecessary tone is therefore present. Full relaxation of the neck and shoulder girdle muscles cannot, of course, be obtained until the breathing has improved but much unnecessary tenseness can be relieved. In some cases the practise of relaxed head and shoulder movements will be of assistance.

Increase of Chest Expansion

This is a very important principle since chest expansion is usually limited either as a result of loss of elasticity of one or both lungs or due to spasm of the bronchiole muscle, or through the presence of adhesions. Chest expansion can nearly always be increased by the use of breathing exercises. In the majority of chronic lung conditions better expansion will be gained by training the patient first in expiration. Where elasticity is lost, fuller expiration may be obtained by showing the patient how to give pressure on the chest by the use of a broad webbing belt, how to assist air exit from the lungs by relaxation of the chest and by movements of the trunk. The second step in gaining better expansion is to teach the patient to use more fully those areas of the lung which are not being used to the best capacity. In most cases breathing is taking place at the upper part of the chest, so that by use of manual pressure the patient should be taught to use all parts of the lower lobes. Full expansion cannot be obtained if thoracic joints are limited in range, hence mobilising exercises may be taught, such as easy relaxed movements of the trunk, isolating where possible to the dorsal spine if the general condition of the patient is suitable. Once taught these can be advantageously combined with breathing. In addition relaxed movements of head and arms should be included.

Correction of Faulty Breathing

This again necessitates the use of breathing exercises. The patient is taught to use all parts of the lung, special emphasis being laid on regions which are not being fully exercised. A usual procedure, but one naturally subject to variation, is to train full expiration, then to progress to improving diaphragmatic breathing. When this has been grasped, to teach upper and lower lateral costal breathing and then posterior costal. If necessary this is followed by training unilateral breathing. Training must continue until the patient can use any part of either lung at will. It is usually a considerable time before full control of the thorax is gained and, as near as possible, correct breathing becomes a habit.

Correction of Posture

Unilateral lung conditions tend to lead to the development of a scoliosis, bilateral conditions to high shoulders, faulty carriage of head, kyphosis and in some cases flat chest and protuberant abdomen. In all cases, owing to disturbance of gaseous interchange and hampered action of the lungs, metabolism is impaired, muscle tone and strength is consequently poor and the sense of correct posture is lacking. It may be impossible to gain perfect posture but it can certainly be improved. The patient can be trained to feel what the correct posture is, the postural muscles can be strengthened so that they can hold, without fatigue, a better position and contracted structures may be gently stretched.

Aiding Expectoration

In those cases in which cough, due to increased formation of secretions, is present, it is essential to aid their elimination with the least possible strain and effort on the part of the patient. Ineffective coughing is not only tiring, but it results in raised intra-pulmonary pressure and strain on the lung tissue and heart. The patient has, therefore, to be taught to cough effectively.

In cases where mucus is viscid and adherent, percussion on the chest, together with breathing exercises, usually give the patient considerable assistance; if on the other hand secretions have accumulated in cavities or are deep in the small tubes, then 'tipping' should be added.

Improvement of General Health

This is mainly in the hands of the physician but some help may be given by the use of light general exercises and, where the physician wishes, the administration of artificial sunlight. Improvement of breathing and elimination of stagnant secretions will be followed by improvement of general health.

Chapter II

ACUTE RESPIRATORY CONDITIONS AND PHTHISIS

Pneumonia is an acute inflammation of the interstitial tissue and parenchyma of the lungs. If it is diffuse, involving one or more lobes, it is usually classified as a lobar pneumonia, while if it is localised to scattered lobules throughout one or both lungs it is termed a broncho-pneumonia.

On the whole, though, pneumonia may occur at any age; the disease is one which attacks either young children or elderly people.

LOBAR PNEUMONIA

In the majority of cases the organism responsible for the inflammation is one or other of the many varieties of the pneumococcus. The micro-organisms may reach the lung from those harboured in the nose and throat by inhalation from the air, or by the blood stream from a pneumococcal process elsewhere. Whether or not they actually cause inflammation depends partly on their virulence but also very largely on the resistance of the patient, which varies with age, general health and the condition of the lungs. The very young and the very old have a low resistance to the pneumococcus, as do those who are undernourished or debilitated. If there is chronic disease of the bronchi or lungs, or congestion due to chronic cardiac disease, the lung tissue will offer a poor resistance to the micro-organisms.

The micro-organisms are usually inhaled into the terminal bronchioles and alveoli at the hilar region and inflammation starts at this point and spreads peripherally. The pleura is almost always involved in the process and lobar pneumonia is therefore accompanied by pleurisy.

Changes in the Lung

The changes are identical with those of all inflammatory processes. The capillaries in the alveolar walls and septa become dilated and congested,

138

consequently inflammatory exudate causes oedema of the walls and interstitial tissue, while much fluid passes into the alveoli driving out the air and causing a state of congestion. The exudate produced as a result of the action of the pneumococcus is typically fibrinous, it therefore clots and the alveoli become filled with a solid substance consisting of fibrin, plasma, red blood cells, leucocytes, lymphocytes and pneumococci. Thus within two or three days of the onset of the condition the lobe is solid, dry and airless—consolidation has occurred.

Before resolution can take place the solid exudate must be softened and this, all being well, is the next stage. Leucocytes, lymphocytes and monocytes invade the exudate, the leucocytes and monocytes tackle the pneumococci ingesting them so that they rapidly disappear, damaged cells are carried away to the bronchial lymph glands by the lymphocytes, while the fibrin is dissolved by the proteolytic enzyme liberated by the damaged leucocytes. Resolution can now occur because the softened exudate can be removed. Since the pneumococci have been destroyed the blood vessels will return to their normal size, the alveoli will be cleared partly by coughing up the liquefied exudate, partly by its absorption and partly by the action of the phagocytes.

If the pleura is involved it also shows the changes of inflammation. The membrane becomes hyperaemic and congested and fibrin is deposited on the surface giving it a rough shaggy appearance. Sometimes a serofibrinous effusion occurs into the pleural cavity. The fibrin may organise and adhesions may bind the two layers of the pleura together.

Signs and Symptoms

The patient, early in the attack, complains of severe pain in the area due to the fibrinous pleurisy. This pain is made worse on each inspiration, and consequently an attempt is made to limit respiratory movements of the affected lobe; limitation of movement of the overlying area of the chest is, as a result, often noticeable. To allow fuller expansion of the good lung the patient tends to lie over on the affected side.

Cough develops early, at first it is hard, painful and relatively unproductive. Such sputum as there is is stringy, due to the fibrinous nature of the exudate, and rusty coloured as a result of the presence of broken down red blood corpuscles. Occasionally bright red blood may be present if acutely dilated capillaries rupture. When softening of exudate takes place copious fluid sputum will be expectorated.

As consolidation occurs, dyspnoea, shallow breathing and cyanosis appear. These are the result of anoxaemia since the exudate in the alveoli prevents the normal gaseous interchange, and possibly owing to toxaemia, the respiratory centre does not react to the increased carbon dioxide in the blood by producing deeper inspirations. Pyrexia, raised pulse rate and all the signs of acute toxaemia will be present. If there is poor oxygenation of the blood and toxaemia, delirium may occur.

Complications

Many complications may arise, including cardiac failure, as a result of pulmonary congestion and toxaemia but three particularly concern the physiotherapist—organisation of exudate, abscess formation and empyema

Organisation of the exudate does sometimes occur though the reason in any one particular case is not always clear. If the fibrinous exudate is not softened reasonably soon, fibroblasts will grow into it from the alveolar walls, followed by capillaries, and this granulation tissue will inevitably become changed into fibrous tissue. Thick strands of fibrous tissue pass from one alveolus to the next and eventually the whole area of lung may become solid and fibrous. This condition is known as unresolved lobar pneumonia and is characterised by persistent cough and diminished movements in the corresponding area of the chest wall.

Abscess formation usually only occurs if the patient's resistance is very low or the micro-organisms are particularly virulent. Actual destruction of tissue then takes place, the alveolar walls break down and a cavity filled with pus is formed. Fibrosis tends to occur in the surrounding area.

Empyema may develop if the patient's resistance is low.

PRINCIPLES OF TREATMENT BY PHYSIOTHERAPY

Treatment by physical measures is not indicated in the acute stage where, as in all acute inflammatory conditions, rest and medical treatment are of prime importance. Since the introduction of sulphapyridine in 1938 and, later, of sulphonamides and penicillin, patients have recovered more rapidly and fewer require physiotherapy. Physical treatment, however, may be ordered either when resolution is progressing well, or in cases of unresolved pneumonia, or in lung abscess.

Resolving Lobar Pneumonia

At this stage the purpose of physiotherapy is threefold: first, to gain full expansion of the affected lobe; second, to improve the general condition and resistance of the lungs; third, to aid the condition of the general musculature.

Expansion of the affected lobe should occur as the alveoli are cleared of the exudate and normal movement should return. Re-expansion is, however, sometimes hampered by pleural adhesions. In addition, through fear of pain, there has been voluntary limitation of movement of this part of the chest and this may continue when pain subsides. For these reasons, breathing exercises are valuable. As soon as the patient has some understanding of better breathing as a whole, unilateral breathing exercises are commenced. The sound side of the chest is steadied by the physiotherapist's hand, while the patient is encouraged to expand the affected area against slight manual resistance. This type of breathing is persevered with until the expansion equals that of the opposite side.

Improvement of the general condition and resistance of the lung is gained through stimulating the pulmonary circulation by encouraging deep breathing, both inspiration and expiration. Later, when the patient is stronger, trunk movements may be used in addition to the breathing.

The building up of the general strength is an important point because there is a severe degree of toxaemia attendant on pneumonia and the result of even a comparatively short illness is to leave the patient weak and 'shaky'. The general musculature therefore requires strengthening before the patient is allowed to get up. Special attention to all postural muscles is necessary, of particular importance are the back, abdominal muscles and intrinsic and extrinsic muscles of the feet. Careful progression is necessary as the patient must not be tired.

Unresolved Lobar Pneumonia

Physical treatment is very necessary in these cases, since it is essential to try to prevent the formation of fibrous tissue. Therefore, as soon as it is realised that resolution is not proceeding as it should, an attempt is made to clear the exudate and promote movement of the affected area. If necessary postural drainage may be given, but great care must be taken as the general condition of the patient is poor, deep 'tipping' and heavy percussion should be avoided. Unilateral breathing exercises are started at once and given several times a day. As soon as the patient is fit enough, he is taught to give his own manual pressure.

Though unilateral breathing is by far the most important, double-sided expansion exercises should also be given so that general thoracic mobility is improved and circulation aided.

Gradually active exercises are introduced as in the preceding cases.

Abscess Formation

Though a lung abscess may be the result of lobar pneumonia it more often occurs in broncho-pneumonia, inhalation of septic material or as a result of septic embolism. Consideration to this condition will therefore be given later in this chapter.

Empyema.

This will be considered later (see page 146).

BRONCHO-PNEUMONIA

Broncho-pneumonia is nearly always secondary to some other condition. It may follow whooping cough, measles, or one of the other infectious diseases of childhood. Occasionally the inhalation of septic material during operations on the nose, mouth or throat may cause an attack. The condition is very closely associated with bronchiectasis, since plugging of the bronchioles with infected material and consequently local collapse is liable to set up an acute inflammatory condition of the small tubes.

It is the lobules rather than the lobes which are affected in this type of pneumonia, and usually lobules scattered throughout one or both lungs. There is an acute inflammation of the walls of the bronchioles with destruction of the epithelium and pus formation. The surrounding alveoli become filled with inflammatory exudate and small areas of consolidation therefore occur. If a bronchiole becomes completely blocked by pus, air cannot enter the alveoli distal to the obstruction and collapse of the lobule occurs. Thus a characteristic feature of a broncho-pneumonia is the presence of areas of consolidation and areas of collapse. Recovery is very rarely straightforward, it is usually slow with consequently great likelihood of organisation of the exudate with patches of fibrosis. The walls of the bronchioles nearly always show some degree of permanent damage since destruction of the epithelium is followed by fibrous tissue formation with weakening and dilatation of the tubes.

The signs and symptoms differ from those of lobar pneumonia in that the onset is slower, the temperature rising more slowly but once elevated being more erratic and continuing for much longer. Pain is not usually so marked since the pleura is not necessarily involved if the affected lobules are not near the surface. The sputum is purulent and not rusty-coloured like that of the lobar type. The patient on the whole is more ill and the toxaemia is much more severe since pus is invariably formed.

If physiotherapy is ordered it will follow the same lines as in the preceding type but will be more slowly progressed. Since both lungs have usually been involved bilateral breathing exercises will be used, but very careful observation and palpation will help to decide if any special areas of either side require more detailed attention.

LUNG ABSCESS

An abscess in the lung may complicate either lobar or broncho-pneumonia. It is probably more often the result of the inhalation of a foreign body or some septic material from the upper respiratory tract. Inhalation of such material is not necessarily followed by abscess formation because if the cough reflex is active the substance should be expelled, but there are circumstances where the reflex is depressed. Thus, for example, both morphia and anaesthetics depress the cough reflex and if substances are inhaled under these conditions they tend to be retained; hence in operations on the mouth, nose or throat under general anaesthesia, there is danger of inhalation and retention of septic material and consequently of the development of an abscess. Another possible cause is the impaction in a pulmonary vessel of a fragment of a septic thrombus from elsewhere in the body; this will readily cause infection of lung tissue.

In nearly every case the abscess forms at the periphery of the lung and hence lies near either the interlobular or costal surfaces, in these cases the pleura is also very often inflamed. Sometimes the abscess is a closed cavity filled with pus, usually toxic irritation causes proliferation and a fibrous capsule forms around the cavity. Such an abscess is not uncommonly the result of a septic embolus. If the abscess follows broncho-pneumonia or is due to inhalation it more often communicates with a bronchus, though this does not necessarily imply free drainage because the mucosa of the bronchus may be swollen and congested.

According to whether the abscess can drain or not, so symptoms vary. A typical history is that of a rise of temperature and pulse, pain (if the pleura is affected) and a dry unproductive cough. If no communication exists the patient becomes increasingly ill, there is evidence of toxaemia and, in time, marked clubbing of the fingers. In many cases the initial symptoms are followed by the sudden coughing up of a large quantity of greenish-yellow sputum which, if secondarily infected by certain micro-organisms from the mouth, will have a foul odour. The appearance of this sputum indicates that the abscess has now made communication with a bronchus. Should there be really good drainage the condition may undergo spontaneous cure but unfortunately this does not often happen. Usually free drainage is blocked by the inflamed mucous membrane, and general ill-health toxaemia and cough with expectoration continue. The main object of treatment is to destroy the micro-organisms and to promote free drainage and so gain closure of the abscess cavity. For this reason penicillin therapy, bronchoscopy and postural drainage are the methods chosen.

Physiotherapy consists of supervising postural drainage. A very careful study of the X-ray film must be made so that a position can be chosen which ensures that the pus will flow from the cavity into the bronchus normally supplying that area. If the pus is thick and does not drain easily percussion to the thorax should be used. Since drainage is so important the patient should take the suitable position every four hours and, where possible, lie in the position for half to one hour at a time. It is often considered wise to avoid breathing exercises because on inspiration the effect of the lowered intra-pleural pressure will be to enlarge the abscess cavity. If breathing exercises should be ordered, diaphragmatic breathing only, and with the emphasis on expiration, should be given.

If medical treatment does not prove effective, operative treatment is usually necessary. The most usual procedure is excision of the area of the lung since in this way involvement of a larger area of lung tissue is avoided and fear of septic embolism removed. Pre- and post-operative physiotherapy will be necessary to avoid the complications of post-operative collapse of the remaining areas of the affected lung, postural defect and limitation of arm movements.

PLEURISY

Inflammation of the pleura may be a primary condition or secondary to disease of the underlying lung, occasionally it is due to direct spread from neighbouring areas such as the ribs or pericardium.

Three main types of pleurisy may be recognised: dry pleurisy, pleurisy with effusion and empyema. Other cases of pleural effusion exist but in these cases the effusion is usually the result of mechanical factors and is not due to inflammation or irritation of the pleura, for example in both cardiac and renal diseases fluid may collect in the pleural cavity.

DRY PLEURISY

A dry pleurisy is a common accompaniment of lobar pneumonia. Chill and exposure may apparently be its cause, but in these cases it is very probable that there is a tuberculous infection of the underlying lung which is so slight that it has failed to give rise to symptoms. It is an important point to remember that most cases of dry pleurisy which are not part of a lung disease have this underlying tuberculous factor.

As a result of irritation, the pleura becomes congested, both parietal and visceral surfaces being involved. Dilatation of the blood vessels results in an exudate which is fibrinous in character, fibrin is therefore deposited on the adjacent surfaces giving them a rough, shaggy appearance. If the fibrin is not rapidly absorbed organisation, by the growth of capillaries and fibroblasts from the pleura, will occur and dense adhesion formation may result, seriously hampering the action of the lung.

Pain, cough, absence of movement of one area of the chest and elevation of temperature, pulse and respirations are features of dry pleurisy. Breathing is painful and shallow because the patient is frightened to take a deep breath. Pain is usually severe and stabbing in type, made worse on coughing and breathing, since on inspiration the tense, inflamed pleura is stretched by the movement of the chest wall. Movement is diminished since it is voluntarily inhibited through fear of pain. Irritation of the visceral layer of the pleura results in a dry painful cough, though expectoration may be present if pleurisy is due to lobar pneumonia.

PLEURISY WITH EFFUSION

An effusion of sero-fibrinous fluid may occur at once or may follow a dry pleurisy after a few days. It is most common when inflammation of the pleura occurs in tuberculosis of the lung, lung abscess, bronchiectasis and pneumonia. Occasionally it follows a primary dry pleurisy when an unsuspected tuberculous lesion of the neighbouring area of lung tissue will be the cause. The fluid may escape into the pleural cavity while quantities of fibrin are deposited on the adjacent surfaces of the pleura. Often the fibrin organises and adhesions form, bridging the pleural layers and localising the fluid. If there is much fluid the lung retracts and, if the visceral layer of the pleura is covered with fibrin, it may not be able to re-expand because the fibrotic pleura contracts.

Pain is, in this type of pleurisy, less pronounced because the fluid reduces movement of the ribs and consequently repeated stretching of the pleura is considerably lessened. On the other hand dyspnoea is much more severe as pressure is exerted on the lung. The chest wall may bulge and become immobile due to the accumulation of fluid.

In most cases the fluid will gradually absorb, but there is some danger of deposit and organisation of fibrin with consequent adhesion formation, and thickening of the pleura, with limited re-expansion of the lung.

OUTLINE OF TREATMENT BY PHYSIOTHERAPY

Neither type of pleurisy calls for early physiotherapy, particularly if the condition is apparently primary. Medically, both types are best treated by general rest in bed and local rest of the chest by means of strapping in the position of expiration. If fluid is present it will usually in time absorb, and only if it is excessive and causing much loss of aerating surface or if it fails to absorb over several weeks, is aspiration carried out.

If the pleurisy is part of pneumonia, physiotherapy will be carried out as previously indicated for cases of this condition. If the condition is primary then prolonged rest and, if possible, sanatorium treatment are necessary in order to prevent the unsuspected lung lesion from becoming active, therefore breathing exercises are undesirable.

EMPYEMA

Pus may form in the pleural cavity as a result of infection of the pleura by micro-organisms directly, or by spread from the lung. Occasionally a lung or sub-phrenic or liver abscess may rupture into the pleural cavity, or micro-organisms may invade as a result of traumatic conditions of the chest.

One of the commonest conditions to be accompanied by pleurisy is pneumonia. If an empyema develops during an attack of lobar pneumonia, its onset is usually after the severe stage of the illness, temperature and pulse then unexpectedly rise again. If it occurs in a case of broncho-pneumonia it usually shows signs during the acute illness. If the pus is streptococcal in origin it is thin and there is little fibrin, consequently few adhesions form. The pus tends, in these cases, to spread over the whole pleural cavity since it is not localised by adhesions. If the pus is pneumococcal in origin it is usually thick and there is much fibrin. If the two layers of the pleura are in contact, adhesions tend to form and these may wall off the pus, forming a type of abscess. On the other hand if the layers are held apart by fluid, a layer of fibrous tissue forms on the surface of the visceral and parietal pleura. This becomes thick and hard and as it contracts tends to hamper the movement of the lung and chest wall.

Since the pus, in this condition, is contained within a completely closed cavity, the patient will appear and will be very ill. There will be a hectic temperature, dyspnoea, pain in the chest, and all the symptoms of toxaemia.

The main object of treatment is to evacuate the pus as soon as possible so that re-expansion of the lung can occur, the empyema cavity is obliterated and dense adhesion and fibrous tissue formation with permanent hampering of respiratory function, is prevented. Evacuation of pus cannot, however, always be obtained as soon as the condition is diagnosed.

The patient may be already suffering from a lung affection which has seriously reduced his vital capacity and drainage of empyema may produce a further and fatal lowering. If the pus is thin and adhesion formation has not occurred, to open the pleural cavity will mean massive collapse of the lung and shift of the mediastinum. If time is allowed the pus will invariably thicken and as it thickens adhesions also form causing the layers of the pleura to become adherent and the pus to become a localised abscess. For these reasons rib resection may not be undertaken at once but the patient tided over the intervening period by repeated aspirations and penicillin therapy.

As soon as loculation of the pus occurs a rib resection is most often carried out, the pus is evacuated and air-tight drainage instituted.

In cases of tuberculous empyema rib resection is not usually carried out. If there is no secondary infection it may be possible to close the empyema by encouraging expansion of the lung. The fluid is, in this case, drained either by aspirations or pleural wash-outs. If the underlying lung is diseased and the pleural cavity secondarily infected it is usual to perform a thoracoplasty so resting the lung and closing the cavity. Aspiration or intercostal drainage of the empyema may be necessary between the stages of the operation, but drainage is to be avoided where possible because so often a sinus results, the drainage track failing to heal.

As soon as drainage is instituted, physiotherapy should be commenced. Its main objects are to gain re-expansion of the collapsed area of lung tissue beneath the empyema cavity, to prevent the development of thoracic deformity and to ensure full range of arm movements. Details of this treatment are given elsewhere (see *Physiotherapy in Some Surgical Conditions*).

Occasionally a chronic empyema develops either because drainage has been inadequate or because re-expansion of the lung has proved impossible owing to much thickening of the pleura or the establishment of a fistula connecting the lung and pleura. In the latter case the suction effect of a negative intrapleural pressure will be lost. In these cases, an attempt may be made to close the empyema cavity either by stripping the thickened pleura or by a modified form of thoracoplasty.

PULMONARY TUBERCULOSIS

Pulmonary tuberculosis is nearly always the result of invasion of the lung by the tubercle bacilli through inhalation either from dried sputum, infected droplets of sputum, or by infected material taken into the mouth. Once inhaled, the bacilli may travel along the bronchi being inhaled from one into another or may be ingested, but not destroyed, by polymorphonuclear leucocytes and carried by them into the lymph spaces.

The reaction of the bronchi and alveoli to the invasion is similar to that of any other tissue. The presence of the bacilli acts as an irritant and provokes an inflammatory reaction. Within a very short time the micro-organisms are ingested by leucocytes which in their turn are absorbed by macrophages. Lymphocytes form a ring round this little mass of cells, their function being to destroy the toxins liberated by the tubercle bacilli.

The complete group of cells form a microscopic cluster known as the tuberculous follicle. Several of these may fuse together to form a nodule about the size of a millet seed and known as the miliary tubercle. These tubercles are avascular and in addition the bacilli produce toxins which cause necrosis of cells, consequently the cells at the centre of the tubercle break down and form a cheesy mass. This process is known as caseation. Nearly always the caseated material subsequently softens. In a great many cases toxic irritation stimulates the fibroblasts to increased activity and a fibrous capsule therefore forms around the tubercles, in this lime salts are deposited. Healing may then be said to have taken place by fibrosis and calcification.

Whether or not healing occurs depends very largely on the resistance of the patient and the severity of the invasion, as well as on whether the attack is a primary one or a re-infection.

A primary invasion nearly always causes the formation of a small caseous area in any part of the lung, often near the periphery. The bacilli travel in the lymph stream to the hilar lymph glands which consequently become infected. This is known as the primary complex. If the resistance is reasonably high, healing of both caseous patch and lymph glands occurs by fibrosis and calcification, if resistance is low or invasion severe, a rapid spread may occur by the bronchi or blood stream and death ensues.

A second invasion produces rather different reactions. It practically always affects the apex of the lung, often the right, and evokes an acute local reaction. The reaction is characterised by an excessive but local-ised necrosis of cells and therefore caseation. The caseated material rapidly softens and, as bronchi are often involved, cavity formation is likely. Spread to hilar lymph glands is very rare. The result of this second infection depends on resistance and type of invasion. If resistance is high it is possible that the caseated patch may heal by calcification without cavity formation. More often the softened material is coughed up, a fibrous capsule forms around the resultant cavity which is eventually calcified, but a certain amount of infected material may remain in the cavity and may at some time, if resistance is lowered, be a source of further trouble. If, on the other hand, resistance is low or invasion occurs in those not previously affected, the process is less localised, the micro-organisms spread and widespread cavitation occurs. There appears, in these cases, to be little attempt at fibrosis or calcification.

In all cases the pleura over the affected area tends to become involved, with adhesion formation and thickening which may render attempts at artificial pneumothorax ineffective.

THE PART PLAYED BY PHYSIOTHERAPY IN TREATMENT

The main objects of treatment are to rest the damaged lung, to raise the resistance and so assist the fight against the micro-organisms, and to obtain closure and healing of the cavities. How these objects are fulfilled depends on the severity of the condition and cases may be roughly grouped into those who require medical treatment and those for whom some form of thoracic surgery will be necessary. Physical measures are mainly required for the second group, though some little help may be given to the medical cases.

Cases Treated Medically

These patients will include early cases or those who are too advanced to warrant any operative measures. The main treatment for these is rest. For early cases absolute rest in bed, usually for several months, is essential. Since rest should be complete and at first the patient should neither wash nor feed himself, he is best nursed in a sanatorium or hospital where he can lie out in the open air all day. Rest will give nature a chance to bring about arrest of the condition, but resistance may be raised by seeing that the patient is given plenty of good food, vitamins and fresh air. During this stage physiotherapy is not usually advocated but a few weeks after the patient has ceased to run an evening temperature resumption of activity is very gradually allowed. Then physiotherapy can play a useful part in planning the graduated active work from simple bed exercises to walking and eventually to quite strenuous activity. Only in the very later stages are breathing exercises begun and then they are bilateral with special emphasis on diaphragmatic breathing.

Surgical Cases

For those patients who do not improve with rest treatment or for others too advanced to be successfully treated in this way, rest for the affected lung may be more successfully obtained by temporary or permanent collapse therapy. Temporary collapse may be obtained in certain cases by the introduction of air into the pleural cavity or by a rib resection, separation of the lung and pleura from the ribs and admission of air into the space so formed.

These measures obtain an artificial pneumothorax and physiotherapy is not usually required. There are many occasions when an artificial pneumothorax cannot be induced owing to dense pleural adhesions which fix the lung to the chest wall. If the adhesions are in the form of fibrous bands a thoracoscopy may be performed and the adhesions divided, if the pleura is thickened and adherent, the lung and pleura may be separated from the chest wall by a thoracotomy. In the later case physiotherapy is necessary to ensure that spinal deformity does not follow the rib resection and postural exercises will therefore be given.

Should the base of the lung be particularly affected a phrenic nerve crush or a pneumoperitoneum will be carried out. In the latter case air is introduced into the peritoneal cavity and the diaphragm therefore raised.

Permanent collapse may be considered if other measures prove unsatisfactory or if there is much fibrosis and cavitation, provided the other lung is not too seriously affected. In this case a thoracoplasty performed in stages causes a permanent sinking in of the chest wall. For these cases pre- and post-operative physiotherapy are essential.

Two particular points require emphasis, first, postural training is essential since a bad deformity will develop if care is not taken; second, diaphragmatic breathing must be taught. This is because the base of the lung is very rarely affected but, following the operation, is likely to collapse due to accumulation of secretions. It is essential that this should not happen since vital capacity, already low before the operation, will drop still further following the thoracoplasty and the ability to use the base of both lungs may well make a very great difference to the patient's chances of recovery. Diaphragmatic breathing should therefore be carefully taught before the first stage of the thoracoplasty, and practised immediately after. Provided the other lung is unaffected, expansion of this may also be encouraged.

Chapter III

CHRONIC RESPIRATORY CONDITIONS

CHRONIC BRONCHITIS

Chronic bronchitis is a chronic inflammatory condition of the lining membrane of the larger and medium-sized bronchi, usually occurring as a result of infection. It is most common in middle-aged and elderly people, particularly those who live in industrial areas in a cold, damp climate. Occasionally chronic bronchitis may follow repeated acute attacks, but more often it is the result of lowered resistance of the bronchial tree, so that the mucous membrane succumbs easily to bacterial invasion from sources such as the nasal sinuses, antra or tonsils. The lowered resistance may also be the result of some organic change in the lung, such as diminished elasticity which lessens the thoracic movements causing slowing of circulation and stagnation of secretions; alternatively resistance may be lowered by pulmonary congestion due to mitral stenosis or incompetence.

Chronic bronchitis may also be the result of continued irritation of the bronchi by some chemical or mechanical irritant such as gases or dust and smoke.

Pathological Changes

As a result of chronic inflammation, hypertrophy of the mucous membrane occurs, the blood vessel walls are thickened and fibrous tissue is formed. The whole lining of the larger tubes usually becomes covered with a thick viscid mucus. This results in a narrowing of the walls of the tubes and consequently extra strain is thrown on the muscles of respiration if air is to be got in and out of the tubes. If the condition continues, unrelieved, degenerative changes occur, atrophy succeeds hypertrophy, the mucous cells, lymphoid tissue, and ciliated epithelium are replaced gradually by fibrous tissue and consequently the protective function of the membrane is lost. The degenerative changes tend to spread to the muscular and even to the outer coat, cartilage may be replaced by fibrous tissue, and muscular tissue loses its tone and elasticity. The walls of the bronchi are thus weakened and their natural elasticity lost. The weakened tubes easily dilate and cavity formation may result.

Signs and Symptoms

The outstanding features of chronic bronchitis are cough, dyspnoea and diminished respiratory movements.

The onset is usually insidious. Each winter the patient suffers from a chronic cough, and as the years pass the cough continues for a longer time until eventually it is present the whole year round. This cough is worse at night, disturbing the patient's sleep. Expectoration varies with the state of the bronchial walls. Often the sputum is thin and viscid but when the walls become smooth and atrophic the cough may be quite dry. During acute attacks the sputum is often muco-purulent.

Dyspnoea is always a feature, partly because there is loss of elasticity and therefore diminished expiration and inspiration and partly because the thick mucus hampers air entry and exit into the smaller tubes. These facts mean extra work for the muscles of respiration to overcome the resistance of the inelastic lungs and the narrowed tubes. More stimuli reach the brain and there is therefore a change in respiratory rate and rhythm.

In long-standing cases cyanosis may be present. As emphysematous changes occur, pulmonary congestion arises and consequently a greater quantity of reduced haemoglobin is present in the blood stream.

Gradually respiratory movements decrease. Since elasticity is lost the tubes cannot lengthen fully as the chest enlarges in inspiration, and on expiration little recoil occurs. Loss of elastic recoil leads to diminished movements in the thoracic joints. In an attempt to assist breathing, the accessory muscles of respiration are brought into play, the neck and shoulder girdle muscles become tense, and breathing is almost entirely apical. Over-use of the accessory muscles of respiration may give rise to pain in the upper part of the chest.

As a result of diminished movement of the diaphragm digestive and circulatory disturbances appear.

TREATMENT BY PHYSICAL MEANS

No cure is possible for sufferers from chronic bronchitis but their condition can be considerably improved, and acute attacks can often be warded off. There are four main points in the treatment. Attempts should be made to *reduce the thickening of the mucous membrane*. This is dealt with by the physician, drugs being used in an attempt to achieve this object. It has been found that cortisone is occasionally successful.

The patient must be *taught to cough effectively*. These patients tend to struggle to clear the tubes by a continuous cough without pausing for inspiration. This throws a strain on the heart and vessels and succeeds in making the patient giddy and distressed with no good effect. There are two points to stress therefore. First the patient should breathe in, cough, breathe and cough, and the reason and value of this should be explained. Secondly, the cough must be a deep one not simply a throat cough, the patient is therefore taught to do a short expiratory 'grunt'.

If mucus is adherent and difficult to cough up percussion is valuable in order to loosen it. There is usually no need to tip the patient and percussion is best done in side lying and lax sitting with the arms and head supported since both are good positions in which to practise breathing following the percussion.

Control of respiration is most important. Since there is often considerable peri-bronchial fibrosis the lungs are more difficult to move, therefore there is overuse of the intercostals and accessory muscles of respiration and consequently dyspnoea. It is necessary, therefore, to train the patient to use the diaphragm more fully and consciously to relax the intercostals and accessory muscles of respiration. This training must be extensive since it is not enough to be able to control breathing while in half lying position or sitting in a chair, but the patient must carry this through to all activities, standing and walking in the street, going up stairs, and doing housework. Training may therefore start in half lying and side lying. The patient is taught to sigh the air out of the chest contracting the upper abdominal wall, then after a brief pause to relax the abdominal muscles and let the air be sucked into the chest concentrating on the filling up of the lower part of the lungs. Progression is made to teaching the same exercise while standing, the arms resting on an object such as the back of a chair. The patient is taught to relax the head and shoulders and then practise the breathing so that this can be done if necessary when he is out walking. Further progressions in this way are made.

Training in general relaxation and especially in relaxation of the upper chest are essential since this reduces tension in all muscles and so lessens dyspnoea. In addition it is hoped that there may be associated relaxation of the bronchial muscle. Training should start in half lying and side lying and progress to sitting and even to standing as far as is possible.

Simple easy movements of the neck, shoulders and dorsal spine are an adjunct to the treatment. They are valuable because the chest wall itself tends to become stiff and the posture is poor. They may be done in such a way as to assist relaxation and expiration. Thus relaxed trunk dropping forwards in the sitting position may be combined with breathing and will not only increase movement in the spine and thorax, but will also assist expiration and relaxation.

Another very important point, though one not strictly in the physio-therapist's province, is the *removal of fear and anxiety*. In this the physio-therapist can help by encouraging the patient to talk and stressing the importance of mentioning any fears he has to the physician. If there are home and financial difficulties these should be reported.

EMPHYSEMA

The word emphysema means inflation, and aptly describes a state of the lungs in which the alveoli and alveolar ducts are distended and their walls atrophied. It is a condition which occurs in elderly people, particularly men. A variety of causes may be responsible for the changes. There is possibly a hereditary weakness of the lung tissue, and in this case any factor which causes a forcible overdistension of the alveoli may result in permanent dilatation. A chronic cough is therefore a possible cause. A partial obstruction of a bronchus may produce the condition, because, whereas inspiration widens and lengthens the tubes, so tending to over-come the obstruction, expiration produces a diminution in the lumen and consequently increases the obstruction. Air can therefore be drawn into the tubes distal to the partial block, but, once in, is difficult to expel, and the alveoli therefore become increasingly distended with air. A partial obstruction of this type may be due to chronic bronchitis or to prolonged attacks of asthma.

An emphysematous condition of part of a lung may be compensatory. If one lobe is removed, the remaining lobes expand and fill up the space in the thorax, the expansion being brought about by the drop in intra-pleural pressure consequent to the reduced lung volume.

There is a senile type of emphysema in which degenerative changes occur in the alveolar walls, but the alveoli are not distended and the lung is small, this is therefore not a true emphysema.

Changes

Continual stretching of the alveolar walls results in atrophy and thinning and in time the septum separating one alveolus from the next breaks down and disappears. Instead of a great number of alveoli, they are now few but very large in size. Two serious complications arise from this stretch-ing and breakdown. In the first place, the elasticity of the lung is greatly reduced. This means that the lung fails to recoil adequately when the muscles of inspiration relax, the chest wall, therefore, tends to remain in the position of inspiration. Gradually changes occur in the soft tissues and the shape of the chest alters till it takes on permanently the 'barrel-shaped' appearance in which the antero-posterior diameter equals the transverse, the costal angle is greater than a right angle, the ribs are more horizontal and the intercostal spaces are wider. With diminished recoil of the lung, expiration is decreased and a greater effort is required to produce both expiration and inspiration. The accessory muscles of respiration are brought into action and dyspnoea develops. In the second place the capillaries in the alveolar walls are stretched and their lumen diminished while those in the septa are completely obliterated. Thus the pulmonary capillary bed is markedly reduced and considerable obstruction to the pulmonary circulation arises. This obstruction results in increased work for the right ventricle, so that hypertrophy follows, and in time evidence of heart failure appears.

Signs and Symptoms

The chief clinical signs of the condition are dyspnoea and cyanosis. At first the patient is dyspnoeic only on exertion, but his capacity for exercise grows less and he is eventually dyspnoeic even at rest. This dyspnoea is partly due to the difficulty in expiration, the result of loss of elastic recoil of the lung, with therefore greater quantities of residual air and less diffusion of gases between the alveolar air and that in the bronchial tubes. It is also partly the result of the loss of aerating surface and diminished interchange of gases between the alveolar air and the blood. It is also due to the extra muscular effort required to move the inelastic lungs and the stiffened thoracic joints.

Congestion in the pulmonary circulation leads to cyanosis since a much greater quantity of reduced haemoglobin will be present in the blood stream.

Cough is not characteristic of emphysema but, as a result of lowered resistance, chronic bronchitis is a common complication, and when this occurs a cough will be present.

The 'barrel-shaped' chest, the kyphotic dorsal spine, the short neck and high shoulders and the diminished chest expansion, are all characteristic features of an advanced emphysema.

OUTLINE OF TREATMENT BY PHYSIOTHERAPY

No cure can be expected or obtained, but a certain degree of help can be given to the patient. Treatment aims at preventing recurrent attacks of bronchitis, assisting expiration and increasing the thoracic mobility. Whatever steps are taken to achieve these objects, they must be taken with the full understanding that the patient readily becomes dyspnoeic and that there may be some heart involvement. For these reasons carefully taught relaxation and breathing exercises, together with easy simple exercises are all that can be given.

Relaxation and breathing exercises. The patient must first be made comfortable. As he is usually elderly and dyspnoeic, the half lying position, with a pillow under the knees, the back and head well supported, and arms resting on pillows is usually most suitable. General tenseness is then reduced by the practice of relaxation carefully taught, special attention being paid to face, neck, shoulders and chest. Once reduction in tone is obtained, instruction in breathing may begin. Since the main object is to increase the power of expiration the patient is taught how to reduce the size of the chest and so how to drive more air out. Great emphasis is laid on ease of expiration and consequently the patient is asked to 'sigh' the air out rather than 'hiss' and force it out. As the patient learns to sink the ribs and upper abdomen expiration will naturally lengthen and mobility increase. Progression may be made by giving firm but gentle pressure on the sides of the chest at the end of expiration and, if suitable, the patient may be taught to do this with a strap, a careful watch being kept to see that the shoulder girdle muscles are not tensed. Still further progression is obtained by combining expiration with forward and side bendings of the trunk. Though the emphasis should definitely be on expiration, it is advisable to try to obtain better expansion of the large basal areas of the lung since so much of the expansion is apical and obtained by the accessory muscles of inspiration. The patient is therefore taught to use the diaphragm more effectively and here his acquired ability to relax the neck and shoulder muscles is useful. On no account should he be allowed to force the upper abdomen up but he should contract it, as he has been practising, on expiration and then relax it and allow it to come up on inspiration. Progression of this work may be to practise diaphragmatic breathing in sitting, standing and walking until it becomes a habit. In the meantime, lateral costal expansion and posterior costal are attempted, gently and with no forced effort.

When some improvement in breathing is gained, very gently, and step by step, simple mobilising and postural exercises may be added, taking care that dyspnoea is not produced. It should be possible to raise the exercise tolerance slightly if the addition of exercises is slowly and carefully carried out.

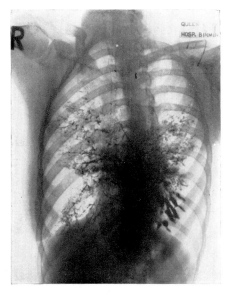
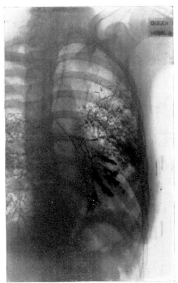

PLATE VII. BRONCHIECTASIS

(a) Showing involvement left lung   (b) Showing involvement middle
                                          and lower lobes

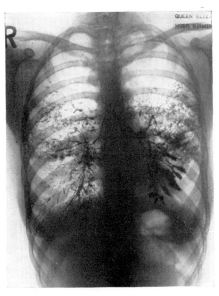

(c) Showing involvement both lungs

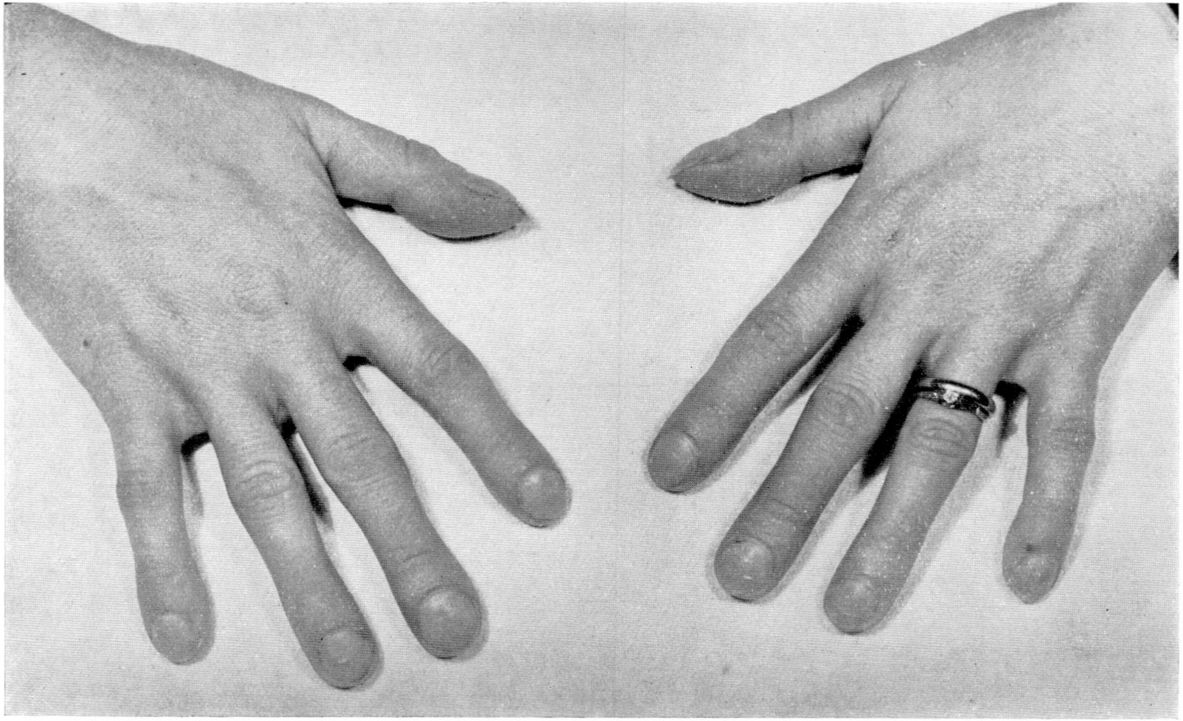

PLATE VIII. CLUBBING OF FINGERS IN BRONCHIECTASIS

BRONCHIECTASIS

Bronchiectasis is a condition of dilatation of the bronchi or bronchioles with stagnation of secretions and consequently a tendency to secondary infection and pus formation. The bronchiectasis may be widespread, affecting the tubes of both lungs or all lobes of one lung, or it may be localised to a small number of bronchi possibly in one lobe only. It is found more commonly in the lower lobes, particularly the base of the left lung, possibly because the left bronchus is so placed that it is more readily compressed by any enlargement of mediastinal lymph glands (see Plate VII). The dilatations vary in shape. If they occur in the larger bronchi they are often cylindrical, while in the smaller tubes they may be saccular.

CAUSES

Bronchiectasis may be congenital but it is much more often the result of obstruction of a large or small bronchus. Such obstruction may be caused by the mechanical pressure of a growing neoplasm or enlarged tuberculous gland. In children the very narrow tubes can be readily obstructed by plugs of mucus during an attack of measles, whooping cough or broncho-pneumonia. Immediately following an abdominal or thoracic operation, when secretions are increased and the action of the cilia and the cough reflex are depressed, there is particular danger of the formation of a mucous or muco-purulent plug and obstruction. If a bronchus is completely blocked the air distal to the block will be gradually absorbed and the lobule, segment or lobe will, therefore, collapse. The negative intra-pleural pressure will, as a result, be increased, and a greater traction force will be exerted on the affected area. This acts on the tubes proximal to the block and these are no longer protected from this force by surrounding air-filled alveoli. The tubes, therefore, tend to dilate and this tendency will be most marked if they are already weakened by inflammation and infection.

CHANGES

In early cases not due to obstruction by infected material, no changes in the epithelium are present. There is simply an area of dilatation surrounded by solid airless lung tissue. Usually, however, there is some degree of chronic inflammation with infiltration of the bronchial walls and surrounding fibrosis. In many cases, sooner or later, secondary infection occurs. Either the original block was formed by septic material and infection spreads to the walls of the bronchus or secretions accumulate and become infected. Infection results in a destructive inflammation and the lining is destroyed, the elasticity lost, the wall of the tube weakened so that the dilatation is increased. Infection spreads to the surrounding tissue and fibrosis occurs and as the fibrotic tissue shrinks, further traction is exerted on the tubes. As the walls become increasingly damaged they lose their sensitivity to the presence of secretions which therefore tend to accumulate, decompose and become purulent. Infection therefore spreads and cavities may form. On any change of position the purulent material may move and come in contact with healthier mucous membrane, stimulating the cough reflex and so being coughed up. Sometimes the movement is impeded by swelling of the mucous membrane. Pus cannot then be drained away and there will be toxic absorption, spread of infection and greater danger of the formation of septic emboli.

Signs and Symptoms

While there is dilatation and low grade chronic inflammation only, no symptoms may be present though there is a great liability for recurrent attacks of bronchitis or broncho-pneumonia. From time to time haemoptysis may occur from rupture of vessels in the congested mucous membrane. Once infection is established and pus is formed, cough and offensive sputum are the outstanding signs. Cough is often associated with changes of posture since these cause accumulated pus to leave the cavities and come into contact with healthy mucous membrane, so initiating the cough reflex. Sometimes, therefore, the cough is not very noticeable during the day but is marked on getting up in the morning and on assuming a lying position at night. Turning over in bed may precipitate an attack of coughing and the patient may find that lying on the affected side lessens coughing, since in this way pus tends to remain in the cavities. The cough may be accompanied by a copious expectoration of foul-smelling sputum, yellowish-green in colour, and the breath has then an offensive odour.

On examination of the chest and the respiratory movements, some flattening of the thoracic wall over the diseased lobe may be noticed and movement may be diminished in this area. Usually vital capacity and chest expansion are decreased.

Since the patient is continuously absorbing toxins and suffering periods of ill-health due to acute bronchitis or broncho-pneumonia, the general health is poor, loss of weight, night sweats, evening pyrexia may be present and clubbing of fingers can sometimes be seen (see Plate VIII). Posture is consistently poor.

OUTLINE OF TREATMENT BY PHYSIOTHERAPY

The tendency is for the disease to spread since toxic absorption and displacement of pus lead to infection of other areas, while plugging of bronchi with subsequent collapse lead to wider dilatation. The constant absorption of toxins is harmful to the patient's general health and resistance, while some danger of pyaemia and cerebral abscess exists. The most satisfactory treatment is therefore removal of the affected area or of the affected lobe, but this is not always possible. The younger the patient and the less the symptoms, the better the chance of successful operation. Treatment by physical measures varies according to the nature of medical or surgical treatment.

Non-operative Cases

There are usually patients over thirty who are either unfit or unwilling to submit to an operation. It may be that the condition is too extensive to allow of surgical procedures. The object in these cases is to raise the resistance of the lung tissues and keep the cavities as clear of secretions as possible. In this way toxic absorption will be less and attacks of bronchitis may be warded off.

Physical treatment can materially help by means of postural drainage, breathing exercises, and light general exercises. Postural drainage must be carried out at least twice daily for the rest of the patient's life, consequently it is necessary to teach the patient the correct positions to be used, and how to attain them easily and in comfort. A careful study is made of the bronchogram, and the drainage positions are chosen accordingly. If no bronchogram is available, correct positioning may be carried out by means of choosing positions and noting those which produce maximum expectoration. Once the positions have been selected they should be tried out, and if they result in little sputum, agility exercises and percussion may be added.

Breathing exercises will assist the circulation to the lungs and bronchi. For this purpose deeper breathing should be encouraged using the chest as a whole. To help loosen pus, localised deeper breathing is taught, particularly encouraging a longer expiration—this breathing being best practised while lying in the drainage position. If the affected lobe is expanding less fully than the healthy areas, localised pressure expansion exercises are taught, training the patient to give his own pressure either by hand or by strap. Instruction in breathing should not be considered complete until the patient can use any part of either lung at will.

General exercises are chosen to fulfil several purposes. They may be agility exercises to loosen mucus and create slight breathlessness and therefore deeper breathing. Some will be chosen for their effect on posture, others to maintain the mobility of spine and thorax. In the case of adults the exercises should not be too heavy and must be well taught so that they can be continued at home. Ideally the patient should receive a course of three to four weeks' treatment and should then continue at home, reporting at intervals of three to six months.

Operative Cases

These will usually be children or young adults who have the condition affecting one or two lobes while the remainder of the lung is healthy. A partial or complete lobectomy is the operation of choice though very occasionally a pneumonectomy or thoracoplasty may be necessary. All cases require pre-operative physiotherapy in order to gain the patient's confidence, to drain the cavities so that the lung may be as dry as possible, to establish a sense of good posture, and gain the best possible control of respiration. Physical treatment is again necessary immediately following the operation to prevent collapse of areas of the sound lobes of the affected side, to maintain good posture and full range of arm movements and to gain full expansion of the remaining lobes. (For fuller details of the treatment see *Physiotherapy in Some Surgical Conditions.*)

BRONCHIAL ASTHMA

The asthmatic patient suffers from recurrent attacks of dyspnoea during which expiration is particularly laboured. The attacks are the result of spasm of the smooth muscle of the bronchi and swelling of the mucous lining with increased secretion of mucus. These spasmodic changes cause a partial obstruction of the tubes and consequently extreme difficulty in expiration. Inspiration is not so difficult because, as the chest expands, the smaller bronchi increase in diameter and the obstruction is at least partially overcome but, as the negative intrapleural pressure decreases on expiration, the lungs and thorax recoil, the bronchi decrease in diameter and the obstruction is, if anything, increased. Since air can be drawn in, but not expelled, the alveoli become increasingly distended with air, and dyspnoea and cyanosis result. When spasm ceases, mucus is coughed up, the bronchi relax and breathing becomes normal once again.

These attacks occur most frequently in childhood though sometimes they commence later in life. In many cases no definite cause can be given. It is probable that the broncho-constrictor centre is unusually sensitive and reacts abnormally to stimuli. The centre may then be 'set off' through irritation of the vagal nerve endings by protein substances inhaled or ingested. Such substance may be in the dusts in the house, the coat of animals, or in the factory; it may be the pollen of plants or it may be in certain foods such as eggs, milk, or shell fish.

There may be irritation by the products of bacterial infection in the upper respiratory tract, or the lungs.

In most patients, and particularly when the attacks commence in childhood, there is a strong psychological factor, the centre being abnormally sensitive to psychical stimuli. It has been noted that the attacks occur more often when the home surroundings are uncongenial or there is absence of a stable background. Attacks are more frequent when parents show anxiety in front of the children or when they discuss the attacks before them.

Changes

Changes of muscular spasm and swelling of mucosa are present during the attack but, at first, the chest will return to normal when the attack subsides. Later, however, if the attacks are frequent or of long duration, hypertrophy of the mucous membrane gradually takes place and, in addition, marked thickening of all coats of the smaller bronchi results. These changes serve to make matters more difficult when spasm of the hypertrophied muscle occurs. In time, continued overdistension of the alveoli will lead to atrophy of their walls and areas of emphysema result. Occasionally excessive mucus may plug the smaller tubes and areas of collapse may also be present.

Signs and Symptoms

The attacks come on most frequently during the night but in really severe cases they may occur at any time. Sometimes there are premonitory signs, the patient feeling restless and experiencing a sense of constriction in the chest. As the attacks develop and the sense of constriction increases, the patient sits bolt upright and if possible holds on to some object in order to bring the accessory muscles of respiration more adequately into play. Long expiratory efforts are made, interrupted at intervals by short spasmodic inspiratory movements. As more and more air is sucked in and less is expelled, the patient becomes cyanosed, the face is pale and anxious, and the skin sweats profusely. There is wheezing as the air is passed in and out through the excess mucus. The attack usually terminates with a bout of coughing when much fluid sputum is coughed up.

These attacks last a varying length of time but in some advanced cases they may continue over several days, the patient, unable to eat or sleep, is exceedingly ill and there is always the possibility of death as a result of the strain on the heart. This state is often spoken of as status asthmaticus.

All patients suffering from asthma but particularly young children, show defective posture. This is most often a general 'slump' in which the head is poked forward, the dorsal spine is kyphotic, the pelvic tilt increased, producing a lordosis, and the chest narrow and flat. There are often also knock-knees and flat feet. This poor posture is probably very largely the result of the instability of the nervous system and the mental attitude of fear and anxiety. The anxious child is the child who tends to stoop and who fails to stand erect to face the world. In addition interference with full oxygenation of the blood leads to imperfect metabolism and impaired tone and strength of the muscles.

PHYSIOTHERAPY FOR ASTHMA

There is no doubt that much improvement can be gained by the use of physiotherapy, provided this goes hand in hand with other measures. Very little is gained by any treatment if the management of the child at home is unsuitable. Since the physiotherapist is likely to see the parents more frequently than the physician does, she may be asked to re-inforce the advice which, without doubt, will have already been given. It is essential that a perfectly normal life should be led. If the child is allowed to consider itself unusual and abnormal, the attacks will be more frequent and a cure is unlikely. Schooling and play should be as little interrupted as possible, the parents should be instructed that under no circumstances should the condition be discussed in front of the child, nor should any anxiety be shown during an attack. If the mother shows anxiety, the child will lose confidence in her, fear will develop and the attacks will be more frequent and prolonged. Once the co-operation of the parents has been gained much can be done for the child. Whether the patient is an adult or a child the principles of treatment are the same, but naturally methods must vary with the age.

Relaxation. To train relaxation is vitally important, particularly in adults who less easily forget the attacks and who therefore tend to remain tense and anxious. As in most chest cases, instruction in general relaxation is necessary but particular attention is paid to the muscles of the neck, face, shoulder girdle and chest. Relaxation must be taught between attacks, then, if the patient has premonitory signs relaxation may be practised and the attack warded off. One of the best methods of gaining relaxation of these areas is by performing relaxed movements. For example, in forearm support lax sitting head dropping forwards and sideways and easy rolling are useful movements; in standing the arms may be raised to reach upward and then relaxed, while in sitting the trunk may be dropped forwards. In the adult, attention is drawn throughout to the 'feeling' of relaxation; once the idea is grasped the same relaxation may be gained in sitting up in bed—the position the patient will adopt if, during the night she feels an attack coming on.

Diaphragmatic and lateral costal breathing. There is little doubt that in most cases of asthma the ability to use the diaphragm properly and to expand the basal area of the lung is lost. It is almost impossible to perform diaphragmatic breathing if the chest is tense and the neck muscles in vigorous action. The patient has, therefore, to be taught to keep the upper thorax still and to use the diaphragm. Considerable supervision of small children is necessary to ensure that the whole abdomen is not pushed up during inspiration by hollowing the lumbar spine. For this reason, the method of placing a paper boat or tiny shoe on the abdomen and telling the child to let it rise and fall has dangers, it is better to let the patient place the fingers on the area between the diverging costal margins and try to swell out round the lower ribs, letting the fingers of the two hands separate gradually. Once the ability to use the diaphragm has been learnt, then the patient may be taught what, in addition to the practise of relaxation, she can do to ward off an attack. It will be explained that provided the diaphragm is used it does not matter how quickly she breathes, consequently she is taught to take the sitting position and practise quick diaphragmatic breathing so that she can put this into effect in the event of the onset of an attack.

Expiration. Relaxation and diaphragmatic breathing are the two most important measures but an important step is to help the patient to gain a longer expiration so that emphysematous changes do not occur. Attention is drawn to an attempt to reduce the size of the thorax during expiration, once this is mastered then longer expiration may be gained by manual pressure on the thorax. Subsequently, expiration to counting, to the saying of nursery rhymes or to reading may be added. A child will take an interest in seeing how high he can count before pausing to take a breath.

Exercises. Simple exercises will be added gradually, to aid expiration, to mobilise stiff thoracic joints and to improve posture. The latter is most important and a very careful training of posture is required, the methods varying with the age of the patient. Illustrations of such exercises will be found clearly set out in the pamphlet issued by the Asthma Research Council.

Later Treatment

The eventual object of treatment is to gain a good habit of breathing in all daily activities and to increase the ability to perform exercise producing normal dyspnoea, without provoking an attack of asthma. To fulfil this object the amount of active exercise is gradually increased, while a very close watch is kept on the method of breathing during the activity. In addition, correct breathing is trained during walking, running and climbing stairs, until eventually the patient breathes correctly as a habit. Training begins by teaching diaphragmatic breathing in standing and then while 'marking time'. So many steps are taken on inspiration and one or two more on expiration; this may then be progressed to actual walking, speed being increased till the patient is running, still using diaphragmatic breathing. Walking upstairs may be taken in the same way, beginning slowly, two steps up to inspiration, three to expiration, one to pause in breathing, then gaining speed by increasing the number of steps to each inspiration and expiration. Particularly for children, once diaphragmatic breathing and longer expiration have been taught, class work should be used. This is necessary because these patients can then receive less individual attention with less apparent emphasis on 'asthma', consequently the children enjoy exercises without considering themselves abnormal.

PART FOUR

DISORDERS OF
THE NERVOUS SYSTEM

Chapter I

INTRODUCTION—SIGNS AND SYMPTOMS OF NEUROLOGICAL DISORDERS

Damage may occur in many ways to any part of the nervous system. Lesions of the Central Nervous System are irreparable because nerve cells do not regenerate and the fibres of the brain and spinal cord have no neurilemma. If the peripheral nervous system is affected, recovery is possible because nerve fibres, which possess a neurilemma sheath, will regenerate (provided their cells of origin are intact). A lesion of part of the brain or spinal cord, however, does not necessarily mean permanent loss of function, for other parts may take over the work of the damaged area. This is particularly seen in lesions of the cerebral cortex.

DISTURBANCE OF FUNCTION

The amount of disturbance of function which follows any lesion depends not only on the extent of damage, but also on the mode of onset, the degree of shock and the particular cells and fibres involved.

The mode of onset influences the extent of the disturbance. Sudden onset always produces more widespread symptoms than will eventually be present. This is because, later, cells and fibres which were not at the time completely destroyed, will recover. In addition a sudden lesion is nearly always accompanied by oedema of surrounding tissue and widespread vascular disturbance. In time oedema (causing pressure on healthy tissue) will be absorbed and circulation will be restored to normal. A lesion which occurs insidiously may spread considerably before any marked symptoms appear. A spinal tumour, for example, may be very large before it is discovered.

Shock. Sudden and severe damage to the brain or the spinal cord is followed by complete cessation of function of that part of the nervous system. Such a condition is known as cerebral or spinal shock. If the patient lives, some recovery of function will occur. Failure to recover is only present where actual pestruction of nerve tissue has taken place. In cases of severe cerebral haemorrhage the patient commonly immediately becomes unconscious, the limbs are flaccid and no voluntary movement is present. If the patient survives, considerable recovery of function almost invariably occurs. In total transection of the spinal cord, immediately following the trauma, complete loss of all function below the level of lesion is present. In time, however, involuntary movements and tone return, though voluntary movement will never recover.

Fibres and cells affected. Some cells and fibres of the nervous system appear to be more readily affected by disease processes than others. The cells of the cerebral cortex degenerate, when deprived of oxygen, in a much shorter time than do those of the spinal cord. As a whole, cells suffer much more from a deficient blood supply than fibres. The virus producing acute poliomyelitis has a special affinity for the anterior horn of grey matter of the spinal cord, while that producing Herpes Zoster attacks the ganglion of the posterior nerve root. In neuritis it is the nerve fibres and rarely the cells which are affected, and certain poisons attack the motor fibres while others affect the sensory fibres.

SIGNS AND SYMPTOMS OF NEUROLOGICAL DISORDERS

There are many signs and symptoms of disease of the various parts of the nervous system. The particular features of any one disease may be difficult to predict because fibres and cells are so closely packed together that a lesion rarely affects one system only. Certain features do, however, stand out and should be looked for by the physiotherapist when the patient is examined. A list of these is given below:

> Paralysis
> Alterations in tone
> Involuntary movements
> Inco-ordination
> Alterations in electrical reactions
> Muscle atrophy
> Diminished or lost sensation
> Paraesthesia
> Pain
> Circulatory impairment

It will be realised that there are many signs and symptoms which are important to the clinician but do not so closely concern the physiotherapist, thus eye symptoms are very important as is the state of reflex activity. With the exception of reflex activity, which has some bearing on physiotherapy, these signs and symptoms will not be discussed.

PARALYSIS

A patient is usually said to be paralysed when he is unable to perform voluntary movement of the affected part of the body. There are, however, two types of paralysis. The muscles will be able to contract if the final common pathway is intact, but the patient may be unable to bring them into action because the ability to initiate voluntary movement is lost. On the other hand, the ability to initiate movement may be present but the final common pathway may be damaged and the muscles cannot therefore be stimulated to contract. The former type of paralysis is spoken of as paralysis of movement, the latter as paralysis of muscle.

Paralysis of movement. If the patient is unable to initiate voluntary movement, although the muscles are capable of contracting, the lesion is probably in the pyramidal or extra-pyramidal system. The exact site of initiation of voluntary movement is not yet certain but it is clear that patterns of movement, not individual muscles, are represented in the cerebral cortex.

Movements are often also affected because these systems exert an inhibitory control over muscle tone, and reflex activity. Thus, if these areas are damaged or diseased, tone may become excessive and reflex activity abnormal. The result may well be that, though some voluntary movement is possible, it is not possible for the patient to move one segment only of an affected limb or to perform isolated movements. An attempt to perform such a movement sets in action a whole reflex pattern. Thus, for example, if the spastic hemiplegic patient attempts to flex the fingers, there is usually a movement of flexion of the wrist and elbow, pronation of the forearm and adduction of the shoulder.

In young children born with defects in the motor areas, tone may be so great and may offer so much resistance to attempted movement that the child gives up trying and voluntary movements fail to develop or develop in faulty patterns.

Paralysis of muscles implies that individual muscles or groups of muscles, or bundles of muscle fibres lose their ability to contract. A movement may therefore be weakened or lost. The lesion in this case will be found in the final common pathway. The cells, from which the axons supplying the affected muscles arise, may be diseased or put out of action, or the axons may be affected so that no message can reach the muscle.

ALTERATIONS IN MUSCLE TONE

Tone is said to be the state of preparedness of a muscle to respond to stretch. It indicates that the cells of the anterior horn of the spinal cord are in a sufficient state of excitability to be readily stimulated to discharge if further impulses reach them. This state of excitability is thought to be 'set' by the reticular formation which itself consists of an excitor and an inhibitor part. Increase in excitability means that fewer stimuli are required to cause the cells to discharge, and a decrease in excitability means the converse.

Increased tone. In disorders of the nervous system tone may be increased to the point at which muscles are in a state of tonic contraction, imposing on the patient abnormal postures and preventing isolated movement. This may be due to deficient inhibitor control of the anterior horn cells so that their state of excitability is so increased that they discharge impulses with negligible or fewer than normal stimuli. The increase in tone could also be due to irritation of the excitor reticular formation.

In the former case the inhibitor stimuli may be reduced as a result of damage or disease of the motor areas of the cortex or of the inhibitor part of the reticular formation. This will account for the increase of tone seen in diseases of the pyramidal system illustrated by the spasticity of some cases of hemiplegia and cerebral palsy.

In these cases the spasticity is usually selective and variable. If the anterior horn cells are in a state of increased excitability any afferent stimuli will cause them to discharge, hence slight stretch on a group of muscles, possibly produced by a certain posture, will result in increase in tone in the muscles. In hemiplegia, for example, in the erect posture there is usually increased tone in the flexors of the arm and extensors of the leg. It will be noted that if the muscle is stretched by means of passive movement, tone increases, but if the movement is then arrested or if it is continued until it is nearly completed, spasticity suddenly 'passes off'.

In some cases, probably when the excitor part of the reticular formation is irritated, tone is increased in all groups of muscles of the affected part of the body. This is seen in some cases of paralysis agitans. This type of increase of tone is maintained throughout the whole range of passive movement and to it the term 'rigidity' is applied.

Increase in muscle tone will have a harmful effect on voluntary movement because it acts as a resistance. Moreover, it tends to lead to the development of contractures and deformity and therefore to limitation of range of movement.

Decreased tone. This will result from decreased excitability of the anterior horn cells so that more stimuli are required to cause them to discharge. In certain lesions of the cerebellum, for example, fewer messages reach the cells through the reticular formation and muscle tone is decreased. Disease or damage of the final common pathway must lead to decreased or lost tone because the cells themselves are damaged or the pathway along which they discharge is no longer intact. Tone will therefore be lost in complete lesions of the peripheral nerves.

Any lesion which diminishes sensory stimuli will result in decreased tone. This will account for the reduced tone seen in tabes dorsalis.

Reduction of tone also interferes with voluntary movement since, on the one hand, a greater number of stimuli are required to initiate the movement and, on the other, guiding and controlling of the movement becomes difficult and inco-ordination is present. In addition, the muscles are less prepared to respond quickly to stimuli and the joints are therefore less well protected and more readily subjected to trauma.

INVOLUNTARY MOVEMENTS

Involuntary movements are usually the result of lesions of the cerebral cortex and corpus striatum. They need not necessarily be of motor origin. For example, there are reflex spasmodic contractions of muscles which are the result of irritating lesions of sensory nerves.

Examples of involuntary movements which are the result of disease of the motor mechanisms are often seen. There are the cramps and spasms of spastic limbs. These are excited by cutaneous or proprioceptive stimuli acting on spinal areas no longer controlled by higher centres. Choreiform movements are rapid, jerky movements serving no useful purpose. When superimposed on voluntary movement they render the latter inco-ordinate. These movements appear to be the result of scattered lesions in the cerebral cortex and corpus striatum, possibly the result of irritation by toxins of rheumatic origin. Again the student will meet athetoid movements present in a particular type of cerebral palsy. This type of movement differs from the choreic movement because it is slower and sinuous and leads to peculiar positions of joints which could not normally be attained. Such movements are difficult to explain, but are the result of sudden excesses in tone in certain muscle groups and are due to damage to the basal ganglia.

The rhythmic tremor seen in many cases of paralysis agitans is another familiar involuntary movement. The cause of this tremor is uncertain, it may be that it is the result of rigidity. Increased tension of one group causes a slight stretch on the opposite group which is also hypertonic, so a contraction occurs. This in its turn sets up a contraction in the opposing group and so a rhythmic to and fro movement is the result. If the limb is adequately supported so that increased tension in one group does not occur, then the tremor may cease.

Fasciculation is another example of involuntary movement. It is the result of irritation of cells of origin of motor fibres. In cases of progressive muscular atrophy, for example, these cells are undergoing degenerative changes. Irritation precedes degeneration and so, in muscles not yet showing marked changes, spontaneous contraction of groups of muscle fibres supplied by the axons of these cells is a characteristic feature.

INCO-ORDINATION

Co-ordination might be said to be the ability to perform a smooth purposeful movement with the least possible expenditure of energy. The student will be well aware that to perform even a simple movement at least four groups of muscle must work. These are the prime movers, antagonists, synergists and fixators. Disturbance or improper functioning of any one of these groups leads to inaccuracy of movement and waste of energy. This may be spoken of as inco-ordination.

The correct correlation of these different groups depends upon several factors. First in importance is the cerebral cortex which grades and combines movements to form a more complex action. Second, the cerebellum and corpus striatum are essential. They control the position of the limb, the tone of the muscles taking part, and the rate and regularity of muscular contraction. These sections of the motor system can only produce the right effect if they are kept aware of the position of the body and joints in space, the range of the movement performed and the state of contraction of the muscles. The cerebral cortex is kept aware of these things through the kinaesthetic sense, impulses travelling from muscles and joints through the posterior columns of the spinal cord to reach, eventually, the post-central area of the cortex. The cerebellum is informed of these events through the vestibular apparatus and the anterior and posterior spino-cerebellar tracts. In addition to knowledge of position and contraction the cerebellum will only be able to play its part if it is kept in close touch with the cerebral cortex as it will come into action only at the request of the cerebrum.

Even if all these factors are intact, perfect co-ordination cannot be obtained if the final common pathway is diseased, since then messages from cerebrum, cerebellum and corpus striatum cannot reach the muscles. In addition the different groups of muscles needed to perform the movements must be of normal strength and tone (increase or decrease in tone of any one group must inevitably upset co-ordination). Again the presence of involuntary movements may upset co-ordination.

The term 'ataxia' so often applied to inco-ordination should be applied to those types of inco-ordination which are not the result of muscle weakness, spasticity, or involuntary movements. If these causes are ruled out two types of inco-ordination stand out: sensory ataxia and ataxia of cerebellar origin.

Sensory ataxia is the ataxia which arises as the result of loss of kinaesthetic sense. The patient, if he cannot see the limb, is unaware of its position in space and so is totally incapable of performing a smooth movement, In addition, muscle tone is reduced since there will be less stimuli from the muscles acting on the anterior horn cells. Co-ordination is, therefore. impaired but is considerably improved if the patient uses his sense of sight as a substitute for kinaesthetic loss. This type of ataxia is present in tumours or injuries of the post-central area of the cerebral cortex, in some cases of subacute combined degeneration of the cord, in the later stages of tabes dorsalis, in many cases of polyneuritis.

Cerebellar ataxia. In this type either because correct messages do not reach the cerebellum or because the cerebellum itself is diseased, inco-ordination is present. If the cerebellum is undergoing a pathological lesion, as, for example, in cerebellar tumour or abscess, or in many cases of disseminated sclerosis, rate and regularity of contraction is impaired and marked hypotonia is present. For these reasons there is inability to steady the trunk or limb, so that during the performance of a movement marked swaying occurs. There is inability to control the movement and so it is carried either too far or not far enough. As the object is approached the movement is not adequately slowed to reach the desired point and so a marked intention tremor develops. This type of inco-ordination is not aided by vision, and this is one of the points which enables the student to distinguish between sensory and cerebellar ataxia.

ALTERATION IN ELECTRICAL REACTIONS

All tissues have certain characteristics of electrical excitability, and the results of stimulation are dependent upon the strength, duration, frequency and rate of change in the intensity of the stimulus, and also upon the state of the tissue itself. The two tissues it is necessary to consider are the muscle and nerve fibres. By means of suitable tests, it is possible to gain information about the state of innervation of muscles and of conductivity in the nerve trunks. Tests of excitability are made by applying a stimulus to the main nerve trunks and to the belly of the muscles and observing the response. These tests fall into two main groups; in the first are the qualitative tests, and in the second the quantitative ones.

Qualitative tests. The classical faradic and galvanic test is qualitative since it is not possible to measure the strength and duration of the stimuli with accuracy. It is, however, a useful guide to the state of innervation of the muscle. The faradic stimulus is an interrupted current of short duration and the galvanic stimulus is a direct current of approximately one second's duration. Where the muscle is normally innervated, a brisk contraction is obtained on stimulating either the nerve trunk or muscle belly with an adequate faradic stimulus. A brisk response is also obtained with the longer stimulus of interrupted galvanism.

With degeneration of the nerve fibres the nerve trunk fails to respond to all stimuli, and conductivity is lost within two to three days of any acute lesion leading to degeneration. The excitability of the muscle itself also changes in degenerative lesions of the motor nerves. It becomes increasingly difficult to elicit a contraction with faradism and, by the second or third week, there may be no response, or only a feeble localised twitch with the maximum current available. Meanwhile the response to galvanism is altering and the contraction becomes sluggish and undulating in character. The loss of nerve conduction and faradic excitability, with a sluggish response to galvanism, is known as the reaction of degeneration and is characteristic of a degenerative lower motor neurone paralysis. If progressive fibrotic changes occur in the denervated muscle the threshold of the galvanic stimulus rises and, finally, the muscle may become wholly inexcitable, a state known as the complete reaction of degeneration. Massive ischaemic necrosis of muscle leads to an abrupt and early onset of the complete reaction of degeneration.

In lesions where there has only been damage to some of the nerve fibres, the response will differ as some of the fibres will give a normal response while the response from the remainder will be altered. There is a positive response on stimulation of the nerve, the response of the muscle to faradism is weak or absent, and it is sometimes possible to detect both a brisk, and sluggish component in the response to galvanism. This is termed partial reaction of degeneration.

In recovering lesions it is sometimes possible to elicit contraction of the muscles by stimulation of the nerve trunk before there is evidence of voluntary contraction. On the whole this qualitative test is of little help in detecting signs of recovery.

Strength-duration curve. This test is one of the quantitative methods of assessing excitability, for both intensity and duration of the stimuli can be measured and plotted on a graph. It is desirable to have at least five known selected durations of stimulus. It is found that, as the duration decreases, the strength of the current must increase. In healthy muscle it has been found that the threshold stimulus at one-thousandth of a second duration is in the region of twice the intensity required to elicit a response to a stimulus of one second duration. The differences between the response of healthy and denervated muscle are shown in Fig 5. Provided a sufficient number of points is available, the graph obtained by testing a partially denervated muscle will show a discontinuity in the curve, i.e. the responses of both innervated and denervated muscle fibres are shown. During reinnervation there are characteristic changes in the responses which gradually become more normal.

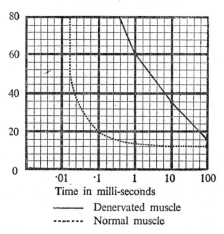

Time in milli-seconds

―――― Denervated muscle

······· Normal muscle

Fig. 5. Strength-duration curve.

Electromyography provides a delicate method of studying changes in electrical potential which are associated with voluntary or involuntary contraction of muscle fibres. The simplest type of apparatus consists of an electrode, amplifier and a loudspeaker. The inclusion of a cathode ray oscilloscope in the circuit makes it possible to observe deflections of the beam produced by the action potentials, as well as to hear the sounds associated with them. Needle or surface electrodes may be used.

As a needle is inserted in healthy muscle, there is a transient outburst of motor-unit activity due to mechanical stimulation of the units through which the needle passes. Otherwise, in healthy, resting limb musculature, there is no detectable activity. Motor-unit action potentials are usually biphasic, associated with a rumbling sound in the loud speaker, and they are evoked by voluntary effort. The frequency of discharge of any one unit rises as effort increases, and other units are also called into play. During the first two to four weeks after a degenerative lesion, e.g. division of a nerve trunk, the insertion type of motor unit potential may be elicited, but there is no motor-unit activity in response to effort. After about two to three weeks, two types of fibrillation action potential appear; those which are evoked by mechanical stimulation, such as the insertion of the needle electrode, and those which occur spontaneously in sporadic outbursts. They are unrelated to any attempt at voluntary movement and occur rhythmically at rates varying from two to ten per second. In a loudspeaker they give rise to sharp clicking sounds.

Electrical reactions give the earliest reliable information about the presence or absence of a degenerative lower motor neurone lesion, and the first signs of re-innervation of muscle are found by electromyography.

MUSCLE ATROPHY

This is a noticeable feature of many neurological disorders. The main reason for atrophy is disuse. If the muscles are not used to the normal amount, metabolism will be decreased and the muscle fibres will therefore gradually shrink in size. The most pronounced atrophy is seen where there is paralysis of muscles and no power of contraction remains. In many of such cases it is not only the final common pathway which is destroyed but the sympathetic nerve fibres are also involved and the circulation, and, therefore, the nutrition to the muscles is reduced.

It is not unusual to find that, if the muscle fibres atrophy, the connective tissue framework of the muscle increases in quantity. This tissue has not the properties of muscle fibres and it has a tendency to shorten, consequently the function of the muscle is increasingly impaired. A muscle which is denervated and untreated for a period of one to two years will almost completely degenerate into fibrous tissue.

DIMINISHED OR LOST SENSATION

Destruction of part of the sensory area of the cortex will result in complete loss of all forms of sensation in one area of the body. Thus, for example, the patient may lose all awareness of one arm. To all intents and purposes the arm may then be considered paralysed because unless he watches the limb, he cannot perform useful movements. Complete severance of the spinal cord would result in loss of all forms of sensation below the level of the lesion.

In partial lesions of the spinal cord some forms of sensation only may be lost. In cases of syringomyelia where a spreading lesion, commencing at the base of the posterior horn, occurs, sensations of heat, cold and pain are lost while others remain intact. Such a condition is spoken of as dissociated anaesthesia, and the actual type of sensation lost depends upon the site of the lesion.

Lesions of peripheral nerves give a varying loss, depending on the nerve. Thus in lesions of nerves which have a large cutaneous distribution there will be a central area of complete anaesthesia, while surrounding this will be an area of partial loss in which tactile loss will be greater than that of pain and thermal sensation. This can be explained by the fact that peripheral nerves in their cutaneous distribution overlap one another, the pain fibres overlapping more than those conveying thermal stimuli.

The effect of sensory loss on reflex action, inco-ordination and muscle tone has already been pointed out in the discussion of disturbances of motor function.

PARAESTHESIA

Abnormal sensations such as tingling, numbness, 'pins and needles', are complained of in a great number of neurological conditions. These sensations may be spontaneous or they may arise as the result of external stimuli. They are due to disease of any part of the central nervous system and are not always explicable. In some cases such sensations are the result of irritation of sensory nerves such as might occur at the beginning of a progressive degenerative condition—they occur very often, for example, in cases of tabes dorsalis and subacute combined degeneration of the cord. These sensations are not uncommon in partial traumatic lesions of peripheral nerves.

PAIN

Pain is most often the result of irritation of pain nerve endings or of afferent fibres conveying pain sensations. Any harmful agent applied to the skin is likely to stimulate the free nerve endings. Impulses will travel along the rapidly conducting fibres and will be accurately interpreted and localised. This type of pain rapidly subsides. Stimulation of pain nerve endings in deeper tissues is usually produced by pressure or stretching. It is conducted more slowly along smaller fibres, and therefore is insidious in onset and persists longer. This pain is much less well localised. Pain from deep tissues is thus often referred to other structures, sometimes at a considerable distance away. The distance to which it can be referred depends on the extent of the area supplied by a segment of the spinal cord. Thus, for example, a lesion in the gluteal muscles may stimulate pain nerve endings so that impulses travel along the afferent nerve fibres to reach the fourth and fifth lumbar and the first sacral segments of the spinal cord. These segments supply an area of skin extending into the thigh, leg and foot and pain may therefore be felt in any part or all of this area.

From the physiotherapist's point of view certain facts which have a bearing on treatment by physical means emerge from the discussion of sensory signs and symptoms.

First, loss of sensation is important. This is partly because, if muscle joint sense is lost, inco-ordination of movement must result, though the use of the sense of sight can partly replace the lost kinaesthetic sense. Lost sensation is also important because lost ability to be aware of objects in the hand, their size and shape and texture, means likelihood of dropping and failure to make use of objects so that the patient ceases to use the limb for everyday activities. Loss of sensation is dangerous because the patient fails to protect himself against harmful stimuli; there is therefore some danger in the application of heat, of constant current, or any other form of physical treatment in which the patient's appreciation of pain and temperature stimuli has, at least partly, to be relied upon.

Secondly, it is essential to remember that pain may be referred. When a patient complains of pain in the limbs without obvious accompanying signs, careful examination must be made to locate the structure involved. The only treatment which can be successful is that in which the affected structure is dealt with. Treatment directed to the area in which the patient complains of pain may be palliative, but produces no permanent cure. It is also important to remember that there is a psychological element in all pain, and that if the patient is frightened, the sensation of pain will be much more intense.

CIRCULATORY IMPAIRMENT

Running in the spinal nerves are non-medullated post-ganglionic fibres of the sympathetic system. The pre-ganglionic fibres originate in cells in the lateral horn of the dorsal and first two lumbar segments of the spinal cord. They pass through the anterior horn, anterior nerve root and white ramus into the sympathetic trunk, to arborise round cells in a sympathetic ganglion. The post-ganglionic fibres arise from cells in a ganglion and join the spinal nerve through the grey ramus. These fibres are distributed to all the involuntary structures of the area supplied by the spinal nerve in which they travel, to blood vessels, hairs, sweat and sebaceous glands. The functions of these fibres may be impaired by a lesion involving the lateral or anterior horns of the spinal cord or by lesions of the spinal nerves.

Disturbances in the conductivity of the sympathetic fibres result in impairment in circulation and glandular activity. Sweat and sebaceous glands fail to function. The blood vessels, no longer maintained in tone through the vaso-constrictors, dilate, and hyperaemia is quickly followed by stagnation of blood with consequent impairment of nutrition and possibly oedema.

If the disturbance extends over a wide area, skin, muscles, joints and bones will all suffer. The skin, deprived of normal nutrition, becomes thin and shiny, the hairs tend to fall out so it appears abnormally smooth. Owing to impairment of glandular activity it becomes dry and hard. While in this altered condition it is easily damaged and slow to heal.

Muscles quickly show the effects of impaired nutrition. A progressive decrease in the size of the fibres takes place and in time they become replaced by fibrous tissue. Once fibrosis has occurred the physiological properties of muscular tissue are lost and contracture is likely to occur.

Impairment of circulation leads to degenerative changes in joints and painful, stiff joints are the common result.

Decalcification of bone is liable to occur. This is not easy to explain but it has been suggested that the much reduced supply to other areas means increased supply to the bones with consequent hyperaemic decalcification.

The circulation of an area may also be reduced by lack of function of the part, although in such cases the effects are not so marked. In patients suffering from marked spasticity and loss of voluntary movement, for example, the natural stimulus of muscle and joint movement is lost and the limbs are often cold and blue. In young children this circulatory defect may prove serious since the growth of the limb will be impaired.

In some neurological disorders the blood vessels themselves are diseased and nutrition may be impaired even to the point of gangrene. This may be seen in some cases of diabetic neuritis.

Recognition of the grave results of impairment of circulation is essential. Should these changes occur in cases of lesions of peripheral nerves, then recovery of function, when regeneration of the nerve takes place is grossly hampered by fibrosed muscle, stiff joints and inelastic skin. These trophic changes can be minimised by physical means aiming at maintaining circulation and nutrition to the affected area.

ABNORMAL REFLEX ACTIVITY

Alteration in reflex activity is a very complicated subject and cannot be dealt with in any detail here. Reflex activity is controlled by higher centres which in some cases actually inhibit, in others damp down and prevent reflexes from becoming excessive. Thus in lesions at cortical level, abnormal reflex activity may occur and abnormal postures, therefore, may be assumed. These may seriously disturb voluntary movement.

In addition, normal reflexes may be exaggerated, diminished or lost.

Exaggerated reflexes. If a reflex such as the familiar knee jerk is unduly brisk, certain possibilities should be considered. It may be because the controlling influence exerted by the cerebral cortex over the reflex centre is decreased or lost and therefore stimuli produce an uncontrolled response. This is the case in lesions of the pyramidal system.

The brisk reflex might be the result of hypotonia in the opposing muscle group. For example, in the case of flaccid paralysis of the hamstring muscles the knee jerk would be exaggerated because, owing to the hypotonic condition, gradual reciprocal lengthening is not shown. On the other hand, reflexes may be exaggerated when the nervous system is intact. Thus in any case where muscle tone is high, as in hysteria, emotional states, hyperthyroidism, deep reflexes will be increased.

Lost or diminished reflexes are not uncommon eventualities. It is clear that any break in the reflex arc, whether anatomical or physiological, will result in lost reflexes. Any lessening in conductivity is likely to produce sluggish reflexes. This accounts for the difficulty in obtaining the tendon jerks in tabes dorsalis and for the absent reflexes in a case of cut peripheral nerves or in acute poliomyelitis.

Reflexes will be absent in cerebral or spinal shock though later they may become exaggerated. In cases of general diffuse rigidity, deep reflexes are difficult to obtain because relaxation of antagonistic groups does not easily occur. On the other hand, it must be remembered that most reflexes can be voluntarily inhibited.

Two reflexes commonly met with in cortico-spinal lesions require additional explanation. There is the 'clonus' or repetitive jerk in which, following a continuous stretch, an intermittent contraction, at the rate of about seven or eight per second, occurs. Increased tone in the particular group of muscles accounts for this. In the case of ankle clonus the calf muscles are stretched, by sharp dorsiflexion of the foot, and respond by contraction. As they relax and the foot swings back the muscles are again stretched and a further contraction occurs. The second is the extensor plantar response, often spoken of as 'Babinski's sign'. Under normal circumstances, except in the infant (in whom the cortico-spinal tracts are not fully myelinated), if the lateral border of the sole of the foot is stroked firmly the great toe flexes. When the pyramidal system is diseased the great toe extends and in severe cases the other toes fan out and the foot is violently withdrawn. In this case the spinal reflex of withdrawal from the stimulus is no longer inhibited by higher centres.

Chapter II

EXAMINATION OF PATIENT SUFFERING FROM DISORDERS OF THE NERVOUS SYSTEM

A diagnosis of all cases sent for physiotherapy is supplied by the physician, but before treatment can be started detailed information is necessary as to the condition of the patient and the stage of the disease. This can only be obtained by a thorough examination carried out by the physiotherapist who will be responsible for the treatment. In a case of disseminated sclerosis the diagnosis does not make it clear whether this particular patient shows spasticity or ataxia as the main sign: yet either of these two states is possible and each requires entirely different physical treatment. Correct re-education of recovering muscles, in anterior poliomyelitis or peripheral nerve lesions, cannot be carried out until an accurate estimate of muscle power has been obtained.

The examination does not need to be a detailed one such as the physician would carry out. It should be directed towards finding out the features of the condition which can be benefited by physical measures, knowledge of which will enable the physiotherapist to give valuable and effective treatment.

It should begin by a brief talk with the patient. Three main objects are gained by this. Firstly, it enables the physiotherapist to make a general observation of the patient while the latter is unaware of this part of the examination. Colour, loss of weight, appearance and manner may all be noted. Secondly, the patient's confidence can usually be gained and his co-operation ensured by a quiet talk. Thirdly, if skilfully conducted, it supplies certain useful data of age, occupation, home conditions and the patient's own history of the onset and nature of the symptoms.

OBSERVATION

A more detailed examination should next be carried out. The patient, suitably clothed, lies on a bed or plinth in a good light. If the lower limbs are to be examined the physiotherapist should stand at the foot of the bed so that both extremities can be seen in the same perspective. Size of muscles, position of the limbs, trophic signs and the presence or absence of involuntary movements are noted.

Size of muscles. Power depends on size of muscles. Alteration in size may either be decrease (atrophy) or increase (hypertrophy). If atrophy is present examination should be made to discover which muscles are affected. Lesion of a motor nerve results in atrophy of the muscles innervated by this nerve. If a joint is injured or inflamed the muscles acting on this joint will be affected. Sometimes atrophy is the outcome of disuse and in this case a diffuse atrophy will be present affecting all the muscles equally in the area.

If hypertrophy is present there may be an increase in the size of the fibres due to more than normal use or an increase in the connective tissue —a false hypertrophy. The two can easily be distinguished by testing the power of the affected muscles, as true hypertrophy results in increased power, while power is decreased in false hypertrophy.

Any suspected alteration in size should be confirmed by measurement. A point, a definite distance above or below a bony landmark should be marked on the skin of both limbs. Measurement must be made exactly at this level. A careful record should be kept of the figure obtained on both limbs and the site at which the measurement was made. Difficulty may be met in estimating variations in muscle bulk when both limbs are involved and comparison is therefore difficult. It is worth while remembering that atrophy causes bony points to become more prominent, also that alterations in size cause alterations in power. The type of individual should also be taken into consideration as the normal size of the muscle groups will tend to correspond with the build and occupation.

Position of the limb or trunk. Close observation should be made as to the position in which the limbs or trunk are held, as a deformity may be seen at any joint but will be particularly apparent in such joints as the knee and ankle. Much may be learnt by a careful observation of the posture.

The hemiplegic patient tends to lie or sit flexed to the affected side. The patient suffering from sciatica holds the hip and knee slightly flexed, while a case of ulnar paralysis shows a partial claw hand.

Trophic signs. A check should be made on the colour, temperature, texture and smoothness of the skin. The nails should be examined and oedema noted. Changes in these factors may indicate an interruption in the conductivity of sympathetic fibres. Scars and unhealed lesions may be seen. These will occur when superficial sensory loss is added to trophic changes. Lesions then occur because the patient is incapable of feeling pain and healing is slow because the nutrition of the tissues is poor.

Involuntary movements. Careful watch should be kept for tremors, muscle spasm and fasciculation. Tremor is usually most marked when the muscles are not actively contracting and the limb is unsupported. Fasciculation occurs most frequently during and after muscle contraction.

PALPATION

Changes in the tissues can often be discovered by palpation. Muscle spasm, increased or decreased tone, contractures, tenderness and variations in limb temperature can all be detected by the sense of touch. For this reason palpation of muscle groups, joints and skin should follow observation.

When the physiotherapist is satisfied that she has discovered all she can by using her sense of sight and touch, tests of motor and sensory function may be carried out.

TEST OF MUSCLE TONE

Muscle tone may be estimated by the degree of resistance offered to a passive movement. The first step in testing is to teach the patient to relax, otherwise voluntary contraction may be mistaken for increased tone. With the patient relaxed each joint is moved passively several times in all possible directions. If tone is increased, note should be made as to whether the increase is equal in all muscle groups or whether it is more noticeable in some groups than others. Again it should be noted whether the resistance is maintained throughout the whole range of the passive movement or whether it yields suddenly towards the end.

If tone appears to be decreased further tests may be carried out if desired. For example, the ability to hold a position depends on the tone of the muscles. The extended arms may be rested on a support, the support is suddenly withdrawn and if the tone in one arm is decreased that limb falls further and recovers more slowly and less fully than the other.

TESTING OF VOLUNTARY POWER

It is essential to have an accurate and detailed knowledge of the state of the muscles in neurological disorders. This is necessary, not only for diagnosis, but also so that treatment can be carried out adequately. The Medical Research Council has suggested a numerical scale so that voluntary power can be simply and effectively assessed on it. The scale is as follows:

EXAMINATION OF PATIENT

0 = no contraction
1 = flicker, but no actual movement
2 = contraction producing movement when gravity is eliminated
3 = contraction against the force of gravity
4 = contraction against gravity and some resistance
5 = normal strength

Descriptions of the technique are to be found both in the Medical Research Council's handbook and in Kendall and Kendall (1949). By recording the results of the test on a chart, the patient's progress can be seen at a glance (Fig. 6, below). Of course, it would be ideal if the same observer

FACSIMILE OF PROGRESS CHART OF A PATIENT WITH A RADIAL NERVE INJURY

Name: A........................ R....................

Dates	5. vii 1951	19. vii	2. viii	16.viii	12.ix	10. x	21.xi	16. i 1952	30.iv	29. x
Types of Contraction	Voluntary									
Brachioradialis	2+	4	4	4+	4+	5-	?5	5	5	5
E. C. Rad. L.	2	3+	4	4+	4+	5-	?5	5	5	5
E. C. Rad. B.	?1	?3	4-	4+	4+	5-	?5	5	5	5
Sulpinator										
E. Com. D.	?1	2+	3+	4-	4-	4	4	4	5-	5
E. Min. D.	o	o		?	?	?2	?4	4	4	?5
E. C. Uln.	o	2+	3+	4	4+	4+	?5	4+	5	5
Abd. P. L.	o	o	2+	3	3+	4	4+	4+	4+	4+
E. P. L.	o	o	2	3	3	3+	4	4	4	5
E. P. B.	o	o	?1	1	3	3+	3+	4	4	5?
E. Indic.	o	o	o	o	o	·1	3	?3+	4	4
Nerve Conduction: Elbow										

Charts are available for different groups and for the upper and lower limb plexuses. In the columns provided, the response to galvanism and faradism can be indicated for each muscle. In this case, voluntary testing only is recorded.

Fig. 6

FUNCTIONAL CHART

NAME......................... CONDITION...........................

Left Side				Function	Right Side			
Date					Date			
				Bend fingers				
				Stretch fingers				
				Oppose thumb				
				Abduct thumb				
				Extend wrist				
				Flex wrist				
				Grasp				
				Grip				
				Pronate forearm				
				Supinate forearm				
				Flex fingers and extend wrist				
				Extend fingers and supinate forearm				
				Flex elbow and medially rotate arm				
				Flex elbow				
				Extend elbow				
				Abduct shoulder				
				Reach and grasp				
				Take hand to mouth				
				Touch back of neck				
				Touch top of head				
				Feed him/herself				
				Comb hair				
				Wash face				
				Put on coat				
				Do buttons				
				Tie shoelaces				
				Pick up mug				
				Use knife and fork				
				Use spoon				
				Write				

Fig. 7

could always examine each patient on successive occasions. This is naturally not always possible, but there should, in fact, be a negligible difference between the results which different workers obtain, provided that they have been trained in a standardised method of testing. It must be remembered that the test is limited, for it does not necessarily show whether the normal pattern of movement is being carried out, nor whether the patient can perform the necessary movements of dressing himself, etc., nor whether he can fulfil the demands made on him by his normal work. The test only enables one to know the state of the individual muscle. Whoever is testing the patient must, therefore, ask him whether he can perform the everyday movements that normal life requires, and how well, how quickly and for how long he is able to carry out his work.

On page 186 another chart (Fig. 7) is shown which is used to assess the patient's ability to carry out certain patterns of movement. This, of course, cannot be looked upon as an infallible proof of what the patient can do. With complete division of the median nerves it may be possible still to flex the fingers and extend the wrist. This finger flexion is purely passive and, if the wrist is fixed in a neutral or flexed position, the finger movement is eliminated. Similarly, in certain cervical lesions of the spinal cord, patients have been able to feed themselves, light a match and do some simple type of handwork in the absence of any activity in the flexors of the fingers where the extensors of the wrist are still active. It must not be thought that these are 'trick movements' which the patient uses. It is, as Wood Jones stated, the observer who is tricked.

ELECTRICAL TESTS

These should be carried out in any case where there is muscular weakness or paralysis. If there is no nerve involvement the reactions to stimulation with faradism and with interrupted galvanism will be found to be normal. A comparison should be made with a normal muscle, preferably the same muscle on the other side of the body. A weak normal response is an indication that, although all the nerves are intact, the muscle fibres are atrophied and are, therefore, not contracting with their usual strength. A sluggish response to interrupted galvanism is an indication that there are at least some denervated fibres in the muscle. If this is accompanied by no response to faradism a complete reaction of degeneration is present showing that the muscle has no nerve supply. If, however, it is found that the sluggish galvanic response partners a weak contraction to the faradic current it can be assumed that only some of the nerve fibres are missing and a partial reaction of degeneration is present.

If the strength duration curve is the method chosen, the curve of the paralysed muscle will be found to be quite different from the normal curve. The two curves can be plotted on graph paper, and the difference between them noted. If regular tests are taken it will be seen that as the affected muscle improves the strength duration curve will gradually alter its shape to become more like the normal.

The most accurate method of carrying out an electrical test is to record the electrical impulses actually passing in the affected muscle and nerve. This is called an electromyograph and is only carried out by a physician or surgeon. (When making electrical tests it should always be remembered that degeneration of nerve tissue, following an injury, is not complete for at least ten days, and no reliable record can be obtained until after that time has elapsed.)

TESTING RANGE OF MOVEMENT

Range of movement in a joint may be limited by many factors. In neurological conditions limitation is most commonly the result of either degenerative changes in joints due to disturbed circulation and dis-use, or adaptive shortening of muscles and tendons occurring as a result of spasticity or flaccidity of muscle. Increase of range is also sometimes seen. If muscles are hypotonic, as for example in tabes dorsalis and cerebellar lesions, then joints can be carried beyond their normal range. Flail joints occur where complete paralysis of all muscle groups acting on the joint has taken place. Since such alterations are not uncommon, each joint should be put through its full range in every possible direction and limitation or increase noted. If range is limited on passive movement, an active movement in the same direction should be attempted. If the active range is less than the passive, muscular weakness is probably present.

TESTING CO-ORDINATION

It is essential for the physiotherapist to be aware of the presence of inco-ordination. It is also necessary to know the cause of this condition, as the method of re-education varies with the cause. The way in which the patient performs the active movement used in the examination of muscle power is carefully watched. Special tests are also given—these may be selected as desired but usual tests are: placing the heel of one foot on the patella of the other leg, or touching the examiner's finger with the patient's finger.

In order to decide whether the faulty movement is due to kinaesthetic loss, or to lesions of cerebellar tracts or cerebellum, the patient should first perform the movement with the eyes open and then with the eyes shut. Any discrepancy should be noted. The type of inco-ordination may also be recognised by noticing other points: does the patient eventually reach his object? Is there a side to side deviation as the object is neared (an intention tremor)? Does the proximal segment of the limb sway as the movement is performed? If all these points are present the lesion is probably a cerebellar one.

TESTING SENSATION

It is not necessary to carry out a full examination of the sensory system but it is essential for the physiotherapist to be aware of the loss of the sensations of pain, temperature and position. Thermal sense should be tested by lightly touching the skin with hot and cold test tubes, the patient's eyes being screened throughout. Pain sensation can be tested by pinprick. In each case accuracy and speed of response should be noted.

Examination of position sense may be carried out by asking the patient, whose eyes are closed, to touch with the fingers of one hand some other part of the body such as the extremity of the other arm. The sense of position of joints can be tested by moving the joint several times passively, then, after a brief pause, asking the patient to state its position.

Providing the patient's condition allows, the examination should be concluded by observation in standing and in walking. Posture should be carefully noted and the gait analysed, as certain lesions show peculiar characteristics of gait. The tilt of the trunk and the abduction swing of the affected leg are well-recognised features in the gait of the hemiplegic patient. The stamping gait of the tabetic, the reeling progression of some cases of disseminated sclerosis and the high-stepping gait of the sufferer from alcoholic neuritis can all easily be identified.

Finally the physiotherapist should study carefully the records of this examination and on them plan the scheme of physical treatment which will be most beneficial to the patient.

BRIEF SUMMARY OF ROUTINE OF EXAMINATION

A. Interrogation

      (i) General appearance and manner. Speech.

      (ii) Age, occupation, home circumstances, history of condition.

B. *Observation in Supported Position*

    (i) Size of muscles.

    (ii) Position of trunk and limbs.

    (iii) Trophic signs.

    (iv) Involuntary movements.

C. *Palpation*

D. *Tests*

    (i) Muscle tone.

    (ii) Muscle power.

    (iii) Electrical tests.

    (iv) Range of movement.

    (v) Co-ordination of movement.

    (vi) Test of sensation, thermal, pain, position.

E. *Observation in Standing*

    (i) Posture.

    (ii) Gait.

Chapter III

PRINCIPLES OF TREATMENT OF NEUROLOGICAL DISORDERS BY PHYSIOTHERAPY

I f a patient survives the initial lesion in a neurological disorder he immediately begins to think of what recovery of function he is going to make. Function will be defective as a result of damage to the cerebro-spinal system but may be further hampered by such factors as abnormalities in muscle tone, contractures and deformities, severe muscle atrophy, impaired circulation, pain, and stiff joints.

RECOVERY OF FUNCTION

Although completely destroyed nerve tissue in the brain and spinal cord cannot regenerate, this does not necessarily mean that lost voluntary movement will not return. Even in severe lesions there is usually some recovery. One or more of the factors listed below may account for this.

Relief of pressure of oedema and exudate on nerve cells and fibres.
Hypertrophy of any innervated muscle fibres.
Hypertrophy of unaffected muscles.
Establishment of alternative pathways.
Stimulation of inactive neurones.
Branching of unaffected axons to innervate denervated muscle fibres.

RELIEF OF PRESSURE

A vascular or inflammatory lesion may not only destroy cells but may result in widespread haemorrhage and oedema causing pressure on nerve cells and fibres, thus putting them out of action for a period of time. Within a few weeks of such a catastrophe oedema begins to subside as fluid is absorbed into the blood and lymph stream. Those cells which have not been permanently damaged are gradually released from pressure and may begin to resume function. This fact accounts for the extensive recovery of paralysed muscles within the first few weeks following an attack of acute anterior poliomyelitis. All the recovery which will result from this absorption of oedema will probably occur during the first six weeks; any recovery which occurs after this will be due to other factors.

Physiotherapy cannot assist this absorption and recovery.

HYPERTROPHY OF REMAINING INNERVATED MUSCLE FIBRES

A skeletal muscle consists of many muscle fibres each of which receives a nerve supply. This supply is by a fibril of an axon of a motor cell. A single cell gives origin to a single axon which splits to supply a number of muscle fibres. The cell, its axon and the muscle fibres it supplies are together known as a motor unit. In inflammatory or degenerative lesions of the central nervous system, not all the motor cells of a region may be affected, consequently, in any one muscle, many motor units may still be intact and able to function. The strength of the muscle depends upon the number and size of its healthy fibres. Thus, for example, immediately following an attack of poliomyelitis a number of muscles may be completely paralysed. During the subsequent six weeks some cells in the anterior horn may be released from pressure and therefore some motor units in these muscles may recover. At the end of this period no further cell recovery is likely, and the muscle fibres innervated by destroyed cells will never again be able to function. It is still possible, however, to strengthen the muscles since strength depends partly on size of fibre. If the remaining motor units are exercised to their maximum capability hypertrophy of the muscle fibres should occur.

The method used to bring about this hypertrophy may vary from country to country and hospital to hospital but the principle is the same. The maximum possible stimulation of the cells of the anterior horn of the spinal cord must be produced so that all available motor units are brought into action. If the stimulus is less than maximal not all the units will be activated and hypertrophy will not result. Maximal stimulation is not given by simply allowing normal use of the limb. It is gained in several different ways.

Maximal resistance. One method of gaining maximal stimulation is to give the strongest possible resistance to the movement produced by the paresed muscle. Resistance should be such that the patient can still move smoothly through range. It may be therefore only the light pressure of the tip of a finger, the force of gravity, or a twenty pound weight, depending upon the initial strength of the muscle.

This method is effective in two ways. On the one hand it activates all available motor units, on the other it increases tension within the muscle and the sensory nerve endings are therefore stimulated. The more afferent impulses reaching the motor centres the stronger will be the excitation of these centres.

Other proprioceptive stimuli. The sensory nerve endings in the muscles may also be stimulated by stretching the muscle before calling on it to contract. Thus the movement starts from the lengthened position of the muscle.

Afferent stimuli may be applied by firm pressure of the physiotherapist's hand. The hand should be firmly applied on the surface in the direction of the desired movement.

Use of 'overflow'. Another method of increasing the excitation of the motor centres is the use of mass movement patterns as advocated by Kabat. In everyday free activities single muscles are rarely, if ever, used, but complex patterns are normal. There are natural patterns of movement in which there is usually a strong rotational element. Thus, for example, is the flexion-adduction pattern of the upper extremity in which the arm is pulled up and across the face from a position in which it lies in an extended and abducted position. This pattern involves, amongst other groups, the forward and upward rotators of the shoulder girdle, the flexors, adductors and lateral rotators of the shoulder, and the flexors of the wrist and fingers. If one component of this group is weak, resistance is given to the strong components of the pattern, the normal muscle groups will be stimulated and spread of excitation to the cells of the motor units of the weakened muscles is likely to occur. Such spread is commonly known as 'overflow' and is often responsible for the initiation of contraction in a weak muscle which fails completely to respond to isolated exercise. It will be noted that this method is only successful if there are strong components available.

Successive induction. Sherrington pointed out that maximal excitation of antagonists was followed by strong facilitation of excitation of the agonists. He found, for example, that immediately after stimulation of the flexor reflex the extensor centre was hyperexcitable. In this case if one muscle is weak, contraction of the antagonist against the strongest possible resistance will result in an increased excitability of the cells innervating the weak muscle and a stronger contraction of the latter will be obtained if it immediately follows the contraction of the antagonist.

Use of eyes and ears. Anterior horn cells are also stimulated through pathways from the eyes and ears. Thus, if maximal bombardment of motor cells is required to bring into action all available motor units, the patient must be encouraged to watch what he is doing and the physiotherapist must make use of her voice to give emphatic commands.

Volition. Motor cells are also normally excited to discharge through pathways from motor centres in the cerebral cortex. These pathways are rarely likely to be completely destroyed and should be used to their maximal capacity. The patient should make a strong effort to perform each movement throughout the treatment session.

HYPERTROPHY OF UNAFFECTED MUSCLES

In some lesions, particularly those of the spinal cord, no recovery is possible. Thus, for example, in a complete transection of the spinal cord, no voluntary power below the level of the lesion can return. In this case the emphasis of physical treatment lies on the restoration of function and independence. The patient with a complete mid-thoracic cord lesion can dress, feed, wash himself, can get up from his chair and bed and can walk, provided he is correctly trained. To ensure this, certain essential muscles must be hypertrophied and the patient must then be taught to use them in the performance of everyday activities. These muscles are the latissimus dorsi, pectoralis major, teres major, serratus anterior, and trapezius by means of which the pelvis and trunk may be moved and indirectly, therefore, the legs. The triceps, by means of which the elbows can be kept strongly braced, should also be hypertrophied.

ESTABLISHMENT OF ALTERNATIVE PATHWAYS

In lesions of the cerebrum and cerebellum some recovery or some development of movement will occur through the establishment of alternative pathways. It is likely that certain primitive patterns of movement are inherent in the mid-brain and spinal cord. Temple Fay makes use of this knowledge in his treatment of children suffering from cerebral palsy. He bases his work on the fact that, in amphibia and reptiles, movements are controlled by the mid- and hind-brain and that in man, centres for movement exist in these areas but that their work is largely taken over and controlled by the cerebrum. If the cerebrum has been irreparably damaged or has failed to develop, the child may be able to learn voluntary movements by development of these primitive patterns of movements.

The various primitive patterns are used in a progressive way. Each pattern is practised first passively, then actively with assistance and then freely until, by constant repetition, the pattern becomes a permanent one. As the movements are constantly and rhythmically repeated, muscles and muscle and joint sense are developed, undamaged cortical motor cells begin to discharge and some co-ordinated movement becomes possible. The first movement used is the 'defence reflex' in which, if a painful stimulus is applied to the foot, the hip and knee flex and the adductors relax so that the knee moves outwards. The physiotherapist applies the stimulus by flexing the toes and turning the foot in. As the hip and knee flexes she guides the movement and at the end passively replaces the leg. The movement is repeated many times, later the child is encouraged to assist. Eventually the child may be able to carry out the movement voluntarily. The movement is first unilateral, then alternate and then bilateral.

The pattern of movement characteristic of the newt is then practised, that is the arm and leg on the same side are passively flexed and the head turned to this side. Later comes the crossed diagonal pattern in which the arm and leg of the opposite side work together. By means of further progression voluntary movement is gradually established.

STIMULATION OF INACTIVE NEURONES

In the central nervous system there are many more neurones than are actually normally in use, and it is seldom that these will all be damaged in trauma or disease. These neurones might do the work of those destroyed but, if they have rarely if ever been in use, the synaptic resistance is high and they need especially strong stimulation to cause them to discharge. Hence without special treatment these 'dormant' neurones may not come into action and latent possibilities of movement are lost.

Any method which excites the cells of the motor areas particularly strongly is of value. Therefore the use of maximal resistance, stretch, skin sensation, eyes, ears and volition are all of value.

The use of mass movement patterns, and reversal of antagonists and possibly of primitive reflex movements will all increase the bombardment of the cells of the anterior horn of the spinal cord.

Many of these methods can be combined, thus Kabat advocates the performance of mass movement patterns against maximal resistance, using the proprioceptive stimulation of stretch, the effect of pressure by the physiotherapist's hand, of hearing through the physiotherapist's voice, and of sight through watching the movement.

BRANCHING OF UNAFFECTED NERVE FIBRES

It has been found that when the nerve supply to a muscle has not been completely cut off, remaining nerve fibres may branch to innervate denervated muscle fibres. It has been suggested that this process is accelerated if the sensory nerve endings of the muscles and skin are stimulated and faradism has been used to achieve this. It may, therefore, be of some value to use faradic stimulation in cases of paresis in which the afferent fibres are intact as in anterior poliomyelitis.

FACTORS HAMPERING RECOVERY OF FUNCTION

Some recovery of voluntary power and independence in neurological disorders may well occur through one or more of the ways previously indicated but such recovery is often hampered by abnormal muscle tone, by the development of contractures and deformity, by stiff joints, by impaired circulation and by pain. These, therefore, require treatment or prevention.

ABNORMAL MUSCLE TONE

Some tone in muscles is necessary for the maintenance of posture and the performance of movement. If tone is excessive it is difficult for prime movers to overcome the resistance offered by hypertonic muscles. If tone is too low, then the guiding and controlling of the movement becomes reduced or lost. In both cases movement, if present at all, becomes incoordinate.

Increase in tone is usually the result of lack of inhibitory control by higher centres and it results, if it is permanent, in typical postures, and absence or abnormalities of voluntary movement. Such movements as do occur are largely of the reflex type, that is, on attempted movement there is simultaneous contraction of all the muscles of one type of pattern. Thus on an attempt to extend the fingers, flexion of the wrist and elbow, with pronation of the forearm and adduction of the shoulder, occurs.

It is, therefore, essential to deal with this if voluntary movement is to be developed or improved. So essential is this that some authorities base their work largely on correction of faulty tone.

Since increase in tone is central in origin the ordinary techniques of heat, massage and training in relaxation cannot be successful for longer than a very brief period following treatment. Certain methods, are, however, available.

Tiring out spasticity. Occasionally it is possible to tire out and so to overcome spasticity. At the Stoke Mandeville centre for paraplegics a specially constructed bicycle is fitted over the bed and the feet are strapped to the pedals. The actual movement of the pedals is brought about by the hands. Spasticity may disappear after a period of passive exercise of the legs on this apparatus.

Facilitation techniques. Many of Kabat's facilitation techniques used to strengthen weakened muscles and activate dormant neurones may also be successful in reducing spasticity. Particularly valuable is the technique based on the principle of reciprocal innervation. During the contraction of one group of muscles, provided that contraction is against some resistance, relaxation of the antagonists occur. The stronger the resistance the greater is the relaxation. Thus the giving of maximal resistance is likely to reduce spasticity. Kabat used this principle in the method of slow reversal of antagonists. Thus to obtain relaxation of a spastic group he uses the procedure of voluntary contraction of this group in its pattern against maximal resistance in the stretched range, followed by an attempt at voluntary relaxation, followed again by voluntary contraction of the antagonist group pattern against maximal resistance.

Reflex inhibition in posture and movement. This is the method advocated by Mrs. Bobath. Its main point is the inhibition of the reflex increase in tone, which imposes on the patient a typical posture, by the use of reflex inhibiting postures. The child is held in the suitable position, at first spasm may increase, but, gradually, if the position is forcibly maintained, spasm passes off. The period for which spasm is relieved is only very short but gradually this increases. Eventually the child will be able to take up the position for himself. If spasm does pass off voluntary movements tend to occur and the child can be encouraged to perform them.

Decrease in tone. This causes ataxia such as is seen in many cases of disseminated sclerosis. The patient is able to perform voluntary movement but this is inco-ordinate because there is insufficient postural fixation and the presence of intention tremor. There may, for example, be ability to move the arms but the patient cannot feed himself because swaying and intention tremor make it impossible for him to get the food into his mouth.

It will be remembered that the decrease in tone resulting in ataxia may be due to decrease of sensory stimuli flowing into the central nervous system or it may be due to lesions in the cerebellar system (see page 173). If the former is the cause, the main object is to increase the sensory stimuli reaching the motor centres. Hence, once more, use is made of alternative pathways and activation of 'dormant' neurones. The patient is trained to see, feel and hear what he is doing. Simple movements are repeated time after time so that synaptic resistance is reduced in the pathways which are still available. Movements are performed in such a position that the patient can watch every step. When possible they are carried out on a firm surface so that a greater amount of sensory stimulation is produced. They are often done in time to counting so that the patient 'hears' the movement. In walking a stick may be used to tap the ground evenly before the feet are brought down, for the same reason.

If the lesion is in the cerebellar system the principle is again the development of inactive but unaffected neurones and the establishment of alternative pathways. Volition is particularly important; the patient must concentrate on what he is doing and make a supreme effort to control the movement. Simple movements are taken and are repeated time after time. The movement is stopped and begun again if any jerk occurs.

In this way maximum stimulation of cerebellar and anterior horn cells will occur.

Facilitatory techniques may also be used for this purpose. Reversal of antagonists often proves most successful in gaining balance control. For example the patient may be unsteady in sitting. He is then instructed to try to prevent the physiotherapist pushing him first in one direction and then in the other. This is repeated constantly and balance tends to become steadier due to the increase in strength of opposing muscle groups. Resistance also may be used because it increases the sensory stimuli reaching the cerebellum from muscles and joints.

CONTRACTURES AND DEFORMITIES

Deformities tend to develop in pyramidal and lower motor neurone lesions, in striatal damage and in children showing circulatory disturbances. They are the result of adaptive contractures where there is muscle imbalance, of contracture of fibrosed joint structures following oedema, or of impairment of growth. It is essential that they should be prevented or they will hamper such recovery of voluntary power as is possible. Splinting, passive movements, massage and elevation to relieve oedema, and strengthening of weak muscles are the methods of choice.

Splinting is valuable because it maintains a good position and prevents contractures, or provides a continuous stretching force if contractures have already commenced. The majority of splints, however, have the disadvantage that they fix the joint and hamper use of the area. In addition, if there is spasticity, unless they fit absolutely perfectly, they stimulate the sensory nerve endings and increase the spasticity. If there are trophic changes they may lead to the development of pressure sores.

When splints are used, therefore, certain rules should be observed. They must fit perfectly and all 'pressure points' must be protected. They must be removable so that joints may be carried through their full range daily, and the skin toilet attended to. In growing children the splints must be checked frequently so that they are always the correct fit. They must be light so that they add no more weight than is necessary to a weakened limb, and they must be of material which will stand up to wear and tear. They should be easy to apply so that they can be taken off at home and re-applied correctly.

Where possible, splints should allow movement of the joint but return it to its correct position, that is, a splint should simulate the action of the paralysed muscles. Such splints are known as 'lively' splints.

STIFF JOINTS

If joints become stiff the recovery of voluntary power is severely hampered. This is often seen in the shoulder of a hemiplegic patient. This stiffness must be avoided, partly by measures which prevent or relieve oedema and partly by the use of passive movements. If passive movements are carried out slowly and carefully in the full range, ligaments cannot become adherent, normal capsular length is maintained and adhesions resulting from circulatory stasis are avoided. In addition the superficial layers of the cartilage are rubbed off so that the cartilage does not thicken. The synovial fluid formation also is increased by movements.

ATROPHY OF MUSCLES

Lack of normal use inevitably results in muscle atrophy and, consequently, as voluntary movement becomes possible, recovery is hampered by loss of power. Atrophy is at least partly prevented by all the steps taken to regain voluntary power. In cases in which there is paralysis of muscles the most satisfactory method is the use of artificial exercise in the form of electrical stimulation, because this maintains the metabolism of the muscle and so the size of the fibres.

CIRCULATORY IMPAIRMENT

Physiotherapy can do a great deal to prevent or relieve the trophic changes which tend to occur in the skin, joints, muscles and bones of patients suffering from neurological disorders. Any of these may affect the recovery of voluntary movement.

The object of physical treatment is to stimulate the flow of blood through the area and thus avoid circulatory stasis and increase the nutrition and tissue drainage. The natural stimulus to the circulation is active movement and where possible this method should be used. Thus all the methods in use to gain voluntary movement are also fulfilling this object. Where one segment of a limb is unable to move, active movements of other segments will help to maintain the circulation.

In some cases active movement is impossible and passive measures are necessary. These are particularly important in the cases in which there is vaso-constriction.

Vaso-dilatation will mean a better blood supply and it is produced by heating the tissues. Heat may, therefore, be used directly to the area affected providing, firstly, that there is no sensory loss and, secondly, that there is not present already a vaso-dilation due to paralysis of the vaso-constrictor nerves. In either of these cases heat should be applied to the region proximal to the affected area, relying on the fact that there will be a gentler effect on the vessels by the warmed blood entering the area and a lessening of the viscosity of the blood so that it flows more readily in the area of stasis. In addition, there will be a stimulation of the venous and lymphatic flow in the proximal area which will indirectly assist the drainage of the affected area.

Choice between the different sources producing heat depends upon such factors as the condition of cutaneous sensibility and the presence of paralytic vaso-dilation. If sensation and vaso-motor control are normal, inductothermy is a valuable means. Massage is a useful way of stimulating the venous and lymphatic flow and, if there is oedema, it should be carried out with the limb in elevation, but it has to be used with very great care if there is hypertonus or if there is complete atonia, as in the first case it can increase spasticity and in the second it might bruise the flaccid muscle fibres.

Electrical stimulation of the sensory nerve endings and the muscles will help the circulation by stimulating the axon reflex and by increasing metabolism and producing a pumping effect. If oedema is present it is also of value. In the presence of hypertonus this method is better avoided but in cases in which there is hypotonia or atonia the surged faradic or interrupted galvanic currents are useful according to whether the lower motor neurones are conducting impulses or not. If there is no oedema and the first sensory neurones are intact, a sinusoidal bath might be effective, through its stimulating effect on the axon reflex and the warning effect of the hot water.

Sometimes chilblains develop and in this case a strong dose of ultra-violet rays or massage with Iodex is often beneficial.

In complete lesions of the spinal cord, vaso-motor control is lost though later some control may be gained through activity of subsidiary spinal centres. For a few weeks following such a lesion there is danger of the development of pressure sores, great care is therefore necessary in nursing and handling the patient and frequent changes of posture are essential. When active movement is permitted constant active changes of posture and vigorous trunk swinging in half suspension will help to re-establish some degree of vaso-motor control.

In treating all patients in whom trophic changes are present, great care of the skin must be taken. It is easily broken down and is slow to heal.

PAIN

Pain will nearly always affect voluntary movement since the patient is not normally willing to move a painful area. Sometimes the pain which limits voluntary movement is arising from the nerve endings in con-tracted ligaments and periarticular structures when these structures are stretched on movements. Sometimes the pain is the result of an active inflammatory process in a nerve sheath or in the meninges of the spinal cord. In the first case the only treatment is to continue gently stretching the contracted structures. Preceding the stretching by heat often helps to make the movement less painful. In the second case voluntary movements which cause pain should be avoided until the inflammation subsides.

RESTORATION OF INDEPENDENCE

In spite of all that can be done, full recovery may not be possible, but much can be done to give the patient independence in spite of loss of voluntary function. Most important is constant practice in the ward or at home of suitable exercises and occupations. The patient can usually be helped considerably by various 'gadgets'. Thus a tie fitted to a special neck band will enable a man to put on his own tie. A shoe, with a previously fitted elastic lace, and a shoe horn, will save the necessity of someone helping the patient to put his shoe on. Firm bars fitted to the bathroom and bedroom walls will help the patient to stand up, sit down and support himself while washing and dressing.

The patient can also help himself by taking care of his own splints, keeping areas of poor circulation warm, being careful not to damage insensitive areas and doing his own passive movements if these are necessary.

Many different methods have been touched on here; some can be combined, others may be used alone. Choice of method depends on a variety of factors, the two most important of which are the age of the patient and the site and extent of the lesion. Students interested in these methods should refer to the literature listed in the Bibliography (see page 379). It will be realised that considerable training would be required after qualification before some of these methods could be put in practice adequately and satisfactorily.

Chapter IV

HEMIPLEGIA. PARAPLEGIA. CEREBRAL PALSY

HEMIPLEGIA

This is a paralysis affecting one side of the body, characterised by loss of movement, spasticity, exaggerated deep reflexes and an extensor plantar response. It is the result of lesions involving the upper motor neurones in the brain or upper segments of the spinal cord and may occur at any age. Hemiplegia occurring in infancy is either the result of birth injury, or occurs in association with one of the specific fevers. In young adults it is likely to be the result either of a rupture of a congenital aneurysm, or of an angioma or of a cerebral embolism due to the breaking off of a small vegetation in a rheumatic or bacterial endocarditis. It may also be due to the disturbance of a clot in any vessel following some surgical procedure. Alternatively it may be the result of increasing pressure or destruction caused by an intracranial tumour or abscess.

In elderly people hemiplegia may be the result of a cerebral thrombosis or haemorrhage. These are most likely to occur when a degenerative condition of the blood vessels is present, and blood pressure is high.

Changes

Whatever the cause, the pathological changes in the brain tissue will be either degeneration or destruction of cells and fibres. Degeneration may be due to a reduction in blood supply because cells, and to a less extent fibres are quickly affected by a reduction in oxygen. The degenerated material is removed by neuroglial phagocytic cells and cystic cavities bridged by fibrous tissue remain. Destruction may be due to a violent haemorrhage which bursts into and lacerates tissue, resulting in complete destruction of some fibres and interference with the blood supply of others. In time the blood clots and organisation occurs followed by shrinkage of the fibrous tissue, thus relieving some of the pressure. The most common site of a vascular disease producing a hemiplegia is in the anterior cerebral or the lenticulo-striate arteries so that the internal capsule, thalamus and corpus striatum are likely to be affected.

Signs and Symptoms

Hemiplegia can be considered in two stages. The first is one of acute onset, the result of embolism, thrombosis or haemorrhage. Since a sudden vascular disturbance has occurred the patient at first suffers from cerebral shock and in many cases the initial stage is one of unconsciousness with flaccidity of all limbs. When the physiotherapist is called in, the patient will have recovered consciousness and movement of one side of the body, but the other side will show flaccidity, complete absence of all voluntary movement, and the presence of an extensor plantar response. Within a few weeks as the patient recovers from shock and cerebral circulation is re-established, or oedema relieved, the onset of the second stage occurs. This is the stage of residual spastic hemiplegia.

Patients who have a cerebral tumour or abscess causing the condition are usually seen in this stage having never gone through the first.

The onset of spasm can be explained by the fact that as the cause subsides only that tissue which is actually destroyed or has degenerated fails to recover, but this destroyed tissue may have been exerting an inhibitory or controlling influence over other neurones. Two groups of symptoms therefore arise: those which are due to destruction usually known as negative symptoms, and those which are due to over-activity of neurones released from control, known as positive symptoms. The exact nature of the symptoms depends on the site of the lesion, but negative symptoms are loss of movement, loss or impairment of speech and in some cases loss or alteration of sensation. Positive symptoms are usually increase in tone, exaggerated and abnormal reflexes and involuntary movements.

Loss of Movement and Speech

The upper half of the face shows little weakness because the muscles are innervated by both hemispheres and the patient is therefore able to raise his eyebrows and open and close his eyes; such weakness as there is usually recovers rapidly. The lower half is, however, much more affected and movements are weakened or lost. Voluntary movements innervated by the motor centres are much more affected than emotional movements which are controlled by subcortical centres. Weakness is nearly always present in the trunk muscles but this is quick to recover. Total loss of voluntary movements in the limbs is rare and in some cases recovery is complete. Many patients, however, show inability to move one segment of a limb and are quite unable to perform isolated movements. Voluntary movements of the affected arm and leg tend to follow a definite pattern. A willed flexion of the fingers, for example, is usually accompanied by flexion of the wrist and elbow, pronation of the forearm and adduction of the shoulder. Sometimes flexion of one limb precipitates flexion of the other; it is not unusual to see that when a hemiplegic patient attempts to flex the leg in walking flexion of the arm occurs also.

In some cerebral lesions the speech centres may also be affected and a motor aphasia may result. This patient is unable to perform the movements of speech. In its mildest degree this takes the form of inability to give names to objects, in more severe forms the patient may be unable to say any words except yes and no, attempting by alteration in the inflection of his voice to make clear what he is trying to say.

Increase in Tone

This is the characteristic sign of an upper motor neurone lesion showing the features previously described. It is selective, claspknife-like in type, and is increased by external stimuli so that handling the limb or irritation by splints or bedclothes tends to increase the spasticity. This selective increase of tone affecting the flexors and adductors of the arm and the extensors and adductors of the leg tends to impose on the limbs a characteristic posture. The arm is held to the side inwardly rotated at the shoulder, the elbow is flexed, the forearm pronated and the wrist and fingers are flexed. The leg is adducted at the hip, extended at the knee with the foot plantar-flexed and inverted, unless the patient is confined to bed and allowed to remain in the position he prefers, when the leg is usually outwardly rotated at the hip and flexed at the knee.

Altered Reflexes

Due to the lessened control over the reflex arc deep reflexes are exaggerated. Knee and ankle clonus are very commonly found and an extensor plantar response tends to persist. The superficial reflexes are absent since these are mediated by the pyramidal system.

Involuntary Movements

Sudden flexor spasms in the leg are a fairly common occurrence and are the result of uncontrolled external stimuli. Very occasionally athetoid movements and tremors may be observed. The corpus striatum is then probably involved.

Posture and Gait

Weakness and spasticity together confer on the patient a characteristic appearance in sitting and standing. Owing to unilateral trunk weakness and the weight of the weakened or useless limbs the patient tends to lean towards the affected side, and in early cases balance is therefore difficult to obtain. In order to bring the extended leg forward and clear the ground in walking the hemiplegic patient leans to the sound side, raises the pelvis on the affected side and swings the leg forward through abduction in a semi-circle.

Circulatory Changes

Though vaso-motor changes are not present, disturbance of circulation occurs through lack of muscular contraction and joint movement. The limbs are therefore cold and blue. In infantile hemiplegia unless steps are taken to aid the circulation the growth of the affected limbs is likely to be seriously impaired.

Loss or Alteration of Sensation

Sensory fibres may be affected if the lesion occurs in areas where these fibres lie especially close to the motor fibres, as in the internal capsule. Some cases of hemiplegia will therefore show complete loss of sensation of the affected limbs. The patient is unaware of the position of the arm and leg, so that if movements were possible they would be completely inco-ordinate.

Pain is occasionally present. If the lesion affects the thalamus a very unpleasant diffuse and persistent pain is experienced in the extremities. Sometimes a hemiplegic patient complains of pain in the shoulders, hip or fingers. This is not due to a lesion of nerve tissue but to the degenerative changes which tend to occur as a result of disuse of joints and consequently circulatory impairment.

PRINCIPLES OF TREATMENT BY PHYSIOTHERAPY

These follow the lines set out in the preceding chapter. In the early stages with acute onset the main object is to arrest the development of those factors which will later hamper recovery. Heat, given without disturbing the patient, and provided sensation is normal, will stimulate the circulation. This may be followed by slow, firm and deep rhythmical massage. Each joint may be moved through its full range once in every possible direction particular attention being paid to the shoulder, hip, fingers and toes. A very careful watch may be kept on the position of the patient in bed. A foot board is useful and firm pillows will provide a support for the hand and will maintain the arm in some abduction.

In this stage while movements are absent and muscles are hypotonic, attempted active movements are best avoided. This is partly because the attempt to perform them worries and fatigues the patient, and partly because such an attempt appears to precipitate the onset of spasticity.

When voluntary movement begins to recover and spasticity to develop, the main object of treatment will be to encourage undamaged mechanisms to take over the work of those damaged. Mass movement patterns using resistance, stretch, eyes, hearing and volition should be tried (see preceding chapter). One of the great difficulties encountered in 'willed movements' is that the harder the patient tries the more abnormal reflex activity comes into play. Some authorities stress, therefore, the importance of reducing excessive tone. The facilitation techniques advocated by Kabat, particularly slow reversal of antagonists or the method of reflex inhibition developed by Mrs. Bobath are worth trial.

It must not be forgotten that stiff joints and deformities are particularly liable to develop in the hemiplegic patient and these will hamper recovery. Some form of heat, passive movements and splints may therefore be necessary to avoid these complications.

It is essential, whatever method is being used, that the patient should become as independent as possible. He must be shown how to get out of bed, to gain balance in standing, to use a stick and to walk with its help. He is taught to feed, wash and dress himself. If recovery is poor and little more can be expected, the patient's independence can often be increased by the use of gadgets. There are many feeding and dressing aids which are invaluable to these patients.

PARAPLEGIA

This is a paralysis of the lower extremities either of the spastic or of the flaccid type.

The site of lesion may be in the cerebral hemispheres, if it occurs in such a position as to affect the cells or fibres of both leg areas of the motor cortex. More commonly the spinal cord or cauda equina are involved. Occasionally all the peripheral nerves to the legs are affected, such a condition occurring in a polyneuritis.

Some of the most common causes, therefore, are spinal tumours, compression due to vertebral diseases such as Paget's disease or tuberculosis, trauma resulting in severe concussion or compression or even complete division of the cord, disseminated sclerosis, and infections causing degeneration of the peripheral nerves. Three types of paraplegia may be recognised: paraplegia in extension, paraplegia in flexion, and flaccid paraplegia.

Paraplegia in Extension

This closely resembles a hemiplegia in the nature of the signs and symptoms. Pressure on, or inflammation and degeneration of, the fibres of the lateral cortico-spinal tracts results in diminished conductivity and the gradual development of loss of movement and spasticity, exaggerated reflexes, and involuntary movements. As in hemiplegia, the legs tend to be held in adduction and extension. The gait is therefore stiff and jerky.

Paraplegia in Flexion

In progressive lesions or in complete severance of the cord, descending impulses from the brain fail to reach the final common pathway. All voluntary movement in the latter case is completely lost and in the former will gradually disappear, the last movements to go being extension of the hips and knees.

On the other hand spinal reflexes remain intact and the flexor withdrawal reflex which is normally inhibited by higher centres becomes established. In progressive lesions flexor spasms occur from time to time, at first, a light touch on the outer side of the sole of the foot provoking a violent flexion of the leg at the hip and knee and a dorsiflexion of the foot and great toe. As the condition advances less and less stimuli are needed to provoke the spasm, irritation of nerve endings in contracted tendons and ligaments or some slight excitement being all that is necessary. Eventually the legs tend to become fixed in flexion and adduction. This type of paraplegia is likely to occur in advanced cases of disseminated sclerosis and in complete lesions of the cord.

Flaccid Paraplegia

Complete severance of the cord or severe contusion results in immediate loss of all function below the level of the lesion, due to spinal shock. No voluntary movement is present in the lower extremities, all forms of sensation are lost, tone and reflexes are absent. A similar condition may occur in cases of polyneuritis accompanied by Wallerian degeneration of all the peripheral nerves to the legs. In cases of complete lesions of the cord when the patient recovers from shock a paraplegia in flexion is likely to supervene. In polyneuritis eventually recovery will occur but flaccid paraplegia will remain over a long period. In both paraplegia in flexion and flaccid paraplegia loss of control of urine and faeces and some paralysis of trunk muscles are likely to be added to the symptoms of the paraplegia.

PRINCIPLES OF TREATMENT BY PHYSIOTHERAPY

Paraplegia in extension. For those cases in which relief of pressure gives hope of improvement the principles of treatment resemble those used in the treatment of the hemiplegic patient. Reduction of spasticity, prevention of stiff joints and contractures, and re-education of movement being the main considerations. Where no improvement can be expected and progression of the symptoms is, in fact, certain, treatment similar to that for cases of paraplegia in flexion is suitable.

Paraplegia in flexion. For purposes of treatment these patients should be divided into those cases in which improvement will occur and those in which improvement is impossible.

In those cases where a serious pressure can be relieved, reduction of flexor spasms and some recovery of function will probably occur, though restoration to the normal is unlikely. These patients should be treated on the same lines as the hemiplegic case but special care has to be taken not to evoke flexor spasm. An attempt to straighten the limbs daily is important. For patients who have no hope of recovery such as those suffering from transverse myelitis and traumatic severance of the spinal cord special measures have to be adopted. The main object of treatment is to restore these patients to the maximum possible independence. To achieve this object certain requirements will have to be fulfilled. Infection must be avoided in the skin, bladder and rectum. The patient's courage and confidence must be maintained. Contractures and deformities in the affected limbs need prevention and the circulation must be maintained in order to prevent gross trophic changes.

Certain muscle groups must be hypertrophied and the patient must learn to balance in sitting, to dress and wash himself, get in and out of bed, chair, and bath, use the toilet and, at least, walk a very short distance using crutches.

Care of skin, bladder and rectum. While it is not the physiotherapist's province to deal with the paralysed bladder and rectum she should be well aware of the fact that distension of these organs is likely to set up stimuli which evoke massive involuntary movements of the legs. On the other hand it is her province in conjunction with the nursing staff to protect the skin. Great care must be taken in the application of splints and bandages, in the moving of the patient and the making of his bed. Established bedsores and trophic ulcers may be treated by infra-red and ultra-violet rays.

Maintenance of good morale. There is naturally some degree of mental disturbance. This is partly due to the physical disabilities and partly the result of slight general infection likely to occur from the bladder and from trophic ulcers. A cheerful atmosphere, bright surroundings and encouragement will go far to restore the patient's confidence and gain his co-operation.

Prevention of contractures and maintenance of circulation. If contractures and trophic lesions are allowed to develop the wearing of calipers is impossible and walking therefore is prevented. Again, if tendons are contracted sensory nerve endings are irritated and flexor spasms become more severe and frequent.

Circulation may be aided by infra-red, hot baths or short wave diathermy but in each case great care must be taken as skin sensation is absent.

To prevent contractures slow, rhythmical passive movements moving in continuity from joint to joint may be given, then flexor spasm decreases and the limbs can be eventually straightened. If these can be carried out in warm water they prove even more effective. When the limbs are straight calipers may be worn; these maintain the extended position and permit walking. Long-continued passive stretching often helps to straighten the legs and overcome flexor spasm.

Patients suffering from severe damage to the cord above the level of the sixth thoracic segment show disturbance of the vaso-motor mechanism and change of posture is likely to cause fainting. Exercises involving swinging of the limbs and changes of position help in regaining control over a period of time.

Hypertrophy of muscles. If the latissimus dorsi, teres major, pectoralis major, serratus anterior, trapezius and triceps can be sufficiently hypertrophied, the patient can be taught to stand and walk even in the presence of paralysed back and abdominal muscles. Progressive strengthening exercises are therefore commenced as soon as permitted by the physician. Exercises done against the resistance of springs and weights, and trunk swinging with the pelvis and legs suspended should form a considerable part of the treatment.

Balance in sitting. The patient must be able to sit unsupported so that he can move the head, trunk, and arms without losing his balance. This is difficult since sensation will probably be lost in all structures of the buttocks and legs. Training therefore begins using a mirror and with support by the physiotherapist. It progresses through the stages of sitting without a mirror, doing simple arm exercises with some support, sitting without support, eventually to ball throwing and catching in unsupported sitting.

Standing and walking. When the patient can balance easily in sitting, progression is made to standing. The legs are usually fitted with calipers and parallel bars are used. Training begins with balance in standing, then the patient is taught how to bring first one leg forward and then the other. Progression is made to the use of crutches, and when the patient can balance and walk a few steps with crutches he is taught how to turn round, how to get into and out of his chair, how to fall and to get up until eventually be becomes almost fully independent.

Flaccid Paraplegia. Those cases which are due to severance of the cord will eventually become spastic. Treatment on the lines of the paraplegia in flexion should be commenced as early as possible bearing in mind that if contractures can be prevented flexor spasm will be less likely to occur.

For those patients in whom the condition is due to a polyneuritis the limbs only will be affected and the distal segment more completely than the proximal. The purpose of physical treatment is to maintain the circulation and nutrition of the extremities, prevent excessive muscle atrophy, avoid stiff joints and deformities and, when recovery begins, aid it in every possible way. To fulfil these objects, heat, massage, electrical stimulation and passive movements may all be used and when recovery commences active re-education is essential.

CEREBRAL PALSY

The term cerebral palsy is applied to disorders of motor behaviour arising from lesions of growing brain tissue. The motor cortex, the basal ganglia, and the cerebellum are the three main areas of the brain which are responsible for the production of co-ordinated voluntary action and a lesion in any one of these parts or its connections with the rest of the nervous system must inevitably interfere with the performance of the movement. According to the site of the lesion a different group of symptoms will be apparent, the most common being spasm and athetosis. Occasionally an ataxic child will be seen and less often tremor and rigidity may occur.

Cerebral palsy is caused by damage to the brain tissue or defect in its development, but there is much discussion as to the reasons for its occurrence. There may be an arrest of development of some area of the brain during intra-uterine life. Occasionally brain tissue may be damaged through disease in the mother or during the first few years of life as a result of thrombosis of cerebral vessels following specific infections, particularly whooping cough. Injury to the head during birth or in early life may also be responsible.

In cases of intra-uterine damage atrophy of the cerebral hemispheres is usually present. The sulci are wider than normal and the gyri smaller, sometimes actual cavities are present and in most cases there is neuroglial overgrowth. This usually appears to affect the pyramidal system giving rise to the spastic condition but may produce changes in the basal ganglia resulting in an athetosis.

The condition is not often diagnosed during the first year of life. Movements in early infancy are not cortically controlled as the pyramidal tracts are not yet fully myelinated. Purposeless movements are normal and incoordination is to be expected. As the balance mechanism is not developed the child has not yet learnt to sit up. If, however, aimless limb waving and ataxia continue after the first year a cerebral palsy will be suspected.

The Spastic Type

The whole body, four limbs, two or even one may be involved according to the extent of the damage. If all four limbs are affected the condition is known as a Spastic Diplegia. Paraplegia is the term used if both legs are involved, while Monoplegia applies to one limb. Spasticity is the outstanding feature.

Groups of muscles affected by spasticity vary but it is usual to find that in the legs the adductors and medial rotators of the hips, hamstring and calf muscles are affected, tending to produce adduction and media rotation of the legs, flexion of the knees and equinus position of the feet. In the arms, the muscles affected are the adductors of the shoulders, flexors of the elbows, pronators of the forearms, flexors of the fingers and thumbs. The thumb usually lies bent across the palm.

There is a variable loss of voluntary movement. Movement is hampered by spastic muscle so that every time the child tries to perform an active movement he meets resistance. Gradually, therefore, he ceases to try and tends to lie inactive and apathetic. For this reason the normal landmarks in a growing infant's life are either late in being reached or are never reached at all. The baby fails to lift up his head when three or four months old, does not try to sit up or crawl and makes no effort to walk at the normal time of twelve or eighteen months. If the child does eventually stand and walk he does so with his legs crossed owing to adductor spasm and on his toes as a result of contracture of his calf muscles. This is particularly apparent in severe cases when a scissor gait will develop.

As in all spastic conditions reflexes are exaggerated, clonus is sometimes present and the plantar response is often extensor. The mental condition varies from complete idiocy to normal intelligence. In all cases there is likely to be some degree of backwardness because, owing to the disability, the child is unable to learn and develop by contact with his environment. The baby who, because of his disability, is unable to grasp objects and carry them to his mouth, is unable to learn the nature of different weights, textures and tastes. The inability to lift the head limits the range of vision.

In some cases sight, speech and hearing are all affected and even less contact with the outside world is then experienced.

The Athetoid Type

The outstanding feature in this group of cerebral palsies is the presence of involuntary movements of a peculiar slow writhing type, which disturb the performance of voluntary actions. If these movements are very severe the child is unable to dress or feed himself, sitting up is difficult and walking impossible. Athetosis of facial muscles and muscles of tongue and deglutition causes grimacing and dribbling of saliva so that the child is often, erroneously, labelled mentally defective. When the muscles of speech are affected it is often almost impossible to understand what the child is trying to say. If a very great effort is made to control and prevent the movements the limbs may then be held stiffly and a condition of masked athetosis results. This tends to give the appearance of spasticity but may be distinguished by the fact that it is not the claspknife type, more nearly resembling the rigidity of extra pyramidal lesions.

Very often hearing and sight are affected but most of these children are exceptionally intelligent and nearly all are educable.

The Ataxic Type

Since in this case the lesion is in the cerebellum the main features will be muscular hypotonia and incoordination. In the performance of voluntary movement intention tremor is present, the gait is a reeling one and the child falls easily.

PRINCIPLES OF TREATMENT BY PHYSIOTHERAPY

Physiotherapy is only a small part of the treatment. Improvement of the child's physical condition will occur when there has been further development of the mental faculties. The child has to pass through the stages which have been missed in infancy and be taught by experience the nature of the world around him. Treatment is best carried out in a special centre where the physiotherapist is part of a team consisting of the physician and surgeon, nursing staff, the school teacher, the occupational therapist, the physiotherapist and the speech therapist.

The object of physiotherapy depends on the type of palsy. In the case of the spastic child the first aim is to prevent or correct deformities by the use of passive movements and splinting or special appliances. The second aim is to teach volitional movement. When the child has gained confidence a test is carried out to discover lost or weakened movements. Different methods are available to teach volitional movement. Either the use of simple rhythmical movements performed first passively, then as assisted active movements and then freely following Phelps' routine or the Temple Fay method may be used. Alternatively Mrs. Bobath's method may be employed (see preceding chapter and Bibliography).

For the athetoid child the lines of treatment vary. The first thing the child has to learn is to relax and elongate the athetoid muscle groups. When this object has been attained voluntary contraction of the opposing groups is undertaken. Treatment usually begins by teaching general relaxation with the child lying on a mattress on the floor. This is followed by a definite attempt at elongating affected muscles and then voluntary contraction of opposing groups. Progression is made by carrying out the same procedure in sitting, standing and walking. Standing, feeding, dressing are all taught on the same lines, the emphasis being on relaxation of all parts of the body during the performance of these activities.

The main purpose of physiotherapy for the ataxic condition is to train co-ordination. It is nearly always possible by constant repetition of simple movements to improve the powers of co-ordination. Treatment is carried out on the same lines as that for cases of disseminated sclerosis showing cerebellar ataxia.

Chapter V

VIRUS INFECTIONS OF THE NERVOUS SYSTEM

Certain viruses have a special affinity for the nervous system, and these are known as neurotropic viruses. These micro-organisms reach the brain and spinal cord by travelling along the axons of the cranial and spinal nerves; they invade the nerve cells, multiply within them, produce pathological changes, then become inactive and die; they seldom attack nerve fibres.

Two great classes of lesions result from these viruses; a non-suppurative encephalitis or myelitis in which micro-organisms destroy cells, as in acute poliomyelitis, epidemic encephalitis and Herpes Zoster, and an encephalo-myelitis in which the primary lesion is a demyelination of nerve fibres.

ACUTE POLIOMYELITIS

This is an acute infectious disease which may be epidemic or sporadic. It has been customary to state that the disease affects young children more often than adults, and for this reason the term Infantile Paralysis has been commonly used. In recent epidemics, however, the virus has attacked nearly as many adults as children. It may be spread by carriers, healthy individuals who harbour the virus in the naso-pharynx or intestine. It appears that once a patient is affected by the condition the virus loses its virulence and there is little danger of infection. Life-long immunity is gained by one attack.

Much discussion arises as to the way in which the virus reaches the central nervous system. It was originally thought that the olfactory nerve was the route, but it is now considered that the micro-organism travels from the intestine along the sympathetic nerve fibres to the spinal cord, and from the naso-pharynx along the fibres of the fifth, ninth and tenth cranial nerves, which innervate this region, to the brain-stem.

The lesions produced by the virus have a certain definite distribution. In the spinal cord the lumbar enlargement is most often attacked, rather less commonly the cervical. The micro-organism has a special affinity for the cells of the anterior horn, though posterior horn and posterior nerve root ganglion cells are also invaded. In the brain, the cells affected are usually those of the nuclei in mid-brain, pons and medulla. The cortex is not often attacked but when it is, the pyramidal cells of the motor area are most usually involved. The meninges are also affected.

Degenerative, followed by inflammatory, changes are produced by the virus. Degenerative changes in the cells may vary from loss of the Nissl's granules and alteration in the nucleus, to rapid and complete disintegration of the cell. Inflammation following the necrosis results in congestion and haemorrhage, the small blood vessels of the congested area are surrounded by inflammatory cells, and phagocytosis of the damaged cells occurs. Neuroglial proliferation causes replacement of lost nerve cells by neuroglial cells. The meninges become congested and the spinal cord swollen and oedematous. When the changes subside there is likely to be atrophy of the anterior horns in the affected region and secondary degeneration of the axons of the destroyed cells. In all but the abortive cases, in which necrosis of cells does not occur, probably because immunity is gained before serious changes have eventuated, muscular paresis or paralysis develops, the extent depending on the degree of cell damage. Extensive destruction of cells may mean complete paralysis of groups or individual muscles, but less widespread damage may put out of action several motor units with consequent paralysis of groups of fibres of one or more muscles, reducing their power accordingly.

Inflammatory exudate and vascular congestion may cause reduced nutrition and pressure on cells, so temporarily rendering them inactive. These cells should show recovery, and paralysis from this cause will eventually disappear.

The outward evidence of the lesion will vary from patient to patient with the site and extent of pathological change and with the speed at which immunity is acquired. It is sometimes possible to divide the signs and symptoms into the pre-paralytic and paralytic stages, though some cases do not show the first, or at least it may be mild and unrecognised, and many do not reach the second, these being the fortunate abortive cases. The pre-paralytic stage, if recognised, shows the features of a major illness. A rise of temperature possibly to 102° or more for a few days, headache, drowsiness and irritability are common features. Vomiting and diarrhoea may be present. Rigidity of the neck and spine is a characteristic feature and may be due to meningeal irritation. Usually during this stage there is a complaint of pain in the back and legs, while muscular tenderness causes the patient to resent any handling. Pain and tenderness are possibly due to involvement of the posterior roots and ganglia.

This stage may subside leaving no residual symptoms, though the patient may remain irritable, emotionally unstable, and excitable for a considerable period owing to the encephalitis. In many cases, however, within a very short period of the onset there may be the sudden appearance of muscular paralysis, varying very much in distribution from case to case but rarely, if ever, being symmetrical. Occasionally the paralysis begins in the lower extremities and spreads upwards involving trunk and respiratory muscles. Even more rarely, it occurs in successive 'crops' over a period of several days, one attack of fever being accompanied by the onset of paralysis of one group of muscles and this being followed a day or two later by a second attack. Muscular tenderness may last for a few days to several weeks, and when it disappears the patient may be said to have entered the convalescent stage.

During the period of this illness certain serious events may occur. If the brain stem is affected swallowing may be impaired and secretions from the mouth and nose may be inhaled into the lungs. A very heavy strain is then thrown on the respiratory muscles and this is the period of danger, since during the acute illness the muscles most likely to be paralysed are those whose nerve cells are fatigued. If the respiratory muscles show weakness and a respirator is required the position is very serious because the secretions tend to be sucked into the lung.

Recovery

The majority of patients recover from the acute illness. The anterior horn cells which have not been destroyed recover from the effects of anaemia and pressure usually within four to six weeks. The number of cells which have been destroyed depends upon the severity of the attack, the degree of immunity, and upon the absence of fatigue during the acute illness.

At the stage of about three months after the major illness, muscles can be grouped according to their condition into those which are completely paralysed, having shown no flicker of contraction; those which are weakened as a result of paralysis of some of their fibres; and those which, though at first paralysed or paresed, have recovered completely. At this time there is little hope for the first group. Recovery of the second will continue over a period of eighteen months or longer. This is not because there will be any further recovery of motor units, but because those units which remain can be hypertrophied. There is a suggestion that not only do the nerve fibres hypertrophy, but also that the neurones enlarge. In addition there is some evidence to show that axons branch to supply nearby denervated muscle fibres.

SIGNS AND SYMPTOMS AFTER THE MAJOR ILLNESS HAS SUBSIDED

If there is residual paralysis the signs and symptoms are those of a lower motor neurone disease; namely paralysis or weakness, atonia or hypotonia, lost or diminished deep reflexes, circulatory disturbances, muscle atrophy and a tendency to the development of stiff joints and deformities.

Circulatory impairment is much more noticeable in some cases than in others. The more extensive the paralysis the less pumping effect there will be on the soft-walled veins and lymphatics and the slower will be the circulation. Stasis will lead to oedema and nutritional changes. Sometimes, however, in spite of a not very extensive paralysis the limb is cold and blue, chilblains develop readily and growth is impaired. This condition is obviously not a paralytic vaso-dilatation, and this impression is confirmed by the fact that the circulation of the limb can be vastly improved by sympathectomy. The explanation may be that the vaso-dilator fibres (axons of cells in the posterior nerve root ganglia) have been paralysed and there is, therefore, unbalanced action of the vaso-constrictors.

Deformities may develop. Their cause may be any of the reasons already discussed in Chapter I: muscle imbalance, adaptive contractures, fibrosis of capsules and ligaments, and impairment of growth. There is, however, in acute anterior poliomyelitis an additional factor. In the acute and the early convalescent stages of the disease there is considerable tenderness in the muscles accompanied by pain on stretching and a tendency to shortening. This shortening is probably a protective mechanism. The limbs are painful to move; muscles, therefore, contract to prevent movement. Adjacent fascia and skin will also shorten.

In this disease if some muscles are paralysed the spasm will be unequal in its effect and the limb may be held in an abnormal position. If, for example, the quadriceps are weak, shortening of the hamstrings is liable to cause flexion of the knee. If the spasm is not overcome adaptive shortening of the hamstrings may develop.

Muscle atrophy will be very marked in completely paralysed muscles because no nerve impulses can reach the muscle. Metabolism in the muscle is therefore negligible. In the course of time fibrous degeneration will occur and fibrous tissue will replace the muscle fibres.

PRINCIPLES OF TREATMENT BY PHYSIOTHERAPY

For purposes of treatment, cases may be divided into three phases, though every case does not pass through each stage. There is the active phase in which the muscles are tender and the neck and back stiff. Many cases are not seen in this stage, possibly some failing to be recognised; there is the second or convalescent stage in which the pre-paralytic symptoms have disappeared and the patient is now left with varying degrees of paralysis; there is the chronic stage in which no further recovery is to be expected and the best has to be made of whatever condition remains.

THE ACTIVE (ACUTE) PHASE

The essential feature of treatment during the acute illness is rest. This is partly because the condition is an inflammatory one and partly because the fate of perhaps hundreds of nerve cells depends upon the absence of fatigue. The cells must not be excited and physical activity is therefore definitely dangerous. During this stage, however, the avoidance of respiratory complications and care of muscles and joints is essential and here the physiotherapist can assist.

Avoidance of chest complications is of supreme importance in patients in whom the brain stem is involved. For these patients the position in bed is vitally important. The semi-prone position is most often used, first on one side and then the other, and the foot of the bed is elevated so that it makes an angle of 15° with the horizontal. This prevents secretions from draining into the lungs. The physiotherapist may be called on to give gentle percussion in this position in order to avoid inhalation of secretions. The elimination of secretions may be difficult and she should be familiar with the use of the mechanical sucker.

Care of muscles and joints. It is important to relieve pain and tenderness and so to prevent contracture of muscles, fascia and skin. The greatest relief seems to be obtained from moist heat, and hot packs are therefore used if equipment is available, care being taken to handle the limbs as little as possible. Gentle passive movements carried just to the point of pain are given to each joint. Pain always becomes less if these methods are used, and gradually full range of passive movement can be obtained. Correct position of the patient in bed is very important in order to prevent the deformities which may result from muscle weakness. The most suitable position is supine with one pillow under the head and a small cushion to maintain the lumbar concavity. A rolled-up towel under the knees will prevent hyperextension at these joints and the feet may rest against a foot-board. This posture may not be possible if there is brain stem involvement or if spasm is present, but it is used as soon as possible and is changed repeatedly to the prone position. In the latter position the feet should be over the edge of the mattress to avoid stretching the anterior tibial group.

The correct position will be ordered by the physician and carried out by the nursing staff, but as the physiotherapist may be applying the hot packs, and will be giving passive movements, she is concerned with seeing that she leaves the patient in the correct position.

THE CONVALESCENT PHASE

When all pain and muscle tenderness have disappeared, pyrexia is absent and the rigidity of the neck and back are no longer present, modification of rest and more active physiotherapy may be allowed. Certain cases with a slight paralysis are now allowed to get up for increasing periods of time; others, owing to paralysis or weakness of trunk or hip muscles, may be confined to bed for a lengthy period. Consideration has now to be given to the general well being of the patient and to the local affection.

The first step is to discover exactly what muscles have been affected and to what extent each is involved. This necessitates a complete muscle test of all voluntary muscles throughout the body. Naturally, the patient must not be tired and the test may therefore have to be carried out over a period of several days. Each muscle is charted according to its strength, using the numerical method of the Medical Research Council. Not only are the muscles tested but a careful note must be made of any pain on stretching the muscles and of any soft-tissue shortening. This may be discovered in the posterior neck muscles, for example, by passively lifting the head forward till the chin touches the chest when the patient is in the supine position.

General treatment. Three main principles are considered: maintenance of interest and co-operative spirit, in fact, keeping the patient happy and interested over a lengthy convalescent period; maintenance of a satisfactory condition of all unaffected muscles and joints; keeping a sense of correct posture both for patients confined to bed and for those up but wearing some form of splints.

Maintenance of general health and interest is a very important point as the length of convalescence and final disability cannot be foreseen. General health may be aided by fresh air, good food, and one or more courses of artificial sunlight to act as a tonic. Provision of some form of diversional therapy by the occupational therapist or physiotherapist will help to keep the patient happy. In addition treatment will be carried out as far as possible by the use of apparatus such as pool therapy or suspension therapy, so gaining the patient's interest and co-operation in the treatment. Very much depends on the personality of the physiotherapist. An important point is her ability to stimulate and evoke the patient's interest and by her own enthusiasm to gain the patient's co-operation.

Maintenance of the general musculature is particularly important for those patients confined to bed, especially since as in some cases in which recovery will never be complete, extra work may be thrown on healthy muscles. General exercises for unaffected muscle groups are therefore essential.

Attention to posture is necessary since the postural sense is quickly lost in patients confined to bed. If the child cannot take the correct position, he should be repeatedly placed in it and encouraged to 'sense' it. For those children who are up and about but wearing such splints as arm abduction frames or walking calipers, re-education of posture in the splints is absolutely essential since such splints tend to upset the normal muscle balance.

Local treatment. This aims primarily at obtaining the maximum possible strength of paresed muscles. In cases in which muscles are completely paralysed an attempt should be made to hypertrophy unaffected muscles to take over their function. Since the final object is the restoration of the maximum possible function and independence it is important to avoid such hampering factors as stiff joints, severe muscle atrophy, deformities and trophic changes.

Paresed muscles may be strengthened by using the measures described in Chapter III, Part IV, (page 192). The method of 'overflow' is not, however, successful if there are no strong components available, and this may be quite possible if there is extensive paralysis. In this case the individual muscles must be exercised using the other facilitatory techniques, such as maximum resistance and stretch. Electrical stimulation may be of value to encourage branching of axons. It has recently been suggested that stimulation of the sensory fibres will increase the activity of the anterior horn cells and stimulate, therefore, the branching of their axons.

In some cases in which passive movements have not been used during the acute stage, and occasionally even when they have, there is some degree of soft-tissue contracture. Particular attention is then needed to overcome this or it will limit movement and cause deformity. The tissues can be softened most effectively through stimulating the circulation by means of hot and cold spraying and soaking in hot water. A full-length bath is a most satisfactory way of carrying this out, particularly for children. After twenty minutes of this treatment the tissues are warm and relaxed and passive stretching can be more easily and comfortably carried out. Any joints which are acted upon by paralysed or paresed muscles should then be carried through their full range in every possible direction, taking care not to overstretch weakened muscles or ligaments.

Attempts must be made to maintain as efficient a circulation as possible. If baths or pools are available they are probably the best method; alternatively a choice may be made between hot water in arm- or leg-baths, sinusoidal or constant current baths, inductothermy or radiant heat according to the condition of the skin and cutaneous sensibility.

A further point which requires attention is the danger of bruising or over-stretching paresed muscles. The patient should not sit or lie for prolonged periods on weakened muscles. If the glutei, for example, are affected, the position should be changed frequently and side lying, prone lying and lying should all be used. Splints should not be tightly bandaged over weak muscles nor should heavy massage be used. Stretching is prevented by the use of splints giving support to the affected muscles in some part of their inner range.

There is some controversy over the question of splints. These are advocated to prevent continuous stretching of paresed muscles and the development of deformities. They have their disadvantages if they restrict the circulation, add considerable weight to weakened limbs and interfere with natural use. On the other hand they may be essential to prevent such disabilities as a dropped foot or a knee which constantly gives way. The essential feature is that they should interfere with function as little as possible, hence 'lively' splints are the ideal; they should be light, and, if worn on the hands and forearms, capable of being immersed in water without harm. They must fit well without obstructing the circulation and, therefore, particularly in the case of growing children, they require constant adjustment.

During this phase of the patient's treatment, lasting probably a period of eighteen months to two years, it is essential that the patient should work hard and co-operate in every way. After the first few weeks following the onset of paralysis there is no danger of damaging the nerve cells by fatigue; exercise may therefore be continued until the muscles show signs of fatigue, when a rest should be given and the exercises can then be started again. The patient can also help by the conscientious carrying out of home exercises, by taking care of his splints, by doing his own passive movements and by keeping the affected limbs warm, dry and clean.

CHRONIC PHASE

This is the phase in which, provided adequate treatment has been previously given, no further recovery can be expected. A careful estimate of the position has now to be made. When it is known what muscles are irreparably damaged and what joints are flail or useless, consideration is given as to what orthopaedic measures may be taken to enable the patient to make the best possible use of the affected area. When such operations as tendon transplantations, or joint arthrodeses have been performed the physiotherapist will be able to help by strengthening muscles and by training them to fulfil their new functions. The patient has to be taught to make the best of whatever disability remains, trick movements being developed and encouraged.

ENCEPHALITIS LETHARGICA

Epidemic encephalitis is an inflammatory condition of the brain rarely seen today. Little is known of the cause though it was thought to be due to a virus which produced degeneration of nerve cells, particularly in the basal ganglia and brain stem, and inflammation with neuroglial proliferation. Some of the first cases were reported in 1917, the condition then spread throughout the world in epidemic form, some years later completely dying out. It did, however, leave behind it a number of cases showing symptoms closely resembling those of Parkinson's disease. To these cases the name post-encephalitic parkinsonism has been given. These patients differ in their symptoms from those suffering from Parkinson's disease in the age of onset which may be at any time instead of only in later years, in the fact that there is a tendency to oculogyric crises in which there are attacks of involuntary movements of the eyes, in a fine flutter of the closed eyelids and in the fact that tremor is often absent while rigidity is more marked. These cases will require the same type of physiotherapy as that advocated for Parkinson's disease (see Chapter VIII, Part IV).

Post-infective Encephalitis

An acute widely disseminated encephalo-myelitis occasionally develops as a sequel to one of the infectious diseases of virus origin, particularly measles. It differs from the other neurotropic virus disorders in that it produces a demyelination of nerve fibres with an inflammatory reaction in neighbouring tissues. Just as the patient appears to be recovering from the original illness there is a recurrence of fever with drowsiness, headache, rigidity of the neck and spine, coma and sometimes convulsions. If the spinal cord is mainly involved, a flaccid paraplegia with disturbance of sensation is likely to occur. Spasticity may follow the flaccidity if the upper motor neurone is involved. Spontaneous recovery is the rule, consequently few of these cases reach the physiotherapy department. If, however, recovery is slow certain sequelae may appear within some weeks or months according to the amount and site of damage. Parkinsonism, hemiplegia, spastic paraplegia or choreiform movements may arise. These will require physiotherapy on the lines discussed for similar conditions due to other causes.

HERPES ZOSTER

Herpes Zoster shows an acute vesicular eruption in the cutaneous distribution of the trigeminal nerve or of any spinal nerve but most commonly in the distribution of the thoracic nerves.

The condition is an acute infection of the posterior nerve root ganglion of the spinal cord, the trigeminal or the geniculate ganglia. This infection is probably the result of a virus producing changes in the ganglia very similar to those produced in the anterior horn by the virus of acute poliomyelitis. Men are slightly more commonly involved than women and the condition may appear at any age though it is more often seen in middle-aged or elderly people.

The changes are those of acute inflammation and degeneration in the affected ganglion. There is hyperaemia, swelling and tiny haemorrhages. The cells undergo degeneration as may also the sensory fibres of the posterior nerve roots.

The condition usually commences with a brief febrile illness lasting a few days. During this period fairly severe pain is experienced in the area in which the cutaneous eruption will appear. A few days later erythema occurs in this area, followed by the formation of vesicles starting at the point where the particular nerve becomes cutaneous and following its course to its termination. Thus in involvement of the ophthalmic nerve, vesicles appear on the side of the root of the nose, the inner end of the eyebrow, up along the forehead and sometimes on the cornea. In the case of a dorsal nerve the vesicles are found along the intercostal space to mid-line. The vesicles are filled with a clear fluid and the skin around is erythematous and swollen. About the fifth or sixth day from the time of eruption the vesicles dry up and scabs are formed, these tend to fall off leaving tiny scars or pigmented areas. Usually as scars form pain subsides but in elderly people pain may persist and may continue as a post-herpetic neuralgia over a year or two, keeping the patient awake and making life almost intolerable. Very occasionally the infection appears to spread across the cord and involve the motor cells and fibres. In this case a paralysis of muscles supplied by this segment of the cord will occur, with loss of tone, diminished or lost deep reflexes and disturbances in circulation.

There is an interesting connection between Herpes Zoster and chickenpox and it is not unusual to find that an attack of the former condition in one person may be followed by chickenpox in another person in contact with the first.

OUTLINE OF TREATMENT BY PHYSIOTHERAPY

It is not very often that the physiotherapist is called in to help in the treatment of these cases. It may be to deal with the muscular paralysis should this occur. If this is so then physiotherapy will be given on the lines indicated for a case of acute poliomyelitis. On the other hand, ultra violet light may be ordered either for its sedative effect during the stage of pain and eruption or for its counter-irritant effect in the case of a post-herpetic neuralgia. In the first case a mild first degree erythema should be given cutting out the short, irritating abiotic rays, in the second case a second degree erythema should be obtained in the area of eruption. Ultra violet light sometimes proves very effective in preventing or eliminating neuralgia but in other cases it may have no effect at all.

MYELITIS

An inflammation of the spinal cord is not necessarily the result of virus infection but in some cases probably is. The changes which occur resemble very closely those of other virus infections. For this reason the condition will be briefly discussed at this stage.

An acute inflammation of the spinal cord is uncommon. When it occurs it may be the result of trauma affecting the spine, virus infection, infection due to a septic embolism or to syphilis. It may occur equally in either sex or at any age. The inflammation may be fairly widely disseminated but more often it is localised to one segment of the cord, then affecting the whole cross section and consequently being known as a transverse myelitis.

The changes are those of acute inflammation, intense hyperaemia accompanied by haemorrhage, oedema, infiltration of the cord by inflammatory cells, thrombosis of spinal vessels with softening of areas supplied by these vessels, degeneration of nerve cells and their axons and an intense neuroglial reaction. Such changes are likely to produce a complete paralysis, below the site of the lesion, of both motor and sensory function. A lesion attacking the lumbar region will therefore give rise to a flaccid paraplegia, loss of deep reflexes, anaesthesia and loss of sphincter control. Should the inflammation involve the cervical region the arms will show a flaccid paraplegia, the legs being spastic and showing upper motor neurone symptoms.

The extent of symptoms will, of course, depend on the severity of the inflammation. In a mild condition paraplegia may not be complete and full recovery may occur. In a severe lesion complete recovery will probably never occur and over a period of months, flexor spasms may develop and a flaccid paraplegia may become a spastic paraplegia-in-flexion with many voluntary movements and much sensation lost and control of sphincters incomplete.

Treatment by physiotherapy will be ordered for patients who survive the period of acute inflammation, the lines to be followed depending on the signs and symptoms. If a flaccid paraplegia is present treatment will be given on the lines of that indicated for acute poliomyelitis; if there is spasticity treatment will be given as for a paraplegia-in-flexion.

Chapter VI

MUSCULAR ATROPHIES

The presence of muscular atrophy is a familiar feature to most physiotherapists. If atrophy due to disuse is omitted, the many other varieties may be classified into five main groups readily recognisable, if such factors as age and method of onset, distribution and type of atrophy are considered.

These groups are:

Motor Neurone Disease
Peroneal Muscular Atrophy
Post-paralytic Atrophy
Arthritic Atrophy
Primary Muscular Atrophy (Myopathy)

In addition, syringomyelia leads to muscular atrophy, though sensory and trophic symptoms are also present.

MOTOR NEURONE DISEASE

The pathological process in all types of motor neurone disease is a primary degeneration of the lower or upper motor neurones or both. The cause of this degeneration is unknown, the origin is not inflammatory nor is there an accompanying inflammatory reaction. It first appears about middle life. All types are characterised by progressive wasting and therefore weakness, by fasciculation, by the bilateral nature of the condition and by the fact that electrical reactions are usually at first normal but gradually the response weakens as atrophy progresses. In the later stages the reaction of degeneration will be present. Three types are seen: progressive muscular atrophy, amyotrophic lateral sclerosis and bulbar paralysis.

Progressive Muscular Atrophy

The motor nerve cells in the anterior horns of the cervical segments of the spinal cord show marked degenerative changes; their number is diminished and those which remain are small and altered in appearance. Secondary degeneration of the axons will consequently occur. Some degeneration of the lateral columns is always present but this is a much less well-marked feature. Occasionally the motor cells of the lumbar enlargement may be affected first, or later.

The first noticeable feature of the condition is usually a wasting and weakness of the intrinsic muscles of one hand. The patient recognises this because the fine movements of the hand become clumsy and he drops things abnormally often. Should he be in a heavy occupation he finds that the hand muscles ache and tire easily. On careful examination atrophy affecting all muscles equally will be noticed if the two hands are compared. At this stage fasciculation is often obvious particularly in the first dorsal interosseous muscle. If it is not seen with the limb at rest, an active contraction or a light flick or tap over the muscle will probably elicit it. Often, widespread fasciculation in the arm and shoulder girdle muscles may be seen. It seems that the spread of fasciculation precedes the progress of muscular atrophy and muscles which show fasciculation will later show wasting.

Atrophy gradually spreads to the forearm muscles; then, successively, to arm, and shoulder girdle. The upper part of trapezius, the latissimus dorsi and serratus anterior are usually involved rather later.

It is quite common to find that, as the condition progresses, deep reflexes in the lower extremities are exaggerated due to involvement of the lateral columns.

As atrophy and weakness of the muscles increase, deformity tends to develop. A claw hand is very likely since the small muscles of the hand are more severely affected than the muscles of the forearm.

Probably about six to nine months after the appearance of the condition in one hand, it commences in the other, progressing in the same manner. Thus, though the lesion is bilateral, it is not symmetrically severe.

Eventually, the condition tends to involve the respiratory muscles and in a few years death is likely to ensue from some respiratory disease. Very occasionally spread is delayed and life may be prolonged.

Amyotrophic Lateral Sclerosis

In this type of motor neurone disease the degeneration affects particularly the pyramidal tracts and even the Betz cells of the motor cortex. Though the lower motor neurone is invariably involved it is attacked at a rather later date in the course of the disease. The anterior horn cells degenerate and disappear and the anterior nerve root is atrophied but many cells may escape, with the result that some motor units remain intact.

Neuroglial proliferation nearly always results in a fibrous replacement of cells and fibres and sclerosis of lateral columns and anterior horns.

In this type therefore, the picture is often that of a slight spasticity of the lower limbs with exaggerated tendon jerks, clonus and an extensor plantar response. At the same time, or a little later, progressive weakness and wasting appears in one upper limb together with fasciculation as in progressive muscular atrophy, but, owing to the sclerosis of the lateral columns, the deep reflexes of the arm are exaggerated and there is an unusual degree of mechanical irritability of the muscle fibres.

Occasionally the symptoms of progressive atrophy in the arms precede those of spasticity in the legs.

These cases usually progress rapidly, often terminating as a bulbar paralysis.

Bulbar Paralysis

In this case a degeneration, exactly similar to that occurring in the anterior horn in progressive muscular atrophy, occurs in the nuclei in the brain stem. Thus the seventh, ninth, tenth, eleventh and twelfth cranial nerves are affected. This condition is sometimes therefore known as a glosso-labio-pharyngeal paralysis. Usually the first symptom is difficulty in articulation, speech being laboured, particularly when the patient is tired. A little later, when the pharyngeal muscles begin to waste, deglutition becomes difficult. Weakness of the soft palate leads to regurgitation of fluids through the nose, while affection of the lip muscles makes dribbling of saliva likely and effective closure of the lips impossible. Gradually as the lips, tongue and cheek become involved, speech becomes unintelligible. Fasciculation will be seen in the tongue, lips and muscles of the chin. The tongue atrophies and the mucous membrane is wrinkled and thrown into folds over it. Under these circumstances death from bronchopneumonia is likely since inhalation of food into the larynx is almost certain to occur at some stage in the progress of the disease.

OUTLINE OF TREATMENT BY PHYSIOTHERAPY

No form of treatment as yet known arrests the progress of motor neurone disease, therefore physical measures cannot hope to do a great deal for the patient, yet cases of progressive muscular atrophy and amyotrophic lateral sclerosis do reach the department of physical medicine. A certain amount of improvement may temporarily occur because it is possible that hypertrophy of unaffected motor units may take place, giving greater strength to the affected muscles. The development of deformities may be prevented and the circulation and nutrition of the muscles and limb as a whole improved. In this condition, unlike poliomyelitis, gross circulatory changes do not occur but in advanced cases the limb is likely to be cold and stiff due to lack of use. Above all, physiotherapy has a definite psychological value. As long as the patient is receiving treatment he does not feel that he is a hopeless case; thus he remains cheerful and co-operative. The physical measures chosen to aid these patients must be carefully selected. They do not follow the lines set out in Chapter II because the disease is progressive and fatigue might hasten the degenerative processes in the spinal cord. Therefore two points must be considered: firstly, physical measures must not tire the patient and, secondly, they must not be unduly stimulating. For this reason electrical stimulation and difficult exercises are to be avoided. The circulation to the limbs may be stimulated by inductothermy or by local application of the constant current. Massage will aid the nutrition of the muscles and may be given in the form of kneading and picking up to all the muscle groups of the shoulder girdle and upper and lower extremities; such manipulations as hacking, wringing and clapping are better avoided nor should the work be prolonged or tiring. If there is any tendency to the development of deformities which would still further hamper the action of the weakened muscles, these should be prevented by the use of passive stretchings. Splints are not very helpful since they only add additional weight to already weakened limbs. Passive movements and massage may be used to reduce spasticity temporarily in the amyotrophic type. Careful active exercise may be employed to retain present strength or even slightly to improve it but it must be well within the patient's capabilities and below the point of fatigue.

It may be noticed that throughout, work for all four limbs is advocated. This is because the condition will progress in spite of treatment but it is just possible that progress might be delayed by maintaining the condition of the muscles.

PERONEAL MUSCULAR ATROPHY
(Charcot-Marie-Tooth type)

This type of muscular atrophy resembles the motor neurone diseases in that it is due to degenerative changes of nervous tissue, but it is also closely linked to the primary muscular atrophies since it is both familial and hereditary.

The cause of the condition is unknown but it appears to be transmitted directly from one of the parents and its onset occurs in the young adult.

The changes are those of degeneration in the anterior horn of the lumbar enlargement and in the anterior nerve roots. In addition, unlike the other types, the posterior column shows degenerative changes and there is sometimes an interstitial neuritis of the lateral popliteal nerves. Thus both motor and sensory symptoms will be present. Wasting and weakness begin in the plantar muscles of the feet, spread to the peronei and to extensors longus digitorum and hallucis, later affecting the calf muscles and the lower third of the quadriceps group. This peculiar distribution leads to the development of deformities, particularly to a severe pes cavus and foot drop. The wasting of the lower third of the quadriceps gives a peculiar appearance to the thigh resembling that of a bottle.

The ankle jerk will be diminished and gradually lost as wasting of the calf muscles progresses. Fasciculation is often seen in the wasting muscles but it is not a constant feature. Electrical reactions remain normal but are weaker than usual.

Considerable impairment of all forms of sensation in the affected area may be present and diminished position sense may give rise to ataxia.

Occasionally a similar condition may occur in the hands and distal one-third of the forearms. In few cases does the lesion progress beyond the lower third of thigh and forearm; it usually arrests spontaneously at this level. Since progress does not occur beyond this point the disease is not fatal to life. It leaves the patient with a certain amount of disability, but it is surprising how slight this disability actually is. There will be a foot drop but this can be adequately dealt with by the use of a drop-foot spring.

Since the condition will cease to progress, the essential feature is to try to prevent the development of permanent deformities and to maintain as much muscle power as possible. The prevention of trophic disturbances and skin lesions is also an important point. Physiotherapy will therefore prove beneficial. Any form of heat should be carefully applied owing to the defective sensibility. Passive movements are particularly important to prevent contracture of plantar fascia, plantar muscles and tendo achillis and to retain mobility in the toes and foot. Careful active work to maintain reasonable strength in all affected muscles may be given and later the patient should be taught the use and care of the drop-foot spring.

POST-PARALYTIC ATROPHY

In those cases in which the innervation of muscles is completely cut off, profound atrophy results. This differs from the preceding forms of atrophy in that it is neither symmetrical nor bilateral except in cases of polyneuritis. The atrophy does not precede weakness; the loss of power occurs first and is followed several weeks later by atrophy which, if recovery does not occur, progresses until the muscular fibres can be no longer recognised. This atrophy is the result of several factors: first, the great reduction in katabolic processes in the denervated muscles; second, nutrition will be impaired in the absence of the pumping effect of muscular contraction on blood vessels, and third, in some cases vaso-constrictor nerves may be involved with gross disturbance of circulation.

Electrical reactions are both quantitatively and qualitatively changed. In cases of complete interruption of the neurones, the reaction of degeneration will be present.

This type of atrophy also differs in that there is no heredo-familial incidence; neither is there fasciculation. On the other hand, while wasting is proceeding, there is often tenderness of the muscles on pressure, a feature not present in motor neurone disease or in peroneal muscular atrophy.

Physical treatment of this type of atrophy has already been dealt with in the discussion of acute poliomyelitis.

ARTHRITIC ATROPHY

This type of atrophy is not directly due to lesions of the nervous system, but since it is probably the result of irritation of sensory nerve endings through arthritic changes in joints, it has been included here.

Atrophy of muscle is usually obvious in all types of arthritic conditions. It differs from other types of atrophy in its distribution since it occurs only in those muscles which are acting on the affected joints.

Not only does it occur in these groups but it is also most marked in the extensor muscles proximal to the joint; thus for example in an arthritis of the knee joint the quadriceps group is more severely atrophied than the hamstring muscles, while in a lesion of the wrist joint the dorsiflexors of the wrist are more affected than the flexors. Wasting of the muscle fibres reduces their power with the result that it may be impossible to obtain full range of extension in the joint, and flexion deformities may develop. A true fasciculation is not associated with this type of atrophy but muscles may be tender on pressure. Electrical reactions will remain qualitatively unchanged but responses will be weaker. Deep reflexes will be present but diminished in strength.

Much of this atrophy is reflex, the result of irritation of sensory nerve endings in the joint; a little will be due to disuse. Prevention may be impossible though rest causing a quicker subsidence of any inflammatory activity and therefore less irritation of nerve endings, will lessen the degree of atrophy. Treatment can only be successful if active work is given for the muscles, but it must be carefully graded.

PRIMARY MUSCULAR ATROPHY OR MYOPATHY

In cases of primary muscular atrophy, no demonstrable change in the nervous system is present. The disease is one in which some congenital defect in the muscle is probably present and pathological changes take place without known cause. Different types of primary muscular atrophy (myopathy) arise but certain features are characteristic of all cases.

There is a strong heredo-familial incidence, the disease being most often transmitted to the males of the family through the unaffected females. The age at which symptoms first appear is earlier than in other muscular atrophies, being either in infancy, childhood or adolescence. Unlike other muscular atrophies, muscles are often enlarged because increase in the connective tissue of the muscles occurs at the same time as atrophy of the muscle fibres. Fasciculation is never seen, neither are the muscles tender on pressure. The electrical reactions remain qualitatively normal though their strength diminishes as power wanes. Tendon reflexes, which at first are normal, gradually diminish and are eventually lost. The distribution of atrophy also differs; instead of affecting the distal segments of the limbs or the muscles of speech, deglutition and respiration, this lesion attacks the limb girdles and the muscles of expression.

The pathological changes occur in the muscle fibres and in the connective tissue of the muscles. In the early stages the fibres are swollen and the nuclei increase in numbers, later the fibres undergo atrophy. Meanwhile the interstitial tissue increases in quantity and fat is deposited within it. According as to which process is most advanced, so the actual muscle increases or decreases in size. Whether atrophy or hypertrophy predominate loss of power invariably occurs and hypertrophy is thus a pseudo, not a true, hypertrophy.

MYOPATHIES

Myopathies are classed according to the muscles affected and the age of onset into three varieties: Pseudohypertrophic type, Erb's juvenile type and the Facio-Scapulo-Humeral type.

Pseudohypertrophic muscular dystrophy. This is the most common variety. It attacks young boys and makes its first appearance in infancy. Certain muscles show hypertrophy while others are atrophied. Pseudohypertrophy occurs in the calf muscles, quadriceps, and glutei, in the lower part of sacro-spinalis and in the deltoids and spinati. Atrophy is seen in the flexors and adductors of the hips and the hamstring muscles, while in the upper extremities the biceps and triceps are sometimes affected; the lower part of trapezius, pectoralis major and serratus anterior are also involved. The result of these changes is a weakness of some movements and the development of deformities. An increasing disability in stance and gait gradually manifests itself. The child whose extensors are weakened and flexors shortened will have a marked lordosis in standing since the pelvic tilt will be increased and the trunk will be thrown back to compensate. Weakness of abductors will cause a waddling gait. A tendency to clumsy walking and liability to fall easily, with difficulty in negotiating stairs will be early symptoms. As the condition progresses, a characteristic rise from the supine position is noticeable and even diagnostic. If the child is placed on the back and then asked to get up, he first rolls over onto his face then gets onto his hands and knees, the hands are then placed on the thighs and he works his way up, by pushing against the thighs, to the erect position, finally achieving it by jerking the trunk backwards. The atrophy of the shoulder girdle muscles results in inability to depress the arms against resistance, so that if the child is picked up he slides through the physiotherapist's hands. Elevation of the arms is reduced, there is absence of the anterior axillary folds, the scapulae are winged and rotate so that the glenoid cavities tend to face downwards. The shoulders fall forward.

The mother's attention is often drawn to the child's condition by the enlargement of the calves and the late attempt to walk or the clumsy gait. In time the connective tissue tends to shorten and, as the calf muscles contract, the child will stand and walk on the toes.

The condition progresses until the child is unable to get about at all; usually he does not attain adult life as lack of activity, and atrophy of pectoral muscles predisposes towards respiratory affections.

Erb's juvenile type. This type appears rather later, usually in adolescence or in early adult life. There is much less often hypertrophy, atrophy being the outstanding feature. The shoulder girdle is affected first and most severely though the pelvic girdle is affected later. Particularly noticeable is the atrophy of trapezius, pectoralis major and serratus anterior, giving rise to the deformity of winging of the scapulae, and resulting in great difficulty in elevating the arms, through abduction or flexion, above shoulder level.

This condition progresses very much more slowly than the previous type and the prognosis is therefore more favourable.

Facio-scapulo-humeral variety. This appears rather earlier than Erb's type but later than the pseudohypertrophic variety. Both boys and girls are affected, and the progress is more rapid. There is a similar condition of the shoulder girdle but as the name implies, the facial muscles are also involved. The orbicularis oris muscle is usually hypertrophied, so that the lips are thick and everted and the child is unable to close them properly. Drinking and whistling are difficult and speech is not clear. Atrophy of the other facial muscles gives a peculiar mournful expression to the face and closure of the eyelids becomes defective.

Eventually the muscles of the pelvic girdle may also be attacked and posture and gait resemble that of the first variety.

Myotonia Atrophica

This is a very rare muscular atrophy showing a distribution differing from that of muscular dystrophy. The wasting occurs particularly in the sterno-mastoids. Less noticeably in the distal segments of the limbs and in addition, in the facial muscles. A feature peculiar to this type is the presence of increased tone and therefore of delayed relaxation following contraction of the muscles.

Associated with this condition are premature baldness, cataract and mental deterioration.

OUTLINE OF TREATMENT BY PHYSICAL MEASURES

Since all these conditions are progressive and for none is there a cure, physical measures are relatively ineffective. The main purpose is to keep the child up and about a little longer than might otherwise be possible. This may be done by preventing the development of permanent deformities such as flexion contracture of the hip joints, shortening of the calf muscles, and pes cavus, and by maintaining the nutrition of the affected muscle groups. The development of respiratory diseases may also be delayed by the use of physical measures. Thus, massage and passive stretchings will be used for the affected muscle groups, breathing exercises for the chest and a light general scheme of exercises may be given to aid the circulation and maintain freedom of the joints of the limbs and trunk. As in motor neurone disease great care is needed not to fatigue the muscles since this would serve to accelerate the process of atrophy.

AMYOTONIA CONGENITA

This should not be discussed under the heading of muscular atrophies, since atrophy is not a characteristic feature, but since it is a primary muscular disease it bears a close relationship to the preceding conditions and will therefore be described at this point. It is a condition of lack of tone in the voluntary muscles noticed soon after birth or in early infancy following some illness. The muscles are small and soft though not atrophied. They fail to harden in contraction and their power is so slight that the child may be unable to hold up its head, sit up, or walk. Reflexes are diminished and the electrical reactions show a weak normal response.

Unlike the other disorders no progression occurs; in fact, over a long period some slight improvement takes place and in time the child may learn to sit up, though without apparatus he may never attain sufficient strength to stand or walk. One danger is that of damage to joints since muscular atonia will allow them to be carried far beyond their normal range, hence grotesque postures can easily be taken up. A second complication is that of contracture. If the infant is unable to stand, he may be propped up in the sitting position and adaptive shortening of the flexors of the hips and knees may occur.

Because of the possibility of improvement, physical treatment is definitely of value. By careful passive movements contractures should be prevented or tissues may be gently stretched if these have already occurred. The nutrition of the muscles may be increased by a light general massage and active exercises may help to speed up the natural improvement of muscle tone and strength. The child can be taught by gradual stages to hold up its head and to sit up unsupported. If this stage is satisfactorily reached, the next step is to gain the standing position and independent walking. For this the use of weight-bearing calipers attached to a light trunk support may be found possible. It is part of the physiotherapist's work to train the child to stand and walk in the apparatus and to teach the mother how to apply it and keep it in good condition. A reasonably good result is likely to be obtained if the child does not succumb to some intercurrent infection.

MYASTHENIA GRAVIS

This also is not a condition of muscular atrophy but it is a condition in which muscular power is weakened without apparent change in the nervous system and for this reason it is described with other primary muscular disorders.

The condition affects women more often than men and the first symptoms are usually seen in early adult life, though it does occasionally appear in the middle-aged. It is characterised by absence of muscular atrophy while at the same time there is rapid fatigue, and inability to contract of voluntary muscles.

The cause is unknown but it is thought that acetyl-choline, normally liberated at the motor-end plate and making the muscle fibre more sensitive to the nerve impulse, is either not liberated or is destroyed too rapidly. The result of this is a weakened muscular contraction. It is quite often found in these patients that a large thymus gland is still present; in fact removal of this gland has been found to have a definite beneficial effect upon the condition.

There is considerable variability in the onset and the symptoms in myasthenia gravis. In some cases, only the muscles innervated by the brain stem are affected, in others limb and trunk musculature is also involved. In the first case the patient finds that as the day goes on she has difficulty in keeping the eyes open and she has to tilt the head back to compensate for the ptosis. Mastication may become increasingly difficult throughout the day; the head may tend to fall forward and the patient may be seen in a characteristic posture, sitting with the chin supported in the hands and the eyes propped open by the fingers. Squint, diplopia, difficulty in speech and deglutition may all be present from time to time.

When the limbs are affected the patient may find increasing difficulty in lifting the arms, in walking or remaining erect at all.

It is difficult to give any prognosis since so much variation occurs. Some cases progress rapidly until they are unable to perform any voluntary action and they may die from failure of the respiratory muscles or disturbance of deglutition. Others may undergo complete arrest while yet others follow a slow chronic course. Temporary improvement for a few hours is obtained by the use of prostigmine but this does not provide a permanent cure. As has already been pointed out improvement is gained in some cases by a thymectomy.

Physical measures can play no useful part but the physiotherapist may be called upon to carry out an electrical test since a peculiar electrical response is obtained in these cases, known as the myasthenic reaction. Normally, the faradic current uninterrupted will evoke a tetanic response of muscle lasting for several minutes until the muscle is fatigued. In these cases relaxation occurs, while the current is still flowing, often in less than a minute, then when the electrode is removed no relaxation is seen.

SYRINGOMYELIA

Though many other symptoms occur in this chronic disease of the spinal cord, muscular atrophy is a constant and outstanding sign and for this reason the condition is dealt with in this chapter. The disease attacks both men and women equally, in adolescence or early adult life, and its cause is unknown.

The essential feature is a proliferation of the neuroglial tissue in the grey commissure and base of the posterior horn of the spinal cord in the dorsal and lower cervical segments. The newly formed glial tissue gradually softens and liquefies and as it is removed by phagocytosis long cavities remain. Sometimes the lesion remains confined to the upper dorsal region, in other cases it appears to spread along the whole length of the cord.

The symptoms of the lesion are the result of pressure and destruction and depend on the extent of the lesion. The first symptoms are usually sensory due to pressure on, or destruction of, the sensory fibres conveying painful and thermal stimuli and tactile sense as they cross in the grey commissure to reach the opposite side of the cord. A dissociated anaesthesia arises since postural and vibration senses are unimpaired. The patient suffers from diminished or lost ability to appreciate thermal or painful stimuli. Consequently scars and ulcers are likely to be seen on the fingers and Charcot's joints may develop. The shoulder joint is most often attacked and is liable to be completely disorganised, since lost pain sensation will allow severe traumata without awareness of damage. As the condition progresses the anterior horn becomes involved and damage to the motor cells will result in a progressive weakness and wasting commencing in the small muscles of one or both hands and spreading in a similar manner to the progress of a progressive muscular atrophy. Very rarely does complete paralysis occur and the patient often retains a surprising amount of use in the hands. Deformities, particularly claw hand, are likely to develop. If the lesion spreads laterally the lateral horn will be involved in the process with involvement of the pre-ganglionic sympathetic fibres. Circulatory disturbances will then arise, the hands become cyanosed and puffy, the skin thin and shiny, the subcutaneous tissues are thickened so that the hand feels soft and boneless to the touch.

A further lateral spread may cause pressure on the lateral columns and a spasticity of the legs will then occur.

An outstanding feature of the condition is the development of a kyphoscoliosis while other deformities, such as spina bifida and pes cavus, are sometimes associated with it. The condition is very slow in its progress and may possibly be arrested by deep X-ray therapy.

Physiotherapy is nearly always ordered, its objects being to prevent deformities, improve the circulation and to bring about hypertrophy of unaffected fibres of the wasted muscles. The treatment therefore resembles that of progressive muscular atrophy but since progress is slower there is not quite the same danger of fatigue and the treatment may often be slightly progressed instead of regressed as in the former case.

Chapter VII

DISSEMINATED SCLEROSIS. SYPHILITIC AFFECTIONS OF THE NERVOUS SYSTEM

DISSEMINATED SCLEROSIS

This is a chronic condition affecting the brain and spinal cord and producing a very wide variety of symptoms. Women are more commonly attacked than men, usually in early adult life though some cases show symptoms as early as the fifteenth or sixteenth year. The cause of the condition is unknown. An attack is often precipitated by shock, worry or some illness which temporarily confines the patient to bed.

During the acute inflammatory phase small segments of the myelin sheath of the nerve fibres of the brain and spinal cord break up into fatty droplets, the axis cylinders usually remaining intact. The whole length of the fibre is practically never involved. Phagocytes remove the debris and neuroglial cells proliferate, with the result that, when the inflammation subsides, a small patch of scar tissue, through which run demyelinated nerve fibres, remains. The size of the scar is invariably less than the original area of inflammation, with the result that, as inflammation subsides, symptoms become less prominent.

The little patches of scar tissue which result stand out clearly defined, pinkish-grey in appearance and irregular in shape. Though a few are found in the grey matter, the greatest number occur in the white, particularly in the optic nerve and optic chiasma, mid-brain, pons and cerebellar peduncles, and in the lateral columns of the spinal cord; less commonly they occur in the posterior columns.

Noticeable characteristics of the lesion are its tendency to exacerbations and remissions and the varying nature of its symptoms. Since the patches of inflammation and scar tissue may occur almost anywhere in the nervous system, the onset differs from patient to patient according to the area first affected. The optic nerve and chiasma are often affected early and blurring of vision may be the first point of which the patient complains. Pain, and tenderness of the eyeballs on pressure will lead to a diagnosis of a retro-bulbar neuritis—a diagnosis which in young people is very often a guide to the recognition of an early disseminated sclerosis. In many cases the eye symptoms last only a few days, then pass off and no further symptoms appear for some months or even years. The next attack may affect the same area or it may attack other areas and new symptoms may arise such as slight frequency in micturition paraesthesia, a feeling of heaviness in one leg which drags a little on walking, exaggerated deep reflexes and loss of the superficial abdominal reflexes.

Later, as more and more inflammatory patches occur and one area of scar tissue fuses with another, consequently compressing many axis cylinders, more marked and stable symptoms will appear.

Later Signs and Symptoms

When the condition is more advanced and symptoms more stable, the characteristics of the disease will depend upon the region of the nervous system showing most sclerosis. Cases then roughly fall into certain groups, though it is necessary to bear in mind that, though the symptoms of one lesion predominate, symptoms of other lesions will usually be present.

For purposes of treatment by physical measures, patients suffering from this disease may be divided into those in whom the lesion is most marked in the cerebellar peduncles and those in whom the incidence is heaviest in the lateral columns. A few will show predominant symptoms arising as a result of lesions in the posterior columns but these are a smaller, less common group.

Many patients show mental changes of which euphoria is the most striking.

In nearly all cases the legs are more affected than the arms or trunk, the fibres to the legs presenting a longer course to be attacked.

Cerebellar Type

The function of the cerebellum is to co-ordinate voluntary movement, to regulate the tone of contracting muscles, to maintain the postural fixation of the limbs and trunk and to augment the action of the motor cortex. It carries out these functions by receiving and sending messages from and to the brain and spinal cord through the cerebellar peduncles. Patches of sclerosis in the peduncles, in the cerebellum or in the cerebellar tracts will interfere with the proper fulfilment of these functions.

There are two outstanding features which arise from this disturbance. These are muscular weakness and hypotonia, and incoordination of voluntary movement. The hypotonia is such that the initiation of voluntary movement becomes increasingly difficult with resultant loss of power to perform movements. Almost complete loss of power in the legs is a not uncommon feature in advanced cases of this type.

Incoordination is the result of the hypotonia and lack of postural fixation. Movements are performed in an uneven manner and a marked side to side deviation is seen as the limb nears its object, known as an intention tremor. Overshooting of the mark is due to the inability of the hypotonic antagonists to slow the movement down sufficiently. In severe cases the whole body may show tremor on the attempt to perform a movement of any one part.

Nystagmus and staccato speech are both evidence of incoordination. Nystagmus, or oscillation of the eyeballs as the eyes are rotated to one side, is the result of inability to co-ordinate the action of the ocular muscles. Staccato speech is the breaking up of the words into separate syllables in order to gain clarity in talking when co-ordination of lips, larynx and tongue is difficult.

The combination of weakness and ataxia produces a staggering gait rather resembling that of the drunken man. The patient holds the arms out ahead ready to grasp any object if she feels she is about to fall. At first this ataxic gait may be only noticed in turning round, or walking round objects or taking stairs, but later increasing difficulty is met until eventually the patient is unable to walk unaided. In these cases the time may come when, the arms and trunk also affected, the patient becomes entirely dependent on others, the incoordination of the arms making even feeding an impossibility.

These symptoms are the outstanding features. Reflexes may be exaggerated owing to lack of tone in antagonistic muscles and, in addition, there is nearly always an extensor plantar response and sometimes some cutaneous sensory impairment indicating minor lesions in the lateral and posterior columns.

The Upper Motor Neurone Type

In these cases the lesions predominate in the lateral columns of the spinal cord, consequently increased muscle tone of the spastic type and exaggerated reflexes are the characteristic features. There is a fairly usual mode of progression of symptoms in these patients. The condition begins with slight increase of tone in the calf muscles and weakness of the anterior tibial group so that the toe is dragged a little along the ground in walking. The leg feels heavy and tires easily. At this stage there will be an extensor plantar reflex and exaggeration of the knee and ankle jerks. Gradually spasticity increases involving extensors of knee and adductors of hip, while increasing weakness of flexors makes flexion of hip and knee difficult. Knee and ankle clonus are readily elicited and the superficial abdominal reflexes are absent. The patient may complain of numbness and vibration sense may be diminished, but there is not usually much sensory loss unless the posterior columns are involved.

Gradually, as more sclerosis develops and the brain is increasingly cut off from the spinal cord, flexor spasms begin to appear. At first these may be only occasional and slight but they gradually become more marked until no appreciable stimulus is required to produce them. Eventually with progressive weakness of power in all groups, the legs fail to extend, remaining in severe flexion. Adaptive shortening occurs, tendon organs are irritated by the contracted state of the tendons and tone is still further augmented.

In many cases weakness of abdominal muscles complicates the picture, making unsupported sitting an impossibility.

Some degree of cerebellar ataxia is likely to be present but movement may be so diminished that it is not appreciable. These patients probably suffer more than those who are primarily ataxic, because the flexor spasms are painful and distressing, while in addition, sores easily develop on prominent bony points which, due to deformity, are abnormally exposed. Bladder troubles are also often present.

Sensory Ataxia

In some cases the posterior columns are more affected, kinaesthetic sense is impaired and cutaneous sensibility diminished. The patient, unaware of the position of his limb, is unable, unless he closely watches, to perform a co-ordinated movement. Walking is ataxic and if sensibility in the soles of the feet is reduced the gait will closely resemble that of the tabetic patient. In these cases Rhombergism will also be present.

There will nearly always be some evidence of involvement of lateral columns and cerebellar peduncles.

PRINCIPLES OF TREATMENT BY PHYSIOTHERAPY

In view of the wide variety of symptoms, extreme care has to be given to the choice of suitable physical measures for each individual case of disseminated sclerosis. In making this choice certain considerations are essential. The first of these is the group into which the particular patient falls. It should be fully realised that many cases cannot be classified into one or other of the above groups since symptoms of all types are present fairly equally, but when such classification can be made choice of treatment is much simpler.

The second consideration is the severity of the condition and whether or not the patient is reasonably likely to be able to return to his normal occupation. It is essential to have some idea as to the immediate prospects, so that the line of treatment can be adequately planned. In more advanced cases it is helpful to know whether the physician is expecting the patient to be kept on the feet, with or without the use of apparatus or sticks or crutches. For those who can never hope to walk again, consideration must be given to methods available to enable them to be as independent as possible in eating, washing and dressing. A further consideration is that of the medical treatment being given. If the patient is receiving artificial hyperpyrexia treatment by T.A.B. injections she should not get out of bed for walking exercises during the ten or fourteen days of the course.

The first step, therefore, is a detailed examination of the patient conducted on the lines set out in Chapter II, Part IV. This should enlighten the physiotherapist on the nature and severity of the main symptoms, the regions of the body affected, the state of the patient's vision, and the degree of independence in the normal activities of life.

Cases in Which the Main Symptoms are of Cerebellar Origin

Mild cases. These patients are usually early cases showing eye symptoms and some degree of ataxia in walking. Muscle tone is poor and power may be a little diminished; difficult movements, especially the more highly skilled activities of the hands, are mildly incoordinate.

The main object of physiotherapy in these cases is to train a better coordination of voluntary movement and to gain a greater strength of muscles. This is carried out on the lines discussed in Chapter III, Part IV, for the treatment of decrease in tone. It is essential to gain the greatest possible number of afferent impulses so that all motor areas including cerebellum, cortex and subcortical areas are stimulated as strongly as possible, therefore maximum resistance, stretch, and touch, sight and hearing should all be used. These may be employed in the special exercises designed by Dr. Fraenkel, but modified, as he did not make use of resistance and stretch. Improvement will certainly occur without the use of these, but they may serve to hasten the progress. Co-ordination of movement appears to improve, particularly with the use of the reversal of antagonists.

Constant repetition is a very important point and the patient's attention must be held closely, because in this way it is hoped that alternative pathways, probably from the cortex, will be established, and 'dormant' neurones activated.

If alternative pathways can be established there is every hope that progress will be maintained for some years in spite of the fact that the disease itself is a progressive one. The prognosis is not of course known and all motor centres may eventually be attacked, while involvement of afferent pathways may decrease the quantity of proprioceptive stimuli which can be used. In these cases alteration in the lines of physical treatment will be needed.

Severe cases. These are people who are unable to stand and walk because hypotonia and deficient power in the leg muscles is such as to make the patient unable to keep the legs straight in standing or propel them forward in walking. Many of these are quite young people who show also incoordination of the arms and trunk, though this is rarely so marked as in the legs.

The first step is to try to get the patient on her feet again. This can sometimes be done by the use of light but strong splints keeping the knees from bending under the body weight, or if the trunk and arm muscles are strong enough, by the use of calipers with trunk straps, and crutches or sticks. To this end physical treatment will consist of carefully graded active exercises for the legs using sling therapy to assist weak movements. Aches and pains in the legs due to fatigue from the effort to perform movements are relieved by massage to the muscle groups. Progressive strengthening exercises should be given to arm and trunk muscles and suitable precision exercises to the arms. The patient is taught to walk in her splints. The physiotherapist should see that the patient is able to interest herself in some sedentary activity.

For very severe cases, where even the arms are grossly incoordinate, an attempt is made to equip the patient with some form of support to the upper arms so that she can feed and wash herself, do a little knitting or coarse fancywork and turn over the pages of a book. If the arm rests on a pile of firm pillows, so that the necessity for postural fixation is avoided, the patient can often do simple things for herself which she would otherwise be totally unable to do. For knitting, the arms may be supported in an ordinary arm sling.

Cases in which the Main Symptoms are of the Upper Motor Neurone

For those patients showing extensor and adductor spasticity and weakness of dorsiflexion of the feet and flexion of the hips and knees the treatment will follow the lines set out for the hemiplegic patient, but as the condition is likely to progress, if the arms and trunk are unaffected, attention is paid to building up these muscles so that the patient can lead an active existence even when walking becomes impossible.

If there are flexor spasms or paraplegia-in-flexion, treatment will follow the lines discussed for this condition in Chapter III, Part IV, particular importance being attached to the attempt to prevent flexion contractures. If the flexor spasms are giving great pain a cordotomy may be performed, the lateral spinothalamic tract being divided. Since pain is then absent it is easier to carry out passive stretchings.

Cases Showing Sensory Ataxia

Treatment is carried out on lines set out in Chapter III, Part IV. Especial use may be made of the sense of sight, since the incoordination is due to impairment of the kinesthetic pathways, but this alone is not effective because there are many occasions when the patient has to go out in the dark; therefore all afferent pathways should be utilised.

In the case of those patients who do not fall into one or other of these groups, treatment will depend entirely on what the patient is capable of doing. It will be a combination of the previous methods.

SYPHILITIC DISORDERS OF THE NERVOUS SYSTEM

Only very few of the nervous disorders are syphilitic in origin. In these, the spirochaete gains entrance to the nervous system through the meninges. Early in the development of syphilis the arachnoid and pia mater are attacked and an inflammatory reaction results, producing changes in the cerebro-spinal fluid and, occasionally, headaches and ocular palsies. With adequate treatment, the meningeal symptoms disappear and a latent period follows. If no further signs of meningeal irritation occur within three or four years, it is usually considered that the spirochaete has been 'turned back' by the meninges and has not attacked the nervous system. If, on the other hand, further symptoms appear, then the micro-organism has probably invaded the brain or spinal cord. Often in this case neurological symptoms do not make their appearance for a further period of five years or more. It is not known what changes are occurring in the nervous system during this period. Two main types of lesions are eventually produced: those attacking the blood vessels and meninges, and those involving nerve cells and fibres. It is possible that the latter are the result of the former, since thickening of the tunica intima with cell infiltration into the tunica adventitia and meningeal connective tissue may cause pressure on cells and fibres, while arteritis will very probably cause diminished blood supply and therefore deficient nutrition to nerve tissue. On the other hand degeneration of nerve fibres and cells does not necessarily follow vascular changes.

Cases of meningo-vascular syphilis do not often reach the physiotherapy department but general paralysis (dementia paralytica) and tabes dorsalis (locomotor ataxia) are occasionally seen. Symptoms of the latter condition are definitely improved by the use of physical measures and for this reason it will be more fully discussed here.

TABES DORSALIS (LOCOMOTOR ATAXIA)

This is a syphilitic atrophy and degeneration of the posterior columns of the spinal cord, from whence the condition acquires its names (tabes = wasting). It occurs more commonly in men than in women and its onset is often about the age of forty, some ten or fifteen years perhaps after the original infection. Its progress is usually very slow and it may spontaneously arrest before very severe symptoms have developed; on the other hand it may progress slowly but inexorably until the patient is so ataxic that he is unable to get about at all. It is extremely doubtful whether antisyphilitic or other measures have any influence on the progress of the disease.

There is still some disagreement on the pathology of Tabes Dorsalis. The changes occur either in the posterior nerve root ganglion, or in the nerve fibres at the point between the ganglion and the spinal cord, or as they lie in the medial part of the posterior column, though in addition changes occur in the posterior nerve root, in the sheath and fibres of the optic nerve, and occasionally in other cranial nuclei. A gradual demyelination of the fibres takes place extending upwards to the first synapse, till eventually the myelin sheath completely disappears. Disintegration of the axons also occurs. At the same time as atrophy is taking place, proliferation of neuroglial cells occurs, consequently neuroglia replaces the parenchyma.

The area of the spinal cord usually attacked is the lumbar and thoracic regions, though occasionally the cervical region may be involved, producing cervical tabes. As a result of the degenerative process there is a gradual disappearance of the posterior columns, and this section of the cord appears flat or even concave instead of showing its normal convexity. The posterior nerve root is small compared to the anterior.

Signs and symptoms depend on the extent of damage to the posterior nerve root, posterior column and optic nerve. The function of the posterior nerve root is to convey all types of sensation into the cord. Short fibres end in the posterior horn or pass anteriorly to form a synapse with the lower motor neurone. Long fibres enter the posterior column conveying sensibility from joints and muscles, from bone and skin. Early symptoms of the lesion are therefore likely to be: pains, loss of deep reflexes, some objective sensory loss, and certain eye defects. As the condition progresses pains may disappear but sensory changes will increase and loss of muscle sense will lead to incoordination.

Pains are often the earliest symptom as irritation preceding degeneration causes impulses in pain nerve fibres. The pains are felt in the trunk and lower extremity since thoracic and lumbar regions of the spinal cord are affected. They are known as lightning pains because they are sharp and stabbing in type, coming on in paroxysms, shooting into the limb at right angles to its long axis. They are felt in the calf, foot and heel particularly, and sometimes in the walls of the thorax. As the condition progresses the pains usually disappear, though in a few cases they may persist.

Tendon reflexes will be diminished and lost as a result of the break in the reflex arc due to the degeneration of short sensory fibres. The ankle jerk is often lost before the knee jerk because it is dependent on the integrity of lower spinal segments. Eventually, loss of the knee jerk will be found and still later the tendon jerks of the upper extremity may be lost.

Objective sensory disturbance is found in the distribution of thoracic segments two to ten particularly, thus analgesia and diminished touch and thermal sensibilities are found on the trunk between the second costal cartilage and the umbilicus, and along the medial border of the arm, forearm and hand. In cases where eye symptoms are present, there is often cutaneous loss in the region of the nose and upper lip. Later, cutaneous loss may become more widespread and complete.

Eye symptoms often appear early in the course of the disease. The pupil contracts, inequality in size often existing in the two eyes. It fails to react to light, only in the very later stages failing to react to accommodation. Atrophy of the iris also often occurs. These changes were described in 1869 by Argyll Robertson and are now known as the Argyll Robertson pupil. It was originally thought that they were due to atrophy of cells close to the Sylvian aqueduct in the mid-brain, but doubt has since been thrown on this hypothesis.

In some cases optic atrophy occurs first in one eye and later in the other. In a fairly short time complete blindness may ensue.

As a result of degeneration in the nucleus of origin of certain of the cranial nerves, ocular palsies are likely to develop, diplopia, squint and ptosis are reasonably common features. Ptosis causes the patient to raise the eyebrows and produce a transverse furrow across the forehead and this, together with the pinpoint pupils and emaciation, give the tabetic patient a characteristic appearance.

Incoordination is seen usually rather later than the foregoing symptoms as the fibres conveying position sense appear to be more resistant to the degenerative process. As position sense deteriorates, movement becomes irregular since the brain is no longer kept aware of the position of the limb in space or the degree of contraction of the muscles. This incoordination is particularly seen if the eyes are shut and when the patient is walking. It is increased by diminished sensation in the soles of the feet which makes the patient unaware of the ground and gives him a feeling as though 'he is walking on cotton wool'. At first he finds slight difficulty in walking straight or negotiating obstacles in his path, later it becomes increasingly difficult to walk in the dark since he cannot then use his sense of sight to replace his lost kinaesthetic sense. Eventually, as long as he remains able to walk at all, he shows a characteristic stamping gait in which he lifts his legs too high, performs unnecessary movements in an attempt to control them, and brings them down rather wide apart to give him a wide base, and unnecessarily hard on the heels to make him aware of the moment when the feet reach the ground. There will come a time when, owing to extreme ataxia, he is unable to walk at all although his muscle power is little affected.

These patients show a positive Rhomberg's sign owing to the kinaesthetic and cutaneous sensory loss, that is, they are more unsteady when standing with the feet together and the eyes shut than in the same position with the eyes open.

Muscle tone is invariably reduced owing to the interruption of incoming messages, consequently the joints may be taken through an abnormally wide range of movement and ligaments are liable to damage. Owing to hypotonia and ligamentous laxity in an already ataxic patient, falls occur readily.

Certain other less common signs may also be present. Owing to sensory impairment, the skin is particularly liable to be damaged and deep penetrating ulcers may be found on the soles of the feet. Spontaneous swelling of joints following some very minor trauma may progress to gross joint changes and complete disorganisation. This is probably the result of unrecognised trauma and inability to experience pain so that the joint is not adequately protected. Occasionally the patient suffers from visceral crises for which no explanation can be offered. Of these, the gastric crisis, in which the patient suffers from pain and vomiting, though abdominal tenderness and rigidity are usually absent, is most common. Some hesitancy in micturition with dribbling of urine and retention are nearly always present. This leads to discomfort which seems to increase the lightning pains, and, more serious still, to infection of the bladder, chronic cystitis and toxaemia affecting the patient's general health and leading to an emaciated and cachectic appearance.

OUTLINE OF TREATMENT BY PHYSIOTHERAPY

Tabetic patients showing ataxia benefit from physiotherapy. Massage may help to improve the nutrition of the muscles, active movements may stimulate their tone, while strengthening exercises may reduce the atrophy which accompanies Charcot's joints, but the really valuable treatment is that provided by precision exercises combined with the use of proprioceptive stimuli and successive induction. The precision exercises were devised by Dr. Fraenkel who found that his tabetic patients improved when treated by simple exercises, constantly repeated. It was thought that the good effect obtained was the result of the improvement of muscular condition, but it is now known that this is not so; but that the improvement is due to the extra work thrown on unaffected nerve fibres and to the bringing into action of 'dormant' neurones and alternative pathways.

The procedure adopted is to examine the patient to find out what movements he can do in a co-ordinated manner. This will indicate the stage at which exercises can be commenced. The exercises are then chosen accordingly. The purpose and method of performance of the exercises is explained to the patient and a clear demonstration given. Stress must be laid on the value of smooth movement so that every effort possible is made to perform the movement with precision. The patient is then placed on a plinth well propped up so that he is able to watch without effort what he is doing. It should be arranged that the limbs can move on a perfectly smooth surface so that friction does not hamper movement and cause inco-ordination. Many patients can perform the movements more smoothly if they are carried out on a marked board to counting. Both patient and physiotherapist may count but it must be done in an even rather sing-song voice to encourage smoothness and avoid jerks. Use of every possible sense to aid co-ordination should be made; thus sight, sound and touch should be employed. To obtain the latter the legs should be free from clothing and to begin with, at least, the heel should make contact with the surface.

Progression is made by passing from a simple movement to a slightly more complicated one, but this is only allowed when the first movement is perfect. Later the same exercises may be practised with the eyes closed. Patients less severely affected may require mainly exercises in standing and walking. The patient is trained in these exercises on the same lines as in the simpler movements, progression being made from walking in marked footsteps, to walking along a line and on a form, to turning round, walking round objects, and negotiating stairs. It is possible with care and constant practice to get a patient, who is almost unable to walk at all, onto his feet and walking unaided once more.

Considerable care is required not to tire the patient as he seldom feels fatigue owing to the diminished sensation, and yet he suffers from the effects of fatigue early because so much energy is wasted in incoordinate movements. A second precaution is to be sure that the patient is not allowed to fall. As previously pointed out he falls easily and this may result in fracture of bones, which are often unduly brittle in this disease, or in the precipitation of a Charcot's joint. In addition, if the patient falls he loses confidence both in himself and in the physiotherapist.

If a Charcot's joint is present it will most likely be the knee which is involved; weight bearing without support should not then be allowed and a plaster splint is usually worn.

Sunlight or heat may be used to help to promote healing of penetrating ulcers and, if so, precautions must be taken bearing in mind the reduced sensibility of the area.

Chapter VIII

SUBACUTE COMBINED DEGENERATION OF THE CORD. AFFECTIONS OF THE CORPUS STRIATUM

SUBACUTE COMBINED DEGENERATION OF THE CORD

This disease is so called because it is a progressive degeneration of the posterior and lateral columns of the spinal cord. It has a close association with pernicious anaemia, although the changes in the nervous system may be well advanced before the onset of the anaemia, or may occur very soon afterwards. The severity of the condition bears, therefore, no relationship to the severity of pernicious anaemia. It is possible that the lesions are the result of an absence of a factor produced in the stomach and stored in the liver, but whether this factor is identical with that responsible for the full development of the red blood corpuscle is not certain.

The disease is seen most commonly in elderly people of both sexes. The lesions usually attack the mid-dorsal region of the cord but ascending degeneration may involve the cervical region and descending degeneration the lumbar. The primary change is a progressive demyelination of the nerve fibres until eventually the myelin sheath is completely destroyed. Later the axis cylinders also disappear. A rather unusual feature is the absence of any neuroglial reaction. In the majority of cases the peripheral nerves are affected, a definite neuritis being present.

There is a characteristic onset, whatever area is most involved. The patient complains of tingling, numbness and a feeling of 'pins and needles' in the tips of the fingers and toes. Numbness of the fingers leads to clumsiness in the fine movements of the hand. Sometimes, as a result of impaired sensation in the soles of the feet, the patient feels as if he is walking on cotton wool. These symptoms are the result of changes in the posterior columns. Gradually some degree of sensory ataxia develops with consequently unsteadiness in gait. Heaviness and weakness of the legs with undue fatigue on walking may indicate early changes in the lateral columns.

On examination it will be found, in many cases, that symptoms of anaemia are present. There are gastro-intestinal disturbances, a yellowish tint of the skin with a bright malar flush, swelling of the feet and ankles, breathlessness on exertion and pallor of the lips and mucous membranes.

The development of signs and symptoms depends on which areas suffer most from degenerative changes. Two particular types usually emerge: a flaccid type and a spastic.

The flaccid variety is the result of peripheral neuritis and presents muscular weakness and hypotonia, loss of deep reflexes and tenderness of the muscles on pressure. Muscular weakness leads to difficulty in walking and early fatigue. Some degree of sensory impairment, ataxia and Rhombergism will be the result of changes in the posterior columns, while an extensor plantar response will indicate the presence of a lesion in the lateral cortico-spinal tracts.

The spastic type will result from lesions mainly attacking the lateral columns, though in these cases considerable changes also occur in the posterior columns. Symptoms characteristic of pyramidal lesions are present; extensor spasticity and weakness of the legs, exaggeration of deep reflexes, a plantar extensor response and sometimes ankle clonus. Some sensory disturbance will be present but spastic weakness may mask the sensory ataxia. Eventually paraplegia-in-extension may change to paraplegia-in-flexion.

The outlook for the patient depends very largely on the type of case. Changes in peripheral nerves are reversible while those occurring in the spinal cord are not. This is due to the fact that regrowth of degenerated fibres is only possible in the presence of a neurilemma sheath. Such a sheath surrounds the axons of the peripheral nerves but is absent from those in the spinal cord. Provided the cause can be alleviated and the condition is an early one, almost complete recovery may occur in the flaccid type though paraesthesia will remain. Little improvement can be expected in the spastic cases though further changes may be arrested.

OUTLINE OF TREATMENT BY PHYSIOTHERAPY

Treatment by physical measures varies with the type. The spastic type will require treatment on the lines indicated either for paraplegia-in-extension or paraplegia-in-flexion according to the stage of the condition.

For the flaccid type with hope of improvement considerably more can be done. The main objects of treatment will be to assist the recovery of power in the limb muscles and to improve the co-ordination.

The first aim is fulfilled by the use of massage to aid the circulation and nutrition of the muscle groups, and by carefully graded strengthening exercises. A voluntary muscle test is carried out for all the muscles of the arms, legs and trunk and re-education will be commenced according to the results of this test. If there is much muscle tenderness, heat may be given and massage modified. Great care must be taken to avoid fatigue.

Training co-ordination requires skilful handling. If the muscles are very weak the usual Fraenkel's exercises may be impossible. In this case, during the performance of assisted active strengthening exercises, great care is taken to insist on the movements being performed slowly and rhythmically with avoidance of irregularities of movement. As power improves Fraenkel's exercises will be gradually introduced, the patient being encouraged to use the sense of sight to replace the lost muscle and joint sense. Later, progression is made to exercises in standing and to walking exercises as in the cases of tabes dorsalis. Even though the changes in the posterior column are irreversible provided they are not too far advanced much improvement can be gained in co-ordination partly by substituting the sense of sight and partly by the hypertrophy of the remaining healthy fibres.

AFFECTIONS OF THE CORPUS STRIATUM

The corpus striatum consists of the caudate and lenticular nuclei, the latter showing an outer part, the putamen, and an inner, the globus pallidus. Afferent fibres reach the corpus striatum from the cerebral cortex, thalamus and mid-brain, while efferent fibres pass to the thalamus, substantia nigra red nucleus and reticular formation of the brain stem. From the red nucleus and the reticular formation messages are conveyed by the fibres of the reticulo-spinal tract to the anterior horn cells and lower motor neurones.

Uncertainty exists as to the exact function of the corpus striatum. It is subordinate to the cerebral cortex and has consequently a reinforcing action on voluntary movement. It is probably responsible for semi-automatic and emotional movements. It exerts a controlling influence over lower centres which in their turn control the tone of voluntary muscles and, in addition, it exerts a steadying influence over the innervation of the lower motor neurone by the upper so that if its influence is removed tremor occurs.

Outstanding features of lesions of the corpus striatum are, therefore, slowing and weakening of voluntary movement, increase of muscle tone, tremors and diminution or loss of emotional and automatic movements. Lesions of the corpus striatum which most often produce symptoms requiring treatment by physical measures are paralysis agitans, chorea and post-encephalitic parkinsonism, the last of these has been dealt with elsewhere (see Chapter V, Part IV).

PARALYSIS AGITANS

This condition, often known as Parkinson's disease, after Dr. James Parkinson who first described it, is a degenerative lesion of the cells of the corpus striatum. The degeneration is probably part of a generalised senile change and often so many cells are affected that minute holes appear as the necrotic tissue is absorbed.

Paralysis agitans invariably occurs in later life usually not earlier than fifty or later than sixty-five. It is about twice as common in males as in females. The condition is characterised by muscular rigidity, tremors, and the gradual slowing and weakening of voluntary and emotional movements.

Tremor is often the first symptom. It consists of a rhythmical alternating contraction of opposing muscle groups at the rate of about four to eight per second. It often ceases during active movement of the part and appears when the limb is at rest, particularly if it is unsupported. The tremor disappears during sleep. Usually it commences in the fingers and thumb of one hand resulting in a 'pill-rolling' movement, spreads to a flexion and extension of the wrist and later may involve all muscle groups of the arm. In many cases the leg of the same side is next affected, particularly noticeable is an alternate flexion and extension movement of the ankle. Next attacked will be the opposite arm and leg. The head may show a flexion and extension or rotatory movement.

Rigidity is practically always present. It differs from the increase in tone of a pyramidal lesion in that it is equal in all muscle groups, and is maintained throughout the whole range of passive movements though full range passive movements are nearly always possible. The muscles yield in a series of jerks, giving rise to the nomenclature of 'cog-wheel' rigidity. Very occasionally this rigidity results in deformities, particularly severe flexion of the fingers and flexion of the trunk.

As a result of hypertonia, fatigue, discomfort and even pain are complained of in the limbs and back, this is also due to the altered position of the joint structures and the abnormal posture imposed on the individual as a result of rigidity and muscular weakness.

Weakness and slowness of voluntary movement are particularly noticeable in the small muscles and fine movements, as a result speech becomes slurred and monotonous, and mastication and deglutition slow and difficult. Movements of the fingers are clumsy, with the result that writing, tying laces or doing up buttons, brushing the hair, gripping a knife or fork all become increasingly difficult. The weakness and slowness are increased by the rigidity which damps down the range of active movement.

Weakness and rigidity are together responsible for alterations in stance and gait. Gradually a bowed position is imposed upon the patient. The head is flexed, the trunk bent, the arms adducted and flexed, forearms pronated, fingers bent at the metacarpo-phalangeal joints and usually straight at the interphalangeal joints, the thumb lying against the palmar surface of the index finger. Knees and hips are slightly flexed. The result of this position is to cause the centre of gravity to fall towards the front of the base and balance is therefore easily upset. Due to the flexed attitude and the rigidity, the patient takes short, shuffling small steps in walking and is unable to stop quickly if someone gets in his way; he may then even take a few steps backward. Owing to loss of semi-automatic movements there is an absence of the swing of the arms in walking, a point unnoted by the patient until his attention is drawn to it.

Weakness of emotional movements together with rigidity give the patient a peculiar masklike expression known as the parkinsonian mask. Blinking is infrequent, the eyes stare, the mouth usually remains slightly open, the face fails to light up in conversation, smiling is slow to develop but also slow to disappear.

Owing to hypertonia reflexes are difficult to elicit but the plantar response will be normal. Sometimes disturbances of the autonomic system occur, there is then excessive salivation, abnormal activity of the sebaceous glands and a flushing of the skin.

The condition is slowly progressive and eventually activity becomes more and more limited until the patient may become completely immobile. The patient remains bright and mentally alert. Intelligence is not affected but there are definite changes in personality, the patient becoming querulous, irritable and inconsistent in behaviour.

OUTLINE OF TREATMENT BY PHYSIOTHERAPY

Though the condition is slowly progressive and no cure is possible as yet, the patient can be helped a great deal by physiotherapy treatment. One of the most important objects is to relieve the aching, fatigue and pain. Since this discomfort is largely due to the hypertonia with consequent impairment of circulation and accumulation of fatigue products, measures which even temporarily reduce tone and promote a freer blood flow will give relief. One of the most effective measures is general diathermy since this causes a slight general rise of temperature with drop in muscle tone, and widespread vaso-dilatation. If this is given in a suitable position, with the patient as nearly lying as is comfortable and all parts of the body well supported with pillows, the patient can practise relaxation immediately following the diathermy without disturbance of the position. The method of contracting muscle groups and then relaxing should be avoided. The most satisfactory way is to think of each group and to try to let some of the tension go. A general massage may follow the diathermy and relaxation practice. This will be carried out deeply, slowly and rhythmically, passing with perfect continuity from one part of the body to another. Abdominal massage will not be omitted since it will help to relieve the constipation so often present.

A second very important object is an attempt to improve the posture of the joints and to prevent deformities. Since faulty posture and deformities are due to muscular weakness and rigidity followed by adaptive shortening of fibrous structures, very rhythmical passive movements may follow the general massage. The movements will be slow and carried out in full range, particular attention being given to the fingers and the head. These movements will be followed by a very careful attempt to strengthen the anti-gravity muscles. Without moving the patient's position contractions of the neck extensors, rhomboids, extensors of the spine, glutei, quadriceps, deltoids and triceps may be taught.

Later pillows may be removed and larger range extension movements performed. Gradually sling and spring work may be added. Very gradual gentle progression may lead to the performance of these exercises in sitting, standing and walking, using a mirror to assist maintenance of good posture.

A third object of physiotherapy, equally important, is to gain quicker, stronger voluntary movements and to substitute for lost automatic movements voluntary movements. Rhythmic, loose, large range swinging movements are necessary here. Great patience is used in teaching relaxed movements. Surprisingly good results are obtained by the use of movements to music, and ball work. Functional movements require special attention and walking to music, learning also to perform voluntary arm swing, is concentrated on. Important also is the practice of fine movements of the hand.

At no time should these patients be hurried or worried. Sufficient time must be allotted to their treatment so that no element of rush enters into the session. Care has to be taken to avoid chill as these patients rarely feel the cold and great attention must be given to the avoidance of fatigue, longer than normal rests being given between exercises. Kabat claims that facilitation techniques are of value in the treatment of these patients. Particularly valuable is the use of mass movement patterns, probably because there will be excitation of inhibitary mechanisms which bring about reduction of rigidity. He finds also that reversal of antagonists and rhythmic stabilisation appear to help the patient considerably. The use of these techniques has not been widely tried out in this country and it is early, therefore, to discuss their value but they warrant trial.

RHEUMATIC CHOREA (SYDENHAM'S CHOREA)

This is an acute toxic infection of the central nervous system, characterised by jerky, irregular, involuntary movements and some degree of hypotonia and muscular weakness. It occurs in females three times as commonly as in males, a very large proportion of the cases appearing between the ages of five and fifteen. Chorea is a manifestation of acute rheumatism and may be complicated by other rheumatic conditions such as endocarditis and erythema nodosum. The precipitating factor appears often to be some mental stress such as overwork at school, shock or fright, bad home circumstances or even illness or trauma. In the cases which reach the postmortem room no very constant changes can be seen. There is usually a hyperaemia, slight degree of degeneration of nerve cells, and an infiltration of lymphocytes around the blood vessels, occurring in the cerebral cortex, corpus striatum and substantia nigra. The condition is insidious in onset.

A few weeks before choreic movements are actually seen the child seems unwell, is irritable, fretful, sleeps badly and cries easily. A mild degree of motor restlessness is seen, there is clumsiness so that the child drops things, and fidgetiness. If asked to do some task the child is inclined to rush at the job and put unnecessary energy into its performance.

Gradually the characteristic movements and muscular hypotonia make their appearance. Usually the movements are sudden, irregular, apparently purposeless, and are often superimposed on voluntary movements rendering the latter incoordinate. In the face these movements are bilateral, a raising of the eyebrows, grimacing, protrusion of the tongue are common movements. The arms are most involved, a sudden jerking of one shoulder or violent extension of the whole arm may be seen. The respiratory movements are often involved and breathing becomes jerky and irregular. Mastication, speech and deglutition may all be disturbed. One particular feature is an irregular waxing and waning in muscular strength, clearly felt if the child is asked to shake hands with the physiotherapist. Again, the involuntary movements normally associated with strong voluntary movements are grossly exaggerated; thus, for example, a vigorous closure of the fist may be accompanied by movements of the whole arm, face and trunk. Co-ordinated work is usually much impaired, sometimes both antagonists and agonists work together or contraction of synergists may be too great for that of the prime movers.

Muscular hypotonia is always present with the result that movements can be carried beyond their normal range. Some degree of muscular weakness may also be detected. Reflexes are usually diminished and difficult to elicit. Irregular action of the heart is another characteristic feature and tachycardia is nearly always present. In some cases, particularly in second or third attacks of chorea, the heart is also affected by the rheumatic toxin and a myocarditis with cardiac enlargement, or an endocarditis leaving some valvular defect will result.

Most cases progress for one or two weeks, remain stationary for several and then gradually subside. Complete cure is rarely obtained under two or three months. Relapses are common and subsequent attacks tend to be complicated by cardiac involvement. An attack during pregnancy is not uncommon in women who have suffered from the condition in childhood or adolescence.

OUTLINE OF TREATMENT BY PHYSIOTHERAPY

Children suffering from this condition are usually kept in bed for several weeks and in the later stages of this period of rest physiotherapy may be started. The main aims of physical treatment are to improve the condition of the musculature and train the child to gain control over the voluntary movements. It is necessary to know whether there is any cardiac involvement in planning the treatment.

The first step in treatment is to gain the child's confidence and a daily visit and chat a few days before physiotherapy is started is helpful to achieve this end. Treatment is introduced gradually, beginning with general massage and relaxation exercises and progressing to the simplest voluntary movements performed rhythmically, often to music. Breathing exercises are given early, the child being encouraged to perform slow inspiratory and expiratory movements to counting. Although the active movements are partly given to strengthen muscles their main object is to gain control. The patient is encouraged to perform them smoothly and without jerks and if jerkiness does occur the movement is stopped, relaxation is practised and then the movement is repeated. Care must be taken if the child is asked to try to lie still for increasing lengths of time because, though the choreic movements can often be controlled and inhibited for a certain length of time, after such an effort they may reoccur more severely. For this reason it is probably better to concentrate on good performance of movements and on learning how to relax. As improvement takes place more complicated movements are added and the child is introduced to games which require some co-ordination, particularly of the forearm muscles and hands. In the very latest stages balance exercises, asymmetrical work, dancing and singing will prove interesting and useful.

Chapter IX

LESIONS OF SPINAL NERVES

A spinal nerve is connected to a segment of the spinal cord by two nerve roots. The anterior root consists mainly of motor fibres, axons of cells of the anterior horn of the spinal cord, the posterior root sensory fibres, axons of cells of the posterior nerve root ganglion. The two roots unite before passing through the intervertebral foramen and issuing as a mixed spinal nerve. Each nerve then divides into anterior and posterior primary rami. With the exception of the dorsal nerves the anterior primary rami unite in various ways to form plexuses from which the main nerves of the limbs are derived. Thus a limb nerve may contain fibres from several segments of the spinal cord.

Each typical spinal or cranial nerve consists of a varying number of nerve fibres in a supporting framework and sheath of connective tissue. Blood vessels supplying the nerve fibres with oxygen and nutrient products form a network in this framework. In a 'mixed' nerve the fibres belong to three groups, motor, sensory and sympathetic.

A motor fibre consists of the axon of a cell in the anterior horn of grey matter of the spinal cord, the fatty sheath of Schwann (myelin sheath), interrupted at intervals at the nodes of Ranvier, and an outer delicate, but tough, homogeneous sheath, the neurilemma. Immediately beneath the neurilemma are oval nuclei embedded in a tiny mass of protoplasm. Each fibre ends by dividing into a number of fibrils, a single fibril terminating in a motor-end plate. By this arrangement one nerve fibre supplies a varying number of muscle fibres. The motor fibres are the largest fibres in the mixed nerve consequently they conduct messages at the greatest speed.

The motor fibre, its cells, and the muscle fibres it supplies, form a motor unit. The pathway the cell and fibre provides is the only way by which messages can reach the muscle fibres. For this reason it is often spoken of as the Final Common Pathway.

Sensory fibres resemble in structure the motor fibres but they are the peripheral part of the single process of the cells of the posterior nerve root ganglion. These axons terminate by special nerve terminations which vary according to the sensations they subserve in skin, muscles, joints and in fact in practically all tissues. Sensory nerve fibres vary in size being always smaller than the motor but larger than the sympathetic fibres. Fibres conveying vibration and joint sense are the largest, those conveying painful stimuli the smallest of the sensory fibres.

Sympathetic fibres differ from the preceding since they have no myelin sheath. They are post ganglionic fibres arising from cells of the sympathetic ganglia, the preganglionic fibres arising from cells in the lateral horn of grey matter of the cord. Their function is to innervate involuntary structures such as the blood vessels, sweat and sebaceous glands. They are the smallest of all the fibres.

If a nerve is completely severed all the fibres will be interrupted and degenerative changes will occur. These changes were first described by Waller, and so to them the term Wallerian degeneration has been applied. Immediately following severance of the nerve, the axons distal to the lesion break up into segments, the myelin sheaths disintegrate into fatty droplets and the debris of both is gradually removed by phagocytic action of leucocytes from neighbouring tissues, leaving an empty tube. The neurilemma for a time at least, remains intact but thickens, its nuclei enlarge and multiply and the protoplasm increases in quantity.

Proximal to the lesion similar changes occur as far back as the first node of Ranvier. Changes occur also in the cells of origin of the damaged fibres. The Nissl granules break up, the neurofibrils disappear, the nucleus is displaced to the side of the cell and the cell body swells.

Regeneration of nerve fibres will take place provided each fibre has a neurilemma, provided there is not too great a gap between the severed ends and providing there is nothing in the way of the growth of the fibre. Then, the proximal end of the axon will grow, throwing out a little tuft of neurofibrils. Those which fail to find a neurilemmal tube disappear, the remainder grow down the tubes at the rate of approximately a millimetre a day.

Complete severance of nerves results not only in Wallerian degeneration but also in serious changes in tissues innervated by the damaged fibres. Muscles will show profound atrophy, this is partly because all tone and power of contraction is lost and therefore katabolic processes are gravely diminished, and partly due to the fact that the blood supply is much impaired, since the pumping action of muscular contraction and joint movement is lost, while more important still, the blood vessels are paralysed and circulatory congestion results. After a lengthy period, if recovery does not occur and maintenance of circulation is ineffective, the muscle fibres will shrink and the fibrous framework of the muscle will thicken and shorten.

Joints suffer also because circulatory impairment, together with diminished or lost sensation, are likely to be followed by degenerative changes in joint structures. In addition circulatory congestion leads to oedema and so to adhesion formation, contracture of the capsule and joint stiffness.

The skin suffers severely if its blood vessels are paralysed and the glands no longer active. Absence of sebum results in a hard scaly skin, deficient sweat means a dry skin, while poor circulation causes a thin atrophic appearance, smooth because the hairs gradually fall out. If the sensory nerve endings are out of action, the skin is very readily damaged and, owing to its poor nutrition, once damaged is not easily healed.

It will be understood that, to a very great extent, the chances of a good recovery following a nerve lesion depend on the condition of these structures.

Types of Nerve Lesions

Seddon has classified nerve lesions into three main types, neurotmesis, axonotmesis and neurapraxia. All these types may be present in the same nerve at the same time. Neurotmesis means 'nerve cut', hence this is a lesion in which the whole or part of a nerve is completely severed and the continuity of fibres and connective tissue interrupted. All messages, motor, sensory and sympathetic will be lost and all severed axons will degenerate. The reaction of degeneration must therefore be present.

In axonotmesis the axons are severed but the tougher connective tissue remains intact. No gap will, therefore, be present and each axon lies opposite its original neurilemma. Degeneration of the fibres distal to the lesion will take place, and the reaction of degeneration will be present but recovery is likely to be quicker and more perfect than in a neurotmesis.

Neurapraxia means 'nerve not functioning'. Although there is no break in the anatomical continuity the fibres cease to conduct messages. Exactly what has happened is not possible to say but it may be that the blood supply has been disturbed and consequently function is impaired. Degeneration does not occur since the axons are still in connection with their cells. A variety of electrical responses may be seen. Usually recovery occurs within a few minutes to several months but in a patchy manner.

Recovery

The rate and extent of recovery depend on two main points—the type of injury and the condition of the muscles, skin and joints. With the first the physiotherapist is not directly concerned, with the second she may play an important part.

The type of injury. The best recovery is likely to be obtained in a neurapraxia where no degeneration occurs. Recovery should be perfect in an axonotmesis but will, of course, take longer, the time depending on the distance of the last structures to be supplied, from the site of the injury.

Results will rarely be so good in the case of a complete neurotmesis. In this instance spontaneous recovery is unlikely because a gap between the severed nerve ends is inevitable. This gap will be filled with blood-clot, exudate and cells and if left alone organisation into scar tissue will occur. In this scar tissue growing nerve fibres will be trapped. Consequently suture of the nerve sheath is essential. Even then, two disadvantages occur; first, some scar tissue must form, second, however carefully the suture is carried out it is impossible to ensure that each growing axon now lies opposite its original neurilemma, hence the fibre may very easily grow down the wrong neurilemma and eventually may reach a wrong termination. This might not be so serious if the severed nerve were entirely motor but it will matter if a motor axon grows to a sensory termination. For these two reasons recovery is less likely to be perfect, especially in the case of mixed nerves. In addition, there will be considerable delay in the start of regeneration, since there may be a period before suture can safely be performed and there will be anything from thirty to sixty days while the fibres grow across the gap and find the neurilemmal tubes. For every day of delay in regeneration there is more possibility of serious changes in the end organs.

The condition of muscles, joints and skin. Changes rapidly take place in all the structures solely supplied by the affected nerve. If nothing is done to minimise these changes stiff joints, grossly atrophied muscles, and damaged and inelastic skin will be the result. Perfect regeneration of nerve will then never produce perfect function. In addition actual resistance to recovery is present since weak, atrophied muscles cannot move stiff joints.

Sites and Results of Injury

Nerves may be injured in any part of their course, though for each nerve there are usually certain particular points at which there is most likelihood of damage.

The roots of the nerves may be stretched or pressed upon as a result of a tumour, extra or intra-dural or a herniated nucleus pulposus, they may be contused in fractures or dislocations of the vertebrae, and even torn from their attachment to the cord by violent stretching injuries. In such cases all structures receiving their innervation from these roots will be affected. The distribution of paralysis and sensory loss will be segmental, that is, certain myotomes and dermatomes will be affected. A myotome is a group of muscles supplied by one segment of the spinal cord, the motor fibres of this segment passing through the anterior nerve root to the plexus and so through one or more limb nerves to the muscles. Thus, for example, injury to the seventh cervical root will affect coraco-brachialis, triceps, anconeus and the extensors of the forearm, though none of these will be completely paralysed since all receive part of their innervation from other segments of the cord.

A dermatome is the area of the skin supplied by a single posterior nerve root. As the limbs develop during foetal life, the dermatomes migrate from the trunk, in the upper extremity becoming mainly parallel with the long axis of the limb, the higher segments distributed along the lateral border, the lower along the medial. In the lower limbs the position is rather different because owing to rotation of the lower extremities, the distribution is arranged in a semi-spiral manner. Much overlapping of dermatomes occur consequently damage of one nerve root rarely leads to loss of cutaneous sensibility (see Fig. 8).

The plexus may be involved in penetrating or blast wounds stretching injuries or inflammatory conditions of surrounding soft tissues. The structures affected will depend on the number of nerve roots entering into the damaged part of the plexus and on the exact site of the lesion. Distribution will not be entirely segmental as more than one segment will probably be involved and not necessarily the whole of each segment.

Nerves derived from the plexus may be damaged in many ways; severance in lacerated wounds, crushing, nipping between fractured bone ends, or stretching as a result of joint dislocations, continued friction as in a roughened groove, or by repeated pressure. Since the nerve contains fibres from several nerve roots distribution is not segmental but, if the nerve is completely severed, all structures solely supplied by that nerve will be denervated. The area of skin supplied by the nerve will not be completely anaesthetic since much overlapping of supply occurs, usually a small central area will show complete loss while around this region will be zones of diminished sensibility.

Diagnosis

It is not part of the physiotherapist's work to diagnose the type of lesion but she may be asked to assist the surgeon or physician by carrying out a voluntary muscle test and by testing the electrical reactions of nerve and

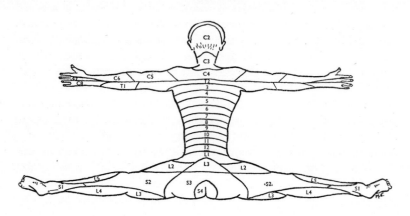

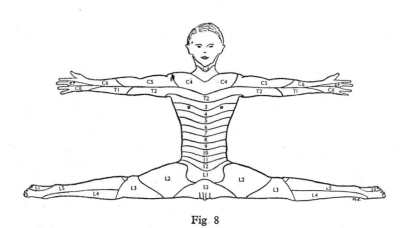

Fig 8

muscle. A decision as to the type of lesion and therefore as to the treatment necessary, will be made partly on these points but also on the nature of the injury, the changes in sensation and the presence or absence of sweating. It is well worth noting that in any one nerve all types of lesion may be present at the same time and that in an axonotmesis not all fibres may be ruptured. If only some fibres are affected it will be the largest which are most likely to suffer and in some cases the tiny sympathetic fibres are the only ones left intact. The presence of sweating on a sweat test, when all other functions of the nerve are lost, will indicate that there is still some conductivity in the nerve and a complete neurotmesis cannot therefore be present.

Voluntary muscle tests are usually carried out by the physiotherapist, since they will need to be performed repeatedly and it is essential that the worker making the first test should also perform the later tests, if any degree of accuracy is to be obtained. The method of charting should be that used by the Medical Research Council. The electrical reactions of nerve and muscle are usually tested after ten to twenty days, when Wallerian degeneration will be complete. This test may be performed by the Physical Medicine Specialist but where he is not available it will have to be carried out by a qualified physiotherapist. Up to recent times the tests were made by the use of the interrupted galvanic and faradic currents, but this was neither a very accurate nor satisfactory method. Tests are now made by the use of strength-duration curves and by electro myography, the latter invariably carried out by the surgeon or physician.

PRINCIPLES OF TREATMENT BY PHYSIOTHERAPY

Cases will roughly fall into two main groups, those in which there is no recovery, and those in which recovery has just commenced or is well on its way.

Cases in Which Signs of Recovery Are Not Yet Present

This group will include cases of neurotmesis, in which as yet suture cannot be carried out or in which suture has been performed but it is too early to expect recovery; axonotmesis in which growth is not sufficient to reach the structures innervated by the nerve, and early cases of neurapraxia. Probably the most important principle is to gain the patient's co-operation and maintain his morale. Almost invariably this will be done if, where it is possible, the rate of the growth of fibres is simply explained, together with the changes which may occur if suitable treatment is not carried out, and if the approximate date at which the first signs of recovery may be expected to appear is indicated. Any slight sign of improvement should be pointed out and all possible encouragement given.

The second principle is to try to prevent changes occurring in the muscles, joints and skin. It is, of course, quite impossible to prevent muscle atrophy, since this is very largely due to absence of function and therefore diminished katabolism. Excessive atrophy and gradual degeneration of fibres with replacement by fibrous tissue can, however, be prevented if the muscle is kept artificially contracting for a period, once or twice daily. This can be done by the use of an interrupted electrical current with a sufficiently long period of flow to stimulate muscle fibres directly, independently of their nerve supply. This treatment will not only stimulate katabolism, but will also have the effect of exerting a pumping action upon the blood vessels and thus will lessen congestion and oedema.

Stiff joints may be prevented if they are exercised in their full range daily. The first step is to test the range on the unaffected limb so that the normal range is known, and then the joint may be firmly grasped, traction exerted and one full range passive movement, in each direction of which the joint is capable, performed. No harmful stretching of paralysed muscles will occur, provided the joint is not carried beyond its normal range. Ideally active movement is best, and this can sometimes be arranged by the use of 'lively' splints, in which a spring simulates the action of the paralysed muscle, then healthy antagonists can contract moving the joint in practically full range while the splint returns the joints to their original position. The danger of stiff joints and degenerative changes in the skin arising as a result of oedema and defective circulation may be slightly lessened by the use of extremely light massage, of short duration, or by the administration of stabile galvanism, provided any loss of sensation is noted and precautions taken. Elevation of the limb is also useful.

The third principle is to prevent the development of contractures and deformities which, if they occur, will hamper recovery. There is a tendency, if a joint is kept at rest, for the capsule to lose its pliability and to contract. The deformity may also be due to the effects of gravity on paralysed muscles, for example, if the extensors of the wrist are paralysed the joint tends to fall into flexion and as no power of active extension is present it remains in this position and adaptive shortening of the antagonistic muscles tends to occur. Shortening of the fibro-elastic elements of the affected muscles may also develop if splinting is maintained too long, with the affected muscles in their short position.

Deformities may be prevented by the use of 'lively' splints where possible. In any case, steps must be taken to support the affected muscles in some part of their inner range, but the support must be taken off several times daily to permit of full range passive movements. Splints must be very carefully checked to see that they fulfil their purposes, that they are light, fit well and are properly applied. This check is particularly important in the case of growing children since splints rapidly become too small.

An important principle is to prevent damage to paralysed muscles, for bruising and continual stretching will retard recovery. Stretching may be prevented by the use of splints and by care in movements, bruising by gentle handling and by the prevention of pressure on a paralysed group.

It is very important indeed to prevent the brain from forgetting the movement which is lost as a result of paralysis. The motor area of the cortex very readily discards a movement which is no longer being performed. When recovery of the muscle occurs much time may then be necessary to re-educate the forgotten movement. This complication is quite unnecessary if the patient co-operates by concentrating on, and thinking of, the movement when the physiotherapist is performing it, so keeping the nerve pathways open, until movement is again possible.

One particular precaution must be mentioned here. If a nerve will have to be sutured, or if suture has already been carried out, the limb will probably be encased in plaster of paris, in the position which approximates the ends of the sutured nerve, for a period varying according to the degree of damage and the type of operation needed, in many cases of about three to five weeks. During this time only those areas not enclosed will receive physiotherapy, but all measures possible should be used to maintain the circulation of the limb and to keep joints moving. When the plaster is removed a different type of splint will be substituted and physiotherapy can then be given as indicated previously, but care must be taken not to stretch the sutured nerve for a minimum period of eight weeks.

Cases in Which Recovery is Beginning

When signs of recovery first appear, there will be some tone in the first muscle to receive innervation by the growing nerve, but no alteration in the other muscles, skin or joints not as yet reached by the nerve. For this reason it is still necessary to carry out all the principles of treatment previously in use, but in addition re-education must now be added. The term re-education covers a wide field. It will be carried out on the same lines as indicated in the convalescent stage of anterior poliomyelitis, though in this case it is the hypertrophy of all the motor units rather than of some only. The cells in the anterior horn have not been active because their axons have been severed, therefore the cells require a greater excitation when the axons have grown again. Facilitation techniques, therefore, may be used to gain maximum excitation of the anterior horn cells.

Trick Movements

A trick movement is one which is performed in some other manner than by the use of the normal prime movers. Such a movement, though often reasonably useful, is rarely so effective or powerful as the normal action. Trick movements are very readily learnt by a patient who loses the use of certain muscles, though he is rarely conscious of how he has acquired them.

If no recovery can be expected, as for example, in some cases of spinal tumour, trick movements are obviously valuable, but if recovery will occur they may be used at the expense of the recovering muscles which will then not be exercised sufficiently. For this reason it is essential for the physiotherapist to recognise the development of these movements, to encourage them where necessary but to prevent them during active re-education and voluntary muscle tests.

Several types of trick movements may be found. One of the commonest of these is the use of other muscles to perform the movement. The use of gluteus maximus to extend the knee, when the quadriceps group is paralysed, is familiar to all physiotherapists. Opposition of the thumb may be produced by the action of the adductor pollicis and the flexor pollicis longus muscles. Abduction and adduction of the fingers may be performed weakly by contraction of the long extensors and flexors respectively.

Another way in which a movement may be produced is by a rebound of the paralysed muscle. This is most often seen when the long extensor of the thumb is paralysed. The patient flexes the terminal joint of the thumb when asked to straighten the tip, then relaxes the flexor, and the terminal phalanx springs back. It is probable in this case that some fibrosis of the paralysed muscle has occurred.

In cases where muscles have several insertions and a double innervation, part may be paralysed while the rest is unaffected. In this case the unaffected part may 'drag' on the paralysed section and movement may be produced. Thus for example in a lesion of the median nerve, flexion of the tip of the middle finger may be produced by the contraction of the fibres of the medial half of flexor profundis.

Occasionally, in spite of complete severance of the nerve, the muscles may still contract. In this case they are probably innervated by another nerve. Such a condition is not uncommonly seen in the hand where in spite of laceration of the median nerve at the wrist, opponens and abductor pollicis are still working. These muscles in this case are supplied by the ulnar nerve. The only possible way of proving this when making a voluntary muscle test, is to anaesthetize the ulnar nerve, then absence of contraction of these muscles will prove the presence of an anomalous nerve supply.

Occasionally a movement may be tricked by another muscle pulling on the origin of the paralysed muscle. A typical example of this is seen in damage to the ulnar nerve in the hand, abduction of the little finger which should be absent may be produced by the pull of flexor carpi ulnaris jerking the pisiform bone.

It is clear that in making a muscle test very great care must be taken to obviate these trick movements or an incorrect diagnosis may be made.

Chapter X

LESIONS OF SPINAL NERVES (*Contd.*)

It would be impossible in this textbook to give a detailed description of every possible nerve injury but if the principles set out in the last chapter are followed no difficulty should be experienced in working out the signs and symptoms and methods of treatment of any particular nerve lesion.

In this chapter the outstanding characteristics of a few of the more common nerve lesions are discussed, together with any special points in relation to causation, diagnosis or treatment.

UPPER EXTREMITY LESIONS

The most common affections of upper extremity nerves are: upper and lower type trunk lesions; cords lesions; and damage to circumflex, radial, median, and ulnar nerves. Much less commonly the nerve to serratus anterior and the musculo-cutaneous nerve are affected.

Upper trunk type (Duchenne-Erb type). This is most commonly a birth injury, though it can occur in adults, and is the result of strong traction exerted between the head and shoulder. It may be simply a mild stretching of the nerve fibres, temporarily affecting their conductivity, or a severe injury such as a complete tear. The exact site of damage varies, the fibres may be torn from the cord within the meninges or damaged before they enter the trunks, but a more common site is at the point where the fifth and sixth cervical anterior primary rami join to form the upper trunk.

The motor fibres of the fifth and sixth cervical segments are distributed to the supraspinatus and infraspinatus muscles, deltoid, teres minor, biceps and brachialis, brachio-radialis and supinator. Consequently there is weakness or absence of power to abduct and laterally rotate the shoulder, flex the elbow and supinate the forearm. The limb hangs limply by the side with the arm medially rotated and forearm pronated. As a result of lost power in the lateral rotators contracture of subscapularis and pectoralis major tends to occur leading to loss of passive abduction and lateral rotation. The cutaneous distribution of the fifth and sixth cervical segments is to the lateral border of the arm, forearm and hand. Usually, however, owing to overlapping of the dermatomes, sensory loss will not be as complete as this, including only a small area in the region of the deltoid and along the lateral border of the forearm.

Recovery depends largely on the severity of the lesion, but is usually rapid though not always complete. In order to prevent contracture the limb should be maintained in abduction and lateral rotation with forearm flexed and supinated. This can be carried out by plaster of paris or a modified abduction frame but, in the first few months of life there is some danger of dislocating the shoulder-joint with this method. For this reason a fairly common practice is to tie the arm behind the head by means of a loop of bandage around the wrist tied to a second loop round the opposite shoulder. After about nine months a firmer splint may be used. The splint is worn until the infant is able to reach up above its head through flexion and abduction. It may then be discarded gradually or may be temporarily replaced by an axillary 'cushion'.

Physiotherapy consisting of massage and careful passive movements is essential, and active movement is encouraged as soon as voluntary power begins to return. Very occasionally if the condition has been neglected, surgical treatment is necessary to divide the contracted structures, this is followed by splinting and physiotherapy.

Lower trunk type (Klumpke's type). Like Erb's paralysis this is usually a birth injury. It may however occur in children and adults. In both cases it is the result of upward traction on the arm. In this type the flexors of the forearm and intrinsic muscles of the hand are weakened or paralysed and the disability if permanent is a very serious one. In a complete paralysis a total claw hand is likely to develop. Cutaneous loss is found along the medial border of the forearm and ulnar side of the hand.

In infants recovery is usually rapid and little splinting is necessary. In adults or infants where the lesion is complete, some form of splint is necessary to maintain slight flexion of the wrist, abduction and opposition of the thumb, and flexion of the metacarpo-phalangeal joints of the fingers. Passive stretchings will be necessary to prevent contracture between the thumb and index fingers, and the development of hyper-extension of the metacarpo-phalangeal joints. Much detailed re-education will be necessary.

Middle type. The seventh nerve or middle trunk is very rarely affected, but, if this should occur, the fibres to the radial nerve are mainly involved and the extensors of the elbow, wrist and fingers therefore weakened.

Brachioradialis is not usually much involved since it receives the majority of its innervation from the sixth cervical segment.

CIRCUMFLEX NERVE

As an isolated nerve lesion, the circumflex nerve may be damaged in fractures of the surgical neck of the humerus or dislocations of the shoulder joint. In the latter case, the nerve is severely stretched in its most fixed position as it passes backwards through the quadrilateral space. The injury is likely therefore to be a neurapraxia or axonotmesis. The nerve fibres may also be damaged as part of a wider lesion affecting the upper trunk or posterior cord of the brachial plexus. The lesion is apparent in the alteration in appearance, the motor disability and cutaneous loss. The rounded contour of the shoulder is lost, as the muscular fibres undergo atrophy, and the acromion process becomes unduly prominent. Gross disturbance of abduction of the arm takes place. Abduction can only occur as a result of trick movements and it is sometimes extremely difficult to analyse these movements. A common way to attempt abduction is to elevate the shoulder and tilt the trunk towards the opposite side, so abducting the arm a short way by means of the thorax. A slightly greater range of movement is sometimes obtained by fixing the head of the humerus in the glenoid cavity by the contraction of supra-spinatus, coraco-brachialis and the short head of biceps, and then laterally rotating the scapula by the action of trapezius and serratus anterior. Again abduction may be reasonably well performed if the movement is carried out in a plane between forward flexion and abduction when considerable help will be obtained from the clavicular fibres of pectoralis major. One usual way of performing abduction in the absence of deltoid is by means of a slight rotation of the arm which puts the long head of biceps in an advantageous position to act as an abductor. Abduction is then produced by this muscle. Forward and backward movements of the arm are weakened since the anterior fibres of deltoid help to swing the arm forward, the posterior fibres backwards. In a complete lesion some cutaneous loss is always present, maximal over the central region of deltoid.

Treatment will follow the principles used in all peripheral nerve lesions but certain points require special attention.

Splinting. A variety of opinion exists on the value and type of splinting for a completely paralysed deltoid and teres minor. Some authorities claim that the natural position for these muscles is with the arm by the side and that stretching of the fibres consequently does not occur in this position, others prefer to rest the deltoid with the fibres in a much shorter position using a light abduction frame holding the arm in about 90° abduction, 40° flexion and 60° lateral rotation. A modification would be the use of a large axillary 'cushion'. It is not usually the physiotherapist who decides the type of splinting to be used but she will be expected to supervise the splint once it has been chosen.

Special points should be considered in this connection. The splint must fit correctly and be properly applied, in the case of a child the mother must be taught how to take it off while keeping the arm in the abducted position and how to re-apply it. The inferior aspect of the shoulder joint must be adequately supported and the arm relaxed on the splint. It is necessary to see that a correct posture is maintained while wearing the splint, since many patients tend to tilt towards the unaffected side in order to balance the weight of the splint, so eventually a scoliosis convex to the affected side develops. Finally it is essential to make certain that the arm is well wrapped up and kept warm.

Re-education. Great care is needed if detailed re-education is the method selected. This is because so many muscles other than the prime movers may be brought into play to perform the movement. It should be borne in mind especially that a great deal of the power of deltoid is used in an upward pull rather than in abducting, and that, to prevent this, latissimus dorsi tends to draw the head of humerus down. If deltoid is very weak its abducting action will be hampered by this action of latissimus dorsi. When re-educating abduction, therefore, the weight of the limb should be taken so that friction is eliminated and fixation by many other muscles is unnecessary. The lying position is most suitable, and if the arm is supported by slings the physiotherapist has her hands free to steady the shoulder girdle so that no muscle contraction is necessary except that of deltoid and supraspinatus. Later, when recovery is well advanced, deltoid has to learn to play its part in co-ordinated movement again.

Arthrodesis. If recovery of deltoid does not occur it may be considered wise to fix the shoulder joint in a position of maximum use, physiotherapy will be necessary after the operation to train the patient to gain fuller range of movement by greater use of the movements of the scapula and clavicle.

RADIAL NERVE

The effect of a radial nerve lesion depends upon the site at which the nerve is damaged. The commonest point of lesion is the radial groove. In fractures of the middle one third of the shaft of the humerus, the nerve is liable to be damaged at the time of injury or later to be involved in the callus formation. This is below the level at which several of the branches to triceps are given off. Occasionally the radial nerve is compressed by crutches as it leaves the axilla below the long head of triceps. Sometimes the nerve may be damaged by crush injuries as it lies between brachio-radialis and brachialis on the anterior aspect of the lower one third of the arm. During fractures of the head and neck of the radius the posterior interosseous branch of the radial nerve may become involved as it passes through the planes of fibres of supinator.

Appearance. On casual glance little will be seen, except perhaps a flatten-ing of the rounded contour of the radial border and posterior aspect of the forearm, but if the patient is asked to lift the arm away from the side, with the forearm pronated, the hand will be seen to drop into flexion while the fingers may appear slightly flexed at the metacarpo-phalangeal joints.

Motor disability. If the nerve is damaged in the axilla and a total paralysis results voluntary extension of the elbow is lost, though it may be partly produced by the force of gravity if the elbow flexors are relaxed. Move-ments requiring strong extension, however, such as hammering are impos-sible. Flexion of the elbow is weakened because of the paralysis of brachio-radialis, on flexion against resistance the absence of this muscle is apparent. Supination of the forearm is weakened, partly due to the paralysis of the supinator but partly because triceps normally acts as a synergist, checking the unwanted flexion action of biceps during supination, and this synergic action is now defective. Extension of the wrist is completely lost as is also voluntary extension of the metacarpo-phalangeal joints though slight ex-tension may be the result of full flexion of the wrist since this stretches the extensor digitorum.

Extension of the thumb is lost but may be tricked, since contraction of the flexor pollicis longus stretches the extensor and then as the flexor relaxes the tip of the thumb springs back. Sometimes a slip of abductor pollicis brevis inserts into the tendon of extensor pollicis longus and in this case on palmar abduction of the thumb slight extension will also occur. Abduction of the thumb is weakened owing to paralysis of the long abductor. The ability to grip is much reduced since the extensors of the wrist act as synergists in the movement of making a fist.

Should the lesion be below the axilla, extension of the elbow will be normal, while if the damage occurs to the posterior interosseous branch only, then supination will be little affected and elbow flexion will be normal, while slight extension of the wrist may be produced by the contraction of extensor carpi radialis longus.

Sensory disability. The radial nerve distributes cutaneous branches in the arm but little sensory loss is noticed as these areas are also supplied by branches from the medial cutaneous nerves of arm and forearm and the musculo-cutaneous nerve. Usually, however, there is a small area of total cutaneous loss on the dorsum of the hand adjacent to the thumb and index fingers.

Special Points in Treatment

Splintage. No splintings for the paralysed extensors of the elbow is necessary but it is essential to support the wrist, metacarpo-phalangeal joints of the fingers and joints of the thumb otherwise adaptive shortening of flexor muscles and lumbricales is likely to occur with permanent disability. A light metal or plaster splint fully supporting the thumb in abduction and opposition, and extending to a point just proximal to the first interphalangeal joint of the fingers may be worn. Special care is then required to see that the metacarpophalangeal joints are not hyperextended or they will quickly stiffen and grave disability will be the result. These joints are better fixed in very slight flexion, when, if the wrist is in a few degrees of extension, no damaging stretching of extensor digitorum will result. Some degree of contracture of the ligaments of the wrist and metacarpo-phalangeal joints appears to occur very easily, thus it is essential to remove the splint two or three times daily in order that the joints are put through their full range.

The most satisfactory form of splint is a Bristow glove or one of its modified forms. It consists of a short metal cock up splint incorporated in a leather support buckled across the posterior aspect of the wrist and dorsum of the hand. Attached to the leather are small springs or elastics which are connected at their distal end to leather cuffs around the fingers and thumb. The patient is able to flex the fingers and thumb, and recoil of the springs or elastic brings them back to their correct position. The great advantage of this splint lies in the fact that the patient can grip effectively and so can usually carry on with his occupation. Functional use means avoidance of stiff joints and maintenance of the circulation.

Re-education will be carried out on the usual lines but special care is needed to restore co-ordination of movement. During the detailed re-education of the extensors of the wrist as prime movers, they have also to learn to act as synergists in flexion of the fingers. Throughout, trick movements must be noted and avoided. Again Kabat's methods may also be employed.

Tendon transplantation. Occasionally, where owing to considerable loss of nerve tissue, recovery is impossible, a tendon transplantation may be performed. The tendon of pronator teres is transplanted into the tendons of extensor carpi radialis longus and brevis; flexor carpi ulnaris into the extensor tendons of the fingers; and flexor carpi radialis into the thumb tendons. Considerable re-education of function is then needed as these tendons have to learn to perform their new function of extension. With repeated practice, however, a very good result is usually obtained.

MEDIAN NERVE

The median nerve is most commonly damaged just above the elbow joint as it lies on the anterior aspect of the lower end of the humerus. In young people a supracondylar fracture is fairly common and a very usual displacement of fragments brings the lower end of the upper fragment forward to contuse the median nerve and brachial artery. The second likely site is at the wrist joint where the nerve lies superficially just lateral and slightly deep to the tendon of palmaris longus. Wounds due to sharp instruments such as glass are very liable to divide the nerve as well as the tendons. Occasionally the nerve is contused at this level during a Colles' fracture.

Appearance. Two particular points are noticeable when the hand is at rest; first, the thumb lies back on the same plane as the palm as a result of the unopposed pull of the extensor pollicis longus and the adductor pollicis; second, there is a hollowing of the lateral and proximal part of the thenar eminence and, in advanced cases, the radial border of the shaft of the first metacarpal can be clearly seen through the skin. One danger of this position of the thumb is the tendency of the soft tissues between the thumb and index finger to contract, so permanently narrowing the space and interfering with the normal use of the hand. In addition considerable changes may be seen in the skin as many sympathetic fibres run in the median nerve.

Motor disability. Much disablement results from a median nerve lesion since the thumb and index fingers are so much affected. Loss of opposition of the thumb is a serious disability as this movement is necessary for gripping. A weak and ineffective movement—pseudo-opposition—may be performed. The adductor of the thumb and the first palmar interosseous muscle flex the metacarpo-phalangeal joint and bring the bent thumb across the palm so that the side of the thumb (instead of the tip) reaches the side of the little finger. Palmar abduction of the thumb is lost as it is largely dependent on the contraction of the abductor pollicis brevis, opponens pollicis and flexor pollicis brevis. Radial abduction is possible as a result of the action of abductor pollicis longus but it is always less in range than that of the opposite side.

A further disability is the inability to flex the terminal joint of the thumb which makes the act of holding objects such as a pen or needle very difficult. Trick flexion must be watched for, if the thumb is radially abducted and the wrist extended, the tendon of the flexor pollicis longus is stretched and it may then cause flexion of the joint.

There is almost complete inability to flex the index finger since both the sublimis and profundis tendons to this finger are out of action, the finger therefore tends to remain in extension and may even become stiff in this position producing the 'pointing finger' of a median paralysis. Flexion of the middle finger is weakened but often slight flexion of the terminal interphalangeal joint is the result of the unaffected fibres of the medial half of flexor profundus pulling on the tendon to this finger.

These various disabilities lead to complete inability to make a firm fist. On attempt at this movement the little and ring fingers curl down fairly well, though even their movement is affected by the absence of the action of flexor sublimis digitorum, the middle finger bends slightly, the index finger and thumb practically not at all, while the thumb fails to fold across the fingers.

Correct voluntary pronation of the forearm is lost, but a trick movement may be performed either by inward rotation of the arm as it hangs by the side or by lifting the arm away from the side with the forearm bent, when gravity will cause the forearm to fall into pronation.

Flexion of the wrist is weakened but not completely lost, since it is carried out by flexor carpi ulnaris and abductor pollicis longus. Usually ulnar deviation occurs during flexion.

Sensory disability. There is some sensory loss over the whole area supplied by the median nerve, the most complete loss usually being found at the tip of the index finger. Often joint sense is also markedly diminished.

Points in Treatment

Splinting. The main purpose in the use of splints is to prevent the thumb falling back against the side of the palm with consequent contracture of the adductor muscle and of skin and fascia. If the thumb is held in the position of palmar abduction and opposition, the hand may be more readily used with consequent prevention of stiff joints and disturbed circulation. For this reason, some form of splint must be devised to obtain a good position. A simple measure is to fix a wrist strap round the wrist, a small leather cuff round the first phalanx of the thumb and connect the two by a strap and buckle in such a way that the thumb is held in the desired position.

Re-education. Great care should be taken to watch for and prevent trick movements during the active work. Special attention will also be needed when recovery is complete to regain normal functional use of the hand.

Prevention of contractures. Daily stretching of the soft tissue between the thumb and index finger should be carried out, while careful full flexion of all joints of the index finger especially are necessary to prevent contracture of the joint capsules and the extensor digitorum.

Sensory disability. It is essential to warn the patient of the danger of damaging the insensitive index finger by heat or by slight abrasions. If such accidents do occur, more than the normal care in the use of dressings should be taken as the atrophic tissues are slow to heal and easily infected.

ULNAR NERVE

The ulnar nerve is most often damaged either at the wrist, due to penetrating injuries, or at the elbow during or after fractures in that region, or as a result of an increasing cubitus valgus. A crush fracture of the medial epicondyle of the humerus may involve the ulnar nerve, or may result in a permanent roughening of the groove for the ulnar nerve, so exposing the nerve over a period of months, even years, to repeated minor friction. A fracture of the lateral epicondyle which unites by fibrous tissue is liable to lead to an increase in the carrying angle, in this case the ulnar nerve which is normally slightly stretched only on extreme flexion of the elbow is now continuously stretched. Occasionally the nerve is damaged as a result of advanced osteo-arthritic changes in the elbow joint. Signs and symptoms of an ulnar lesion may not appear for many years after the initial injury but eventually continued stretching will impair the conductivity of the nerve.

Appearance. The position of the ring and little fingers, especially the latter, is characteristic. Owing to the paralysis of the fourth palmar interosseous muscle and the abducting pull of the extensor minimi digiti brevis, the little finger tends to fall away from the others. In addition, due to paralysis of the medial two lumbricales and consequent unopposed pull of the extensor digitorum the little and ring fingers are hyperextended at the metacarpo-phalangeal and flexed at the inter-phalangeal joints. The flexion deformity is more marked if the lesion is at the wrist since the flexor profundis tendons will then be able to contract and, unopposed by the interossei and lumbricales will flex these joints. This deformity is one to be avoided where possible, since it seriously hampers the grip.

A second characteristic feature is the hollowing between the meta-carpals on the dorsum of the hand, due to the wasting of the interossei. It is particularly noticeable between the thumb and index finger since, in addition to atrophy of the first dorsal and palmar interossei, the adductor pollicis is also involved. In the palm of the hand flattening is noticeable owing to atrophy of the adductor pollicis, lumbricales and the hypothenar muscles, the latter causing also the loss of the normal rounded contour of the ulnar border of the hand.

The appearance of the skin and nails on the ulnar side of both aspects of the hand is striking. Like the median, the ulnar nerve conveys many sympathetic fibres, trophic changes are therefore marked, the skin is thin, smooth, shiny and atrophic, the nails ridged and brittle, while the presence of scars and unhealed lesions give evidence of circulatory impairment and cutaneous sensory loss.

Motor disability. All movements of the hand are clumsy since so many muscles are affected. The ability to make a fist and hold objects in the hand is much reduced. The radial side of the hand in this action is more effective than the ulnar since flexors pollicis longus, sublimis digitorum and pro-fundis digitorum (lateral half) have still an intact innervation. Weak flexion of the proximal interphalangeal and of the metacarpo-phalangeal joints is possible but flexion of the terminal joints of the little and, usually, the ring fingers is impossible.

The action of the thumb is much hampered by the paralysis of the adductor pollicis. This muscle produces both palmar and ulnar adduction. The movement is not completely lost but is seriously weakened. The patient tricks the movement by contraction of the extensor pollicis longus which draws the thumb back and against the palm, while the flexor pollicis longus flexes the tip of the thumb, this action is clearly seen if the patient tries to grip a sheet of paper between the thumb and index finger.

Parting and closing the fingers is hampered by the loss of the interossei. A weak parting is produced by extensor digitorum which extends the metacarpo-phalangeal joints as it separates the fingers. Slight adduction may be produced by the long flexor tendons but the fingers are slightly flexed at the same time. A simple test for the palmar interossei is to link the extended fingers with those of the physiotherapist and to try to grip them, an impossible task if the muscles are paralysed. The ability to per-form 'lumbricale' action by the ring and little fingers is also lost.

The power of opposition of the little finger is missing. Active abduction power is nil unless the lesion is below the level at which the branch to flexor carpi ulnaris is given off, when abduction may appear to occur due to the contraction of this muscle jerking the pisiform bone to which it attaches.

Flexion of the wrist is weakened by the absence of the flexor carpi ulnaris and tends to be combined with radial deviation.

Sensory disability. There is usually total loss of sensation, superficial and deep, in the little finger with rather less complete loss on the ulnar side of the ring finger and ulnar side of the hand. Naturally the extent depends on the level of the lesion and consequently on whether the dorsal and palmar cutaneous branches are involved.

This sensory loss is a great disability, as the patient runs the risk of considerable damage to the skin and underlying tissues of this area.

Points in Treatment

The important point is to prevent the development of ulnar claw hand and so impairment of the functional use of the hand, and yet to allow freedom of use. For this reason the most satisfactory splint is of the 'knuckle-duster" type. This holds the metacarpo-phalangeal joints flexed without interfering with the use of the hand.

The patient must be warned repeatedly of the need to watch the skin and to take care against burns by too hot water, cigarettes, etc.

In carrying out the voluntary muscle test and in re-educating recovering muscle, steps must be taken to eliminate the trick movements which so readily arise.

THE NERVE TO SERRATUS ANTERIOR

Owing to its position behind the main plexus in the neck and upper part of the axilla this nerve is not often injured. It may be damaged in wounds of either neck or chest, or by strain as in carrying heavy weights on the shoulder. A paralysis of the serratus anterior is more often, however, either of unknown origin or due to toxic neuritis of the nerve.

Appearance. With the arm at rest beside the body there is very little change in the position of the shoulder girdle. On careful examination it may be noticed that the unopposed action of the rhomboids and the middle fibres of trapezius has caused a slight scapular shift towards the vertebral column which also results in a slight backward displacement of the acromion. If the arm is now actively raised upward or thrust forward the vertebral border may be seen to leave the chest wall, while the inferior angle instead of moving forward and upward remains close to the vertebral column, even moving nearer towards it.

Motor disability. This varies in a rather inexplicable way from case to case. A complete paralysis of serratus anterior will seriously hamper all arm movements above shoulder level in one patient, while in another abduction and elevation are not markedly impaired though the forward thrusting movement is always limited.

It may be safely said that the serratus anterior muscle steadies the scapula for movements of the shoulder joint, and actively assists movement of the shoulder girdle. After about the first thirty degrees of elevation through flexion or abduction serratus draws the inferior angle of the scapula forward and upward, so producing an upward direction of the glenoid cavity and widely increasing the possible range of elevation. This movement is absent when the muscle is paralysed and elevation movements are therefore severely hampered. In addition, as the arm is thrust forward in pushing movements serratus draws the scapula forward round the chest wall, an action which thus becomes impossible when the muscle is paralysed. Indeed for all co-ordinated movements of the arm serratus anterior plays a part, consequently all movements become less effective.

Points in Treatment

Since deformity is not produced by paralysis of serratus anterior, splinting is of little value. The only value would be to steady the scapula and prevent it leaving the thoracic wall on movements of the arm. It is clearly almost impossible to fulfil this object, and since strapping, plaster or any form of splint are relatively useless they are rarely tried. Re-education may be carried out on the usual lines. Starting positions which fix the scapula should be chosen at first and therefore lying where possible is a good position. Assistance may be given to elevation movements by raising the foot of the bed. Alternatively, facilitatory techniques and mass movement patterns may be employed.

MUSCULO-CUTANEOUS NERVE

A traumatic lesion of this nerve is rare as it has a relatively protected course deep to the biceps muscle. It is more commonly damaged in conjunction with injury to the lateral cord of the plexus or the upper trunk, or lesion occurs as part of an infective polyneuritis.

The outstanding characteristic is weakening of the power of flexion of the elbow. The movement is not completely lost but is performed with the forearm in mid-position by the combined action of the brachio-radialis and the pronator teres muscles. If, however, any resistance is given to the movement such as might be given by some weight in the hand, the movement quickly tires. In this case the trouble lies in the paralysis of coraco-brachialis whose most important function is to prevent the head of the humerus dropping in the glenoid cavity during such an exercise. If absent, on the movement friction occurs between the humeral head and the glenoid cavity, pain and discomfort arise and ability to continue the movement is quickly lost.

Supination is also weakened owing to the lost action of biceps.

Sensory loss is found along the lateral border of the forearm, but is not extensive.

The best method of support is to rest the arm in a large arm sling. The head of the humerus is then supported and does not drop in the glenoid cavity, and the biceps is not stretched. If a sling is worn it is very important to put the elbow through one full range extension movement daily, as the fibro-elastic elements of the biceps very rapidly shorten, and full extension may then become impossible. Supination should also be carried out in full range each day.

Re-education is best carried out in lying so that the downward drag on the humerus is relieved. Care should be taken to maintain the forearm in supination during the re-education of elbow flexion to eliminate trick movement.

LOWER EXTREMITY LESIONS

Any nerve of the lower extremity may be damaged but by far the commonest lesion is of the lateral popliteal nerve at the level of the head of the fibula. The femoral nerve is rarely affected except as part of spinal cord or cauda equina lesion. Disturbance of this nerve is more often seen in an anterior poliomyelitis than in any other condition. The sciatic nerve as a whole may be interrupted by cauda equina lesions, tumours or herniated discs, or by wounds of the pelvis or thigh. A complete lesion is very rare indeed; nearly always if the nerve is damaged it is the lateral popliteal section which is most involved.

THE LATERAL POPLITEAL NERVE

Apart from wounds in the thigh or pressure or stretching within the vertebral canal or pelvis, the lateral popliteal nerve is most likely to be damaged as it lies on the back of the head, and lateral side of the neck of the fibula. In this position it is easily compressed by tight strapping or plaster of paris, or it may be damaged during fracture of this region of the fibula or by some violence applied to the lateral side of the knee joint. If the nerve is completely severed both anterior tibial and musculo-cutaneous terminal branches will be affected, whereas in other cases one or other of these branches only or part of both may be involved. ·

Appearance. Atrophy of the peroneal and anterior tibial group of muscles results in flattening of the normal rounded contour of the antero-lateral aspect of the leg, the anterior border of the tibia becoming unduly prominent and the lateral surface palpable. The foot falls into a position of plantar flexion with a tendency to inversion, the latter due to the unopposed pull of the tibialis posterior muscle. Unless care is taken, the tendo achillis tends to contract and this, in addition to dropping of the forepart of the foot with consequent danger of contracture of the plantar structures, may lead to clawing of the toes and a pes cavus deformity.

Motor disability. The patient is quite unable to dorsiflex the foot or extend the toes, consequently the toes tend to drag along the ground in walking and the patient readily trips over any object. To compensate for this dropping he flexes his knee unduly in walking. The power of eversion is completely lost and the medial border of the foot is not therefore stabilised for the push-off in walking. As the leg is carried forward, the foot is slightly inverted and the lateral border only reaches the ground. The power of inversion is weakened by the loss of tibialis anterior, voluntary inversion being performed only in plantar flexion.

Sensory disability. Considerable sensory loss will be present on the dorsum of the foot and lateral side of leg, this necessitates considerable care in the avoidance of burns from too hot water.

Special Points of Treatment

Splintage is essential to avoid deformity and to prevent the patient tripping and falling. A splint of the 'toe spring' type is desirable, it should be fitted to the lateral side of the shoe to prevent inversion. This enables full use of the ankle in walking but brings the foot back to a right angle after plantar flexion. A plaster splint keeping the foot in mid-position may be substituted at night.

Passive stretching of tendo achillis and plantar structures may be necessary and a very careful watch should be kept to see that deformities do not arise.

In performing a *voluntary test* and in re-educating recovering muscles two special points should be borne in mind. The power of inversion must be tested in dorsiflexion, to avoid the danger of mistaking the movement of inversion produced by tibialis posterior as being due to tibialis anterior. The power of dorsiflexion should be tested with the foot supported midway between plantar flexion and a right angle, as some power might be present which would not be apparent if the foot had to work against the full force of gravity. In this connection, it is well to remember that all testing is best done by making use of middle and inner range and avoiding the resistance of gravity.

It is very essential to watch and re-educate the patient's *posture*, since altered gait is liable to upset the body mechanics and result in disturbances of postural sense. This point should never be neglected in any lesion of nerves of the lower extremity.

MUSCULO-CUTANEOUS NERVE

In this case the power of eversion only will be lost, though there will be little change in the sensory disability. When the foot is dorsiflexed it is also inverted and the danger of a varus deformity is present. Impairment of the use of the foot in standing and walking results from the paralysis of peroneus longus.

ANTERIOR TIBIAL NERVE

Paralysis of the anterior tibial group of muscles results in inability to dorsiflex the ankle and extend the toes. The condition closely resembles that of the complete nerve lesion except that, since the power of eversion is unaffected, the patient tends to evert the foot in standing and walking and may, therefore, develop a valgus deformity. There may be some sensory loss on the adjacent sides of the first and second toes.

MEDIAL POPLITEAL NERVE

This not very common injury may be the result of pressure on or stretching of the nerve roots in the vertebral canal or pelvis, or of wounds in the thigh or popliteal fossa, or may be due to a supracondylar fracture of the lower extremity of the femur with flexion deformity of the lower fragment. Complete severance involves calf, posterior tibial and plantar muscles. Normally considerable trophic changes occur, since the majority of sympathetic fibres to the leg travel in this nerve.

Appearance. Marked atrophy of the calf of the leg with thinning of the foot are characteristics. The heel appears elongated and dropped due to the loss of the support of the tendo achillis. This dropping of the heel, together with the clawing of the toes which follows the paralysis of the interossei and lumbricales, leads to contracture of plantar fascia, ligaments and fibrous tissues of the plantar muscles. A severe degree of pes cavus may arise. The skin of the sole of the foot is thin, atrophic and dry, and there is a tendency to the development of trophic ulcers particularly over the head of the fifth metatarsal.

Motor disability. The most disabling loss is that of plantar flexion of the foot, which means inability to lift the heel in walking and so the development of a shuffling gait with no 'spring'. The loss of the normal heel toe gait is increased by the paralysis of the flexor hallucis longus which plays the most important part in the 'push-off' in walking.

When the weight is off the foot, slight plantar flexion may be performed by the peroneus longus muscle but this can easily be detected since the weak plantar flexion is accompanied by eversion.

There is complete loss of power to flex the toes or to extend the interphalangeal joints of the four outer toes. Inversion of the foot is weakened but is still possible in dorsiflexion by the tibialis anterior.

Sensory disability. Superficial and deep sensory loss on the plantar surface of the foot tends to produce impairment of balance, posture and gait. In addition this loss is dangerous since the sole of the foot is exposed to much friction and trauma. Abrasions and ulcers may, therefore, develop and become septic without the awareness of the patient.

POSTERIOR TIBIAL NERVE

If the posterior tibial nerve is damaged below the level at which its branch to soleus is given off, the calf muscles will be unaffected, the disability will then be the loss of the posterior tibial and plantar muscles. There will still be some disturbance of gait since the toes cannot be flattened against the ground to provide a firm surface for the push-off, nor can the final thrust be gained by the contraction of flexor hallucis longus. Clawing of the toes and pes cavus are still liable to arise.

Points of Treatment

No very adequate means of splinting is available to prevent the onset of deformities. For this reason particular care must be taken to prevent contracture of plantar structures and anterior tibial and extensor tendons.

PAIN IN TRAUMATIC NERVE LESIONS

In an established case of complete nerve lesion pain is not likely; there are, however, cases of partial nerve lesions in which pain is an outstanding symptom. Associated with the pain will be found stiff joints, wasted muscles, decalcified bones and a skin which is pink, warm and sweating profusely.

This condition, known as causalgia, is most commonly associated with lesions of the median and medial popliteal nerves, nerves which convey most sympathetic fibres. In partial lesions of the median nerve, where perhaps the nerve has been struck by a glancing blow with little actual damage, bouts of severe pain may occur in the distribution of the nerve. The whole nerve trunk and the muscles supplied by the nerve may be tender to touch. The patient holds the part absolutely still; this may contribute towards the trophic changes which, in severe cases, are invariably present. The pads of the fingers become thin, the nails ridged and brittle, the skin of the palm of the hand is pink, sweating and glossy. Sometimes the pain is continuous but more often there are acute exacerbations brought on by some factor such as movement or touch.

The explanation of this condition is uncertain. In severe cases there may be irritation of the sympathetic fibres and occasionally the condition is relieved by sympathectomy. In milder cases there may be irritation of sensory fibres by a foreign body or a neuroma may be responsible.

Chapter XI

NEURITIS

Neuritis is an inflammation of one or more nerves, characterised by pain, tenderness, altered sensation and muscle weakness.

Each spinal or cranial nerve consists of a varying number of nerve fibres bound together by a supporting framework of connective tissue. The fibres of a typical nerve are motor, sensory and sympathetic, they vary in size, the motor being the largest, and the sympathetic the smallest, in diameter.

If a nerve is involved in an inflammatory process either the actual nerve fibres or the connective tissue may be affected. Those cases in which the fibres are involved are given the name of multiple peripheral neuritis, or alternately, degenerative or parenchymatous neuritis or polyneuritis. To those in which the connective tissue is the site of inflammation the term interstitial neuritis is applied.

MULTIPLE PERIPHERAL NEURITIS

This type of neuritis can be readily distinguished from an interstitial variety because it is a bilateral, symmetrical condition involving several nerves. The outstanding feature is degeneration of nerve fibres, particularly the distal portion, and consequently diminished motor and sensory function.

Polyneuritis is most often either the result of a deficiency of Vitamin B_1 which appears to be essential to the nutrition of peripheral nerves. Or it is due to toxins which reach the body from without (exogenous toxins) or are produced within it (endogenous toxins), either by the action of bacteria or as the result of errors of metabolism. Endogenous toxins are thought to gain their effect by causing changes in the blood vessels and so reducing the blood supply to the nerves. Toxins, carried round the body in the blood stream, reach the terminal part of the nerves and then ascend along the fibres. Examples of polyneuritis due to deficiency of Vitamin B_1 are alcoholic neuritis, beri-beri and possibly pink disease. Lead and arsenical neuritis are caused by exogenous toxins while diphtheric and diabetic neuritis are due to endogenous toxins.

Pathology

The pathological changes in polyneuritis closely resemble those of Wallerian degeneration, but are rarely so extensive or complete. The medullary sheath breaks up into fatty droplets; the Schwann cells multiply, some acting as phagocytes; the axons tend to split up but seldom completely disappear. These changes are most severe at the distal part of the nerves, though the whole length may be involved.

As a result of these changes function is impaired. At first pain, deep tenderness and paraesthesia are most outstanding, but, according to the degree of degeneration, there will be sensory loss, diminished reflexes and muscle weakness.

In most cases the onset is insidious, the patient complaining of fatigue and aching in the limbs, a feeling of numbness in the hands and feet, and cramp in the calves of the legs and plantar muscles. On examination, deep tenderness is found and deep reflexes are absent or difficult to obtain. If the condition is allowed to progress cutaneous sensibility becomes increasingly diminished, and in many cases postural sense is lost so that if the patient can move at all, he is markedly ataxic. Muscular weakness gradually makes its appearance and progresses until the patient is no longer able to get about. In practically all cases general health is impaired, in some, cardiac symptoms appear, either as a result of toxic myocarditis, or due to involvement of the vagus nerves.

Certain features are more noticeable in one type of neuritis than in others. In lead neuritis the radial nerves are most involved, therefore there are no sensory changes, but the patient suffers from bilateral weakness of the extensor muscles of the wrist and metacarpo-phalangeal joints of the fingers. In alcoholic neuritis degeneration is most marked in small branches of the anterior tibial nerve. Severe cases show numbness and tingling in hands and feet, cramp-like pain in the legs, ataxia, and marked weakness particularly in the dorsiflexors of the ankles. This results in dropping of the feet and a 'high-stepping' gait.

Arsenical neuritis closely resembles the alcoholic type but marked cutaneous hyperaesthesia occurs, and other manifestations of arsenical poisoning, such as skin eruptions, may be found.

Neuritis occurring as a result of diabetes is characterised by pain in the limbs, deep tenderness, and absence of the ankle jerks. In fairly severe cases postural sense is diminished and ataxia is therefore present.

In diphtheric neuritis, a paralysis appears in the fifth or sixth week after infection and is usually more severe in the lower than the upper limbs. There is tenderness on pressure and impairment of postural sense.

Pink disease, like diphtheric neuritis, and unlike other varieties of polyneuritis, occurs in children. In this type of neuritis general symptoms are more marked, the child being irritable, and suffering from lack of appetite, sleeplessness and erythematous rashes. There is hypotonia of muscles, lost tendon jerks and analgesia.

Prognosis. The majority of cases of polyneuritis show complete recovery, provided the toxin can be found and eliminated, and fibrous contactures and deformities have not been allowed to develop. Once the irritant is removed, regeneration of the myelin sheaths and axons will occur. The time of recovery will then depend on the extent of the degeneration.

PRINCIPLES OF TREATMENT BY PHYSIOTHERAPY

The first great essential is rest, in order to prevent over-use of the weakened muscles. During the period of complete rest steps are taken to find and eliminate the toxin responsible and to build up the patient's general strength and resistive powers. It is also important to deal with the local condition, and this is where the physiotherapist can help. During the period of paralysis or muscular weakness it is essential to maintain the nutrition of the muscles and, in fact, of the whole limb. The prevention of deformities and stiff joints is an important object of treatment. As the muscles begin to recover all possible assistance is given to aid their restoration to normal strength. The physiotherapist will carry out these aims as in any lower motor neurone lesion, but certain special points have to be considered. At the beginning of treatment the limbs may still be tender and the patient unable to tolerate massage or the application of splints. Gentle heat and passive movements may be the only suitable physical measures. Great care is taken to support the limbs by pillows and sandbags and to prevent the pressure of bedclothes by cradles. It must also be remembered that there may be some sensory loss and any form of heat or electrical treatment must be used with caution. Treatment is brief, so that the patient is not tired.

INTERSTITIAL NEURITIS

This type of neuritis usually involves a single root or a single nerve and is rarely bilateral or symmetrical.

In many cases no cause for the inflammation can be found, but in some the irritant may be toxins, either spreading directly from some neighbouring focus into the nerve sheath, or carried by the blood stream from the teeth, tonsils or sinuses. In some, cold may be the cause, while others may be the result of trauma, such as pressure, friction or long continued stretching.

Pathology

Inflammatory changes in the connective tissue of the affected nerve are present. The tissue becomes infiltrated with cells, blood vessels are congested and fibroblasts multiply. Some serous exudate occurs. The nerve sheath tends to become adherent to surrounding tissues. In the later stages there is danger of connective tissue overgrowth, which may either press on the nerve fibres, so hampering their function, or may contract, leading to shortening of the whole nerve.

These changes will result in irritation of the nerve fibres and consequently will cause a set of characteristic symptoms. Pain, tenderness and paraesthesia are the result of irritation of sensory nerve fibres. Pain is usually extremely severe and of the burning type. Any movement or position which even slightly stretches the nerve produces a paroxysm of pain. The inflamed nerve is tender to touch, tender points can therefore be found where the nerve is superficial or where it can be pressed against underlying hard structures. Tenderness is also found in muscle groups supplied by the nerve; this is probably the result of muscle spasm and the consequent accumulation of fatigue products within the muscle.

Most patients complain of numbness or tingling in areas supplied by the affected nerve; rarely will there be diminished sensation.

Irritation of motor nerve fibres results in spontaneous contraction of muscle fibres. Sometimes the whole muscle will go into a state of cramp. In many cases slight exaggeration of reflexes will be found, due to the increased irritability of the nerves and consequent hypertonic condition of the muscles.

Muscle atrophy is often seen in cases of interstitial neuritis, but it differs from the atrophy of a polyneuritis because it is the result of disuse and is therefore widespread and not only in those muscles supplied by the affected nerve. In some cases of interstitial neuritis there may be considerable muscle weakness and even flaccid paralysis. This will arise if the inflammatory exudate is sufficient to compress the efferent fibres in the nerve and so impair their conductivity or if the traction or compression causing the inflammation of the nerve sheath has the same effect.

While any nerve may be affected by an interstitial neuritis, those most commonly involved are the great occipital nerve, the femoral, the sciatic and the brachial plexus and its main branches and the facial nerve. Sciatica, brachial neuritis, and facial neuritis will be considered separately.

Prognosis. Most cases of interstitial neuritis recover completely in about six weeks. Occasionally, particularly in sciatic neuritis, the condition becomes chronic, scarring of the nerve with pressure on nerve fibres having resulted from overgrowth of fibrous tissue.

PRINCIPLES OF TREATMENT BY PHYSIOTHERAPY

Treatment for interstitial neuritis due to toxins, virus infection, chill, or for those cases of unknown origin, falls roughly into three stages. There is, first, the stage of acute pain; second, the stage in which pain is beginning to subside; and third, the phase when pain has completely disappeared but the patient is left with general muscle weakness of the part and possibly slight limitation of movement due to disuse.

During the stage of acute pain, as in all cases of acute inflammation, rest is essential. In most cases the patient is confined to bed, the limb is supported in the most comfortable position and kept warm. No physiotherapy is given at this stage, even the application of gentle heat often increases the pain.

As the inflammation begins to subside and pain is less, an attempt may be made to help to promote the absorption of exudate and prevent excessive muscle atrophy. At this stage the application of infra-red usually lessens pain, while constant current applications assist absorption and stimulate circulation. Gentle active movement within the limit of pain will prevent excessive atrophy. It is very important at this stage to watch the effects of physiotherapy. The slightest increase of pain should be followed by temporary cessation of physical treatment.

When pain has disappeared, the object of treatment is to restore the limb to full functional use. This is best obtained by progressive strengthening exercises.

Cases which have become chronic are difficult to treat and many different measures have been tried. Sometimes gentle stretching of the nerve will loosen it from surrounding tissues and overcome its tendency to shorten. If the sheath is adherent to, and pressing on the nerve fibres, injections into the nerve are sometimes used to distend the sheath. Especially tender areas on the nerve trunks may be treated by short wave diathermy or by the constant current. Occasionally a sinusoidal bath is found most effective, though in what way the good results are obtained is not clear. While different measures are being tried out, the limb should be kept in good condition by massage and exercises. For the treatment of interstitial neuritis, due to compression or traction, reference should be made to the section on brachial neuralgia and sciatica.

BRACHIAL NEURALGIA

The term neuralgia is chosen in preference to neuritis because it covers a much wider field. The term signifies pain in the region of the brachial plexus or in the distribution of the nerves originating from the plexus, without giving an indication as to the cause, whereas the term neuritis indicates an inflammation. Brachial neuralgia, even better designated as brachialgia (pain in the shoulder region and arm), arises from a great variety of causes. These may be divided into those in which there is organic change in the nerve roots, brachial plexus, or peripheral nerves and those in which there is no organic change, the lesion being in soft tissues other than nerves and the pain being referred.

CAUSES

One or more roots or nerves of the plexus may become inflamed as a result of a neurotrophic virus. This, however, is not common. Very occasionally, following the injection of diphtheria antitoxin or of vaccines, a severe paralytic neuritis develops. These are illustrations of what might be known as a primary neuritis.

More often inflammation of the nerves is secondary to some other condition. Certain factors may cause compression or stretching of the nerve and this results in inflammation of the nerve sheath. In the cervical spine, tumours, tuberculosis, osteo-arthritis and protruded intervertebral discs may all be responsible. In the region of the brachial plexus a group of abnormalities affecting the thoracic outlet may be responsible. In the arm the ulnar or median nerve may be irritated by pressure or, in the case of the ulnar nerve, by stretching resulting from an increasing carrying angle. Pain may be felt in the shoulder or arm from visceral lesions, as for example, the pain along the medial aspect of the arm in coronary thrombosis and angina. It may also be the result of arthritis of any of the joints of the upper extremity. Lesions in the muscles, ligaments or capsule of the shoulder joint, supraspinatus tendinitis, subacromial bursitis may be the cause of brachial neuralgia and capsulitis. Further, pain may arise from soft tissues of the elbow, forearm, or hand, though these are less often at fault.

DISTINGUISHING FEATURES

The first essential in treatment is the ability to distinguish between the neuralgia due to inflammation of the nerves and that due to involvement of other tissues.

Pain is present in both types of neuralgia. In each it is persistent at rest and on movement, but in the first type it is increased by any movement which stretches or causes compression of the inflamed nerve root or peripheral nerve. In the second type movements which stretch the plexus do not increase the pain but those which exert traction on the muscle, ligament or capsule which is the cause of the trouble will aggravate it.

The site of the onset of pain may help in deciding the type. If the neuralgia is due to lesions of the nerve root or plexus, pain will usually be felt in the neck first; whereas if it is due to a lesion such as a shoulder joint capsulitis, it will first be felt deep in the shoulder.

If the nerve root is involved, pain is usually of two types: a lancinating pain in the cutaneous distribution of the affected root, and a dull burning pain felt in the deeper tissues supplied by this root. Pain which is due to lesions in other tissues is more in the nature of a dull ache.

Tenderness. If the nerve is affected, tenderness can often be elicited by squeezing the muscles supplied by the affected nerve and, if the inflammation is of the plexus or the peripheral nerves, tenderness will be felt over these. Tenderness may also be felt in the posterior neck muscles in lesions of the vertebral column. If the soft tissues are the source of trouble there will be no tenderness in the course of the nerves, but there will be tenderness at the site of the lesion. Thus, for example, if periarticular fibrositis is the cause of pain in the arm, tenderness will be elicited round the shoulder joint and in the muscles acting upon it.

Paraesthesis and numbness. Tingling, a feeling of pins and needles, and a complaint of the fingers feeling numb will only be present if the nerve roots or nerves are affected, since these symptoms are due to irritation of sensory nerve fibres. Their presence in brachial neuralgia is almost always indicative of nerve involvement.

Reflexes may be altered in brachial neuralgia due to compression or stretch, ing. If the sixth nerve root is involved the biceps jerk may be diminished; if the seventh root is compressed or stretched the triceps jerk will be weakened. Reflexes will remain unaltered if the lesion is of other tissues.

Muscle weakness may be present in the muscles supplied by the affected root, particularly if there is prolonged stretching or if the nerve is involved in increasing pressure. In severe cases of disc protrusion, for example, marked paresis may develop. Localised muscle weakness does not occur in the second type, though if the condition is acute there may be diffuse muscle weakness arising from disuse.

Once it has been decided that the neuralgia is the result of involvement of the nerve or of other soft tissues it is necessary to know the exact site and nature of the lesion, since this affects the choice of treatment. The method of finding the site of a soft tissue lesion has already been discussed (see page 108); attention will, therefore, be directed towards the main feature of the lesions causing compression or stretching of the nerve roots or nerves.

Herniated cervical disc. A postero-lateral protrusion of a cervical disc tends to protrude into the bony tunnel through which the cervical nerve issues. This tunnel is narrow and is completely filled by the nerve and a plexus of veins. This additional material, therefore, results in compression of the nerve and veins, with congestion, swelling of the nerve and further compression. The most common sites of disc protrusion in this region are between the fifth and sixth and sixth and seventh vertebrae, thereby compressing either the sixth or seventh cervical nerves.

These cases are usually characterised by a long history of attacks of pain and stiffness of the neck. Eventually one attack is followed by pain radiating into the arm and made worse by coughing, sneezing and certain movements of the neck, particularly extension and side flexion. Paraesthesia is felt segmentally and there may also be weakness of the group of muscles whose main nerve supply is from the affected nerve root. Neck movements are usually limited and the neck is often held stiffly and shows a flattening of the normal concavity.

Tenderness may be present over the lower cervical spine and in the muscles supplied by the nerve.

Osteo-arthritis of the cervical spine. Cervical spondylitis may give rise to brachial neuralgia for several reasons. There may be thinning of the inter-vertebral disc causing narrowing of the bony tunnel for the nerve, there may be thickening of the capsule of the joint between the articular facets, or there may be protrusion of an osteophyte into the tunnel. Any of these may cause compression and inflammation of the nerve. Since the condition is likely to affect a considerable part of the cervical spine, several nerve roots may be involved, and pain and paraesthesia, and muscular weakness if present, are likely to be more diffuse than in the previous case. The condition is usually insidious in its onset. All movements of the cervical spine may be limited and painful. Pain in the neck may radiate up into the occipital region if the upper part of the cervical spine is involved. X-ray evidence of diminished disc space and osteophyte encroach-ment on the intervertebral foramen will confirm the diagnosis.

These two conditions may actually occur together since disc lesions tend to predispose towards osteo-arthritic changes.

Thoracic outlet abnormalities. Various abnormalities are liable to be present at the base of the neck. These give rise to pain, paraesthesia, weakness and sometimes circulatory disturbances in the arm, because they cause a stretching or compression of the trunks of the brachial plexus and the subclavian artery. The trunks of the plexus are prone to stretching because, in the erect position, they are angulated as they pass from the neck into the axilla (see Fig. 9). Any factor which increases the angulation may

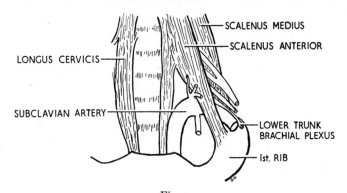

Fig. 9

Diagram to show position of trunks of brachial plexus and subclavian artery in relation to scalenes and first rib

give rise to symptoms arising from traction. A cervical rib may cause trouble because, if present, the seventh and eighth roots or the lower trunk of the plexus lie on it; their angulation is, therefore, increased and as the rib is lifted on each inspiration there is constant friction. Occasionally there are abnormalities in the insertions of the scalene muscles. If the anterior muscle inserts a little further back or the medius a little further forward, the lower trunk of the plexus and the subclavian artery are lifted up between these muscles and compressed. Scalenus anterior may, for unknown reasons, be in a state of spasm, so elevating the first rib and thus increasing the natural angulation of the neurovascular bundle. If the sternal ends of the first rib and clavicle are usually high, while the acromial end of the clavicle drops, the subclavian artery and possibly the trunk of the plexus may be compressed as they pass between the first rib and the clavicle into the axilla.

Drooping of the shoulder girdle alone may produce stretching and, therefore, symptoms. This drooping may be due either to a decrease in normal tone of the elevators of the shoulder girdle or an incorrect posture in which the postural length of these muscles is too great. Fatigue and unaccustomed heavy use of the arms may contribute towards the first factor.

The syndrome which accompanies these abnormalities is different from either of the preceding cases, since although all the trunks may be affected it is most often the lower trunk which is involved. Pain and paraesthesia are found, therefore, along the medial side of the forearm, hand and fingers. If weakness is present it will occur in the small muscles of the hand. Vascular symptoms may also be present. There will then be attacks of coldness, blueness and swelling of the hand, and the radial pulse will be diminished—a sign which is particularly noticed if the arm is dragged down or elevated above the head. In addition there is often aching discomfort at the root of the neck. The syndrome tends to be relieved by raising the arm to shoulder level.

According to the degree of the traction or compression exerted on the neurovascular bundle, so the severity of the symptoms varies. The most intense symptoms are usually produced by the presence of a cervical rib and the least severe by the drooping of the shoulder following fatigue. This latter is probably the cause of the milder syndrome found in the condition known as *acroparaesthesia*. This occurs most commonly in middle-aged women. There is the sudden onset, usually during the night, of numbness and severe pins and needles in the fingers, sometimes associated with pain. Often it is so distressing that the patient, a middle-aged woman, has to get out of bed and rub the hand and swing the arm to get relief. The symptoms quickly subside but may recur during the night. The attack practically always follows a day of hard arm work, the wash day or the day in which much sewing or cleaning has been done.

Ulnar neuritis. The ulnar nerve may be irritated by constant friction if the groove in which it lies at the back of the elbow becomes roughened. It may be subjected to traction if there is an increased carrying angle. In these cases the brachial neuralgia will be limited to the distribution of the ulnar nerve. The pain and paraesthesia will be felt in the ulnar border of the hand and in the medial one and a half fingers. Muscle weakness may be found in the intrinsic muscles of the hand, excluding the lateral half of the thenar eminence and lateral two lumbricales. It may also be noticeable in the flexor carpi ulnaris and medial half of flexor digitorum profundis.

Median neuritis. The most common causes of this type of brachial neuralgia are bony irregularities round the wrist causing friction of the nerve, or compression of the nerve in the carpal tunnel (carpal tunnel syndrome). These will give rise to symptoms usually limited to the distribution of the nerve in the hand (see Plate IX). Occasionally, in severe cases of carpal tunnel compression, pain may radiate up the flexor aspect of the forearm to the shoulder.

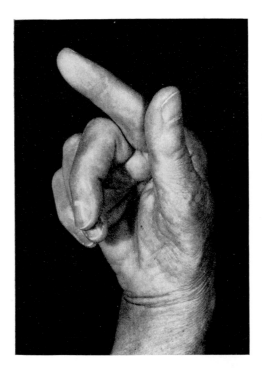

PLATE IX

MEDIAN NEURITIS

(a) Showing pointing fin-
ger on attempted flexion

(b) Same case. Showing
flattening of thenar em-
inence

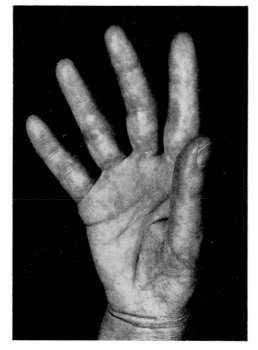

PRINCIPLES OF TREATMENT BY PHYSIOTHERAPY

Treatment of brachial neuralgia depends very largely on the cause.

Primary neuritis due to virus, toxins, etc. Treatment will follow the lines discussed for either interstitial or parenchymatous neuritis (see page 293).

Neuralgia due to a herniated disc. If the disc becomes embedded in the body of the vertebra or shifts even slightly, pressure on the nerve root may be relieved and inflammation should then subside. This may occur spontaneously with rest, and *rest* is therefore the first measure to be tried. If pain is severe the patient is usually treated in bed, with the head adequately supported on pillows and the arm resting in abduction so that the strain on the inflamed nerve root is avoided. As pain subsides the patient is allowed to get up, wearing a large arm sling, and when pain has completely disappeared strengthening exercises for the neck muscles are begun. Training of the correct posture of the head is important. No treatment for the arm is required unless there is muscle weakness, when exercises will be given. If this treatment proves unsuccessful, head traction may be used; this also will be followed by strengthening and postural exercises. Manipulation of the neck under an anaesthetic is occasionally carried out, and again will be followed by strengthening and postural exercises. In a few cases, especially those in whom pain is unbearable or muscle weakness is marked, a cervical laminectomy may be undertaken. Some surgeons allow free movements of the neck after a period of seven to ten days, others order a plastic collar which may be taken off for toilet purposes. In either case any weakness of arm muscles will be treated by exercises and if necessary by electrical stimulation. If the neck is free, exercises will again be used.

Whatever the method of treatment adopted by the physician, the exercises aim at getting a good carriage of the head and strong muscles to support the cervical spine, thus lessening the danger of further herniation.

Neuralgia due to cervical spondylosis. In this type also the chief aim is to relieve pain in the arm by reducing the compression of the nerve root and so relieving congestion. Sometimes intermittent traction will result in stretching of the thickened periarticular tissues or cause slight shifting of the contents of the tunnel. This may be carried out either in the ward or in the physiotherapy department by the physiotherapist. Occasionally gentle manipulation of the neck will relieve pain, possibly because it may break down adhesions or free an adherent nerve root. If these measures are not successful a plastic collar may be ordered.

Improvement is sometimes gained by the use of physiotherapy, which may include traction, short-wave therapy, massage and exercises. Short-wave diathermy is employed in an attempt to soften the thickened peri-articular tissues and so to relieve pain and assist stretching. Massage will improve the nutrition of the atrophied and often shortened muscles at the posterior aspect of the neck. Exercises are used to strengthen the muscles and maintain or increase the range of neck movements. They are particularly valuable to train the patient to hold the head erect. If the head is carried forward the cervical spine is shortened and this may increase compression. As correct a posture of the head as is possible should become a habit. Thus a treatment for brachial neuralgia due to cervical spondylosis might consist of short-wave diathermy, massage, traction, passive movements of the neck, followed by free and resisted active head movements and training in posture.

The arm will only require treatment if there is any muscle weakness or wasting.

Neuralgia due to abnormalities at the thoracic outlet. The first object is to gain a new postural length of the elevators of the shoulder girdle, so that the point of the shoulder is raised and angulation of the neurovascular bundle is relieved. The patient is, therefore, shown the present position of the shoulders, and an explanation is given as to how this position is responsible for her symptoms. She is then taught to take and feel the correct position. Gradually the new position is converted into a habit by constant reminder and by performing simple trunk, head and leg exercises while maintaining the correct position of the shoulder girdle. If there is weakness of the muscles, though often this is not the case, resisted exercises and strong faradism to the elevators of the shoulder girdle should be applied.

If the patient shows intrinsic muscle weakness or circulatory disturbances, physical treatment may be given, but most often these imply some more serious stretching or a compression and surgical treatment is needed to divide the scalenus anterior or remove a cervical rib. If the diagnosis is spasm of scalenous anterior, short-wave diathermy to the neck and training relaxation of the neck and shoulders are both of value. In addition to physical treatment the patient requires advice. Exercises must be practised regularly. Heavy use of the arms should be avoided. Knitting or sewing should not be undertaken for an hour before going to bed. Heavy weights should not be carried and the patient should sleep with a pillow placed behind and below the shoulder so that the shoulder is lifted up and forward. In this way the strain is taken off the neurovascular bundle at the root of the neck.

NEURITIS

Neuralgia due to arthritis of the joints of the upper extremity or lesions of muscle, fascia and tendons. Once more treatment is of the cause rather than of the actual symptoms. Arthritis will be treated according to its type and severity (see Chapter III, Part II). The treatment of soft tissue lesions has already been discussed (see Chapter VI, Part II). The main essential is a very careful examination of the patient to locate the site of the lesion and an equally careful explanation to the patient as to why the shoulder, for example, is being treated when pain is being felt in forearm and hand.

SCIATICA

This is a condition characterised by pain in the buttock and leg. Like brachial neuralgia it may be a primary inflammation of the nerve, or it may be the result of inflammation secondary to compression or stretching, or it may be due to lesions of other tissues.

CAUSES

A primary inflammation is rare, but it may develop as a result of a virus or be due to repeated minor traumata of the nerve. The most common cause is a herniated lumbar disc. One or more roots of the sciatic nerve may also be compressed as a result of osteo-arthritis or ankylosing spondylitis affecting the lumbar spine (see Fig. 10). Spinal neoplasm or tuberculosis may also have the same effect. Pelvic tumours may cause pressure on the sacral plexus.

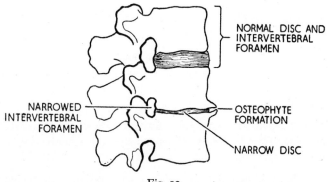

NORMAL DISC AND INTERVERTEBRAL FORAMEN

NARROWED INTERVERTEBRAL FORAMEN

OSTEOPHYTE FORMATION

NARROW DISC

Fig. 10
To illustrate narrowing of an intervertebral foramen in osteo-arthritis

Sciatica is also caused by lesions of the soft tissues of the lumbar region or buttock. One of the commonest sites is in the gluteus medius muscle. This muscle is covered by a tight layer of fascia and any swelling therefore quickly affects the superior gluteal nerve which receives its fibres from the fourth and fifth lumbar and the first sacral segments of the spinal cord. These segments are responsible for the innervation of skin and deeper tissues in the thigh, leg and foot, and pain may, therefore, be felt in these regions.

DISTINGUISHING FEATURES

Pain is present in all types of sciatica. If the cause is primary inflammation or compression, the pain often extends into the ankle and foot, while if it is a soft tissue lesion it is rarely below the knee. If the nerve root is affected, coughing and sneezing will increase the pain. The pain will also vary in type according to its cause (see page 295). Whatever the cause, straight leg lifting is likely to increase the pain, because this stretches all the soft tissues at the posterior aspect of the hip; but if the foot is dorsiflexed when the leg has been raised to the point of onset of pain, then pain will be increased if the nerve or its roots are inflamed, but not if the lesion is in other tissues.

Tenderness will be found in the course of the nerve in a primary neuritis, in the region of the lumbar spine if there is compression of the nerve roots, and often, in both cases, in the muscles supplied by the nerve. This will not be so if the nerve is unaffected, although a tender spot may, for example, be found in gluteus medius.

Paraesthesia will only be present if the nerve or nerve roots are inflamed.

Reflexes will only be affected if the nerve or its roots are involved. If the first sacral nerve root is compressed the ankle jerk may be diminished or lost.

Muscle weakness may be present in the group of muscle mainly innervated by a compressed nerve root. If the cause of compression is a spinal or pelvic neoplasm, muscle weakness usually rapidly progresses to paralysis.

Alterations in posture and gait are liable to occur whatever the cause of the sciatica, but are usually more pronounced if the lesion is one affecting the lumbar spine. Then lumbar scoliosis and sometimes lumbar lordosis may develop.

If it has been decided that the lesion is compression or stretching of one or more nerve roots then it is necessary to examine further to find the cause of the compression.

Osteo-arthritis of the lumbar spine. In this case there has usually been a long history of pain and stiffness of the lumbar region, with a gradual onset of sciatica. There is usually limited movement in this area and pain is felt at some point in every movement. There is often also spasm of the lumbar muscles. In most cases several nerve roots are involved and pain in the leg will not be isolated to one nerve root. Sensory impairment and muscle weakness are not common in this type of sciatica.

Herniated lumbar disc. Herniation occurs more frequently in the lumbar than in the cervical region, because the discs are thicker (see Fig. 11). In fact this lesion is thought to be the most common cause of lumbago and sciatica. The discs between the fourth and fifth and fifth lumbar and first sacral vertebrae are the ones most usually affected. Both the fifth lumbar and first sacral nerve roots cross the fourth disc, and the first sacral crosses the fifth disc also; consequently both these nerves may be compressed or only the first sacral, according to the disc affected.

There is often a history of repeated attacks of lumbago, and one attack may then be followed by radiation of pain into the leg. If the fifth lumbar root is compressed, pain may extend from the buttock down the back of the thigh and lateral side of the leg. Involvement of the first sacral nerve root gives rise to pain, which extends from the thigh down the centre of the calf and through the heel into the sole of the foot. Paraesthesia is often present. In the first case it is usually experienced on the lateral side of the foot, and in the second in the heel and sole (see Fig. 12). Occasionally there is weakness of the peronei and anterior tibial group of muscles. If the first sacral nerve root is compressed the calf muscles may show weakness and wasting and the ankle jerk may be diminished or lost.

On examination tenderness over the lower lumbar spinous processes and lumbar muscles, spasm of sacro spinalis, limited and painful movements (especially in forward flexion), lumbar scoliosis and flattening of the lumbar spine may all be found. Very occasionally symptoms in the leg may occur without accompanying lumbago.

Ankylosing spondylitis. Sciatica is not a common feature of this condition and when it does occur pain rarely spreads beyond the thigh. Once established, ankylosing spondylitis is recognised by the X-ray evidence, the raised sedimentation rate, the stiffness and deformity of the spine and thorax, and the character of the pain, which usually starts rather vaguely in the lumbo-sacral region and tends to spread up the back.

PRINCIPLES OF TREATMENT BY PHYSIOTHERAPY

The principles of treatment depend mainly on the cause.
Primary neuritis. The lines of treatment will follow those indicated for interstitial neuritis (see page 293).

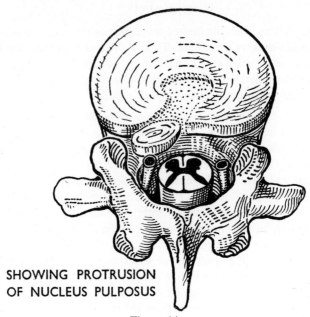

SHOWING PROTRUSION
OF NUCLEUS PULPOSUS

Fig. 11 (a)

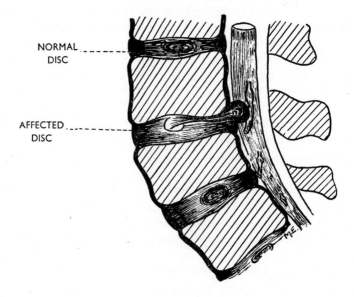

NORMAL
DISC

AFFECTED
DISC

PROLAPSED NUCLEUS PULPOSUS

Fig. 11 (b)

Sciatica due to osteo-arthritis and ankylosing spondylitis. This will follow the lines laid down for these conditions (see pages 87 and 99). If there is any muscle weakness this will be treated by means of strengthening exercises.

Sciatica due to a herniated lumbar disc. The size of a herniated nucleus pulposus usually varies from time to time. This may occur as a result of spinal movements and weight-bearing. In some cases the pressure on the nerve root may be completely relieved. It is because of this possibility that the first treatment tried, if the patient is seen early, is *rest*. Usually the patient is confined to bed for three to six weeks. During this period the strength of the spinal muscles may be maintained by rhythmic contractions of the back and abdominal muscles, and by exercise of latissimus dorsi and trapezius, avoiding movement of the vertebral column. Sometimes the tenderness in the back and leg may be relieved by the use of infra-red irradiation and massage to the back muscles. When the patient begins to get up, exercises to strengthen the spinal muscles, to improve posture, and to gain mobility in the lumbar spine will be given.

One of the most important points in considering the strength of the back is to teach the patient to lift, both from the floor and from above the head, correctly. Trouble in the back often commences following the lifting of a heavy object because so many people lift by extending the back instead of by flexing and extending the hips and knees. No patient should return to his occupation until he can lift correctly.

If rest in bed does not prove successful, traction, manipulation or a plaster jacket may be tried; in either case physiotherapy follows the same lines.

Sometimes none of these means proves successful or if pain is relieved it occurs again later. In some cases the patient may not have reported for treatment until definite muscular weakness or paralysis has developed. In these cases a laminectomy may be carried out for the removal of the protrusion. This may be followed by fusion of this region of the vertebral column or by simple bed rest for twelve to fourteen days. In the case of spinal fusion the patient is immobilised on a frame or a plaster bed for a period of three months and this is followed by a plaster jacket and often, later, by a spinal brace. During the period of bed rest leg and arm exercises are valuable, provided they do not produce movement in the lumbar spine. When the patient is up in jacket or brace, hip exercises and rhythmical back and abdominal contractions may be added.

If the patient is treated by laminectomy and rest in bed for a few days, physiotherapy is more vigorous. The back is temporarily weakened by removal of bone and incision of muscle and therefore requires attention.

The time at which this treatment may begin depends upon the surgeon. Some surgeons prefer to allow considerable time before any systematic course of exercise is started and a period of two to three weeks may elapse before physical treatment is begun. Others advocate early activity and therefore exercise to be begun twenty-four hours to four days after the operation.

When trunk exercises are started, a careful choice of starting positions should be made. Sitting is probably better avoided as it produces most downward compression force on the vertebral column. Lying, prone lying, prone kneeling and standing are suitable as progressive starting positions. The strength of the exercises should be rapidly built up, manual resistance being added as soon as possible.

While strengthening of the back and abdominal muscles is the most important object, it must not be forgotten that faulty posture of the spine and pelvis and limited movement will probably also require attention. The spine will have often been held rigid, in an abnormal posture, for some time before the operation, by muscle spasm due to pain, and this does not right itself immediately after the operation. This is partly because it has become a habit and also because the patient is now afraid to move his trunk in case movement causes pain or damages the sutures. In the course of time, movement will become freer and posture may improve, but the process may be speeded by physical treatment.

Relaxation should be taught in the lying position from the first day after operation and this should be progressed, using the sitting and standing positions. The patient should be taught to lie straight and to be able to feel and take up a good posture. Again this should be progressed to the sitting and standing positions. To combat spasm and rigidity, gentle movement of the spine can be obtained without seriously disturbing the haematoma or the damaged soft tissues. If the lumbar region is affected, small-range pelvic tilting, pelvic rotation and hip updrawing in lying and crook lying are useful movements. Mobilizing exercises should not be begun under four to six weeks.

In many cases, though pain may have been relieved by a laminectomy, muscle weakness and sensory impairment will still be present. These will, in some cases, improve slightly and in others good or full recovery may be expected. In nearly every case there has been a lengthy period before operation has been considered, during which time physical treatment will have been given. If this is so, the exact state of the muscles, in strength and tone, will be known. The physiotherapist will be aware of any sensory loss such as numbness, astereognosis or kinaesthetic impairment. Treatment given before the operation will be continued, modified only by the fact that after the operation the patient is confined to bed for two or three weeks.

Pain is nearly always relieved by laminectomy but any muscle weakness and sensory disturbance present before the operation will be relieved only gradually as the nerve fibres recover from compression. Physiotherapy may therefore be required for the leg muscles as well as for the trunk. The choice of treatment depends on the state of the muscles and may consist of heat to improve the circulation, electrical stimulation to lessen atrophy, passive movements to prevent contractures and deformity, and active exercises to restore power and full function.

Sciatica due to arthritis of the sacro-iliac or hip joints, or to lesions of muscles, tendons and aponeuroses. These cases again require treatment of the cause rather than of the actual sciatica. Treatment of these conditions has already been discussed (see Chapter VI, Part II). It is, as in brachial neuralgia, vitally important that a full and careful examination should be made in order to find the exact site of the lesion. It is also equally important that the patient should have an understanding of the treatment.

FACIAL NEURITIS (BELL'S PALSY)

Interstitial neuritis of the facial nerve differs from other types in the absence of severe pain and the presence of a complete paralysis. This is probably due to the fact that the trunk of the nerve is enclosed for a considerable part of its extent within a bony canal. Oedema of the nerve is therefore likely to result in considerable pressure on the nerve fibres and impairment of their conductivity.

The cause of the neuritis is uncertain; cold and exposure may be responsible for inflammatory changes in the muscles and fascia of the neck, with subsequent spread in the sheath of the facial nerve. In this case inflammation may extend along the sheath into the bony canal. Evidence to support this theory rests on the fact that before the onset of paralysis many patients complain of aching and stiffness in the neck muscles, and pain and tenderness in the region of the pinna of the ear and the mastoid process. Since cases seem to crop up in minor epidemic form during the autumn and early winter it is suggested that the condition may be an infective one. Doubtless some cases are the result of a mild geniculate herpes, the inflammation of the geniculate ganglion spreading to the sheath and fibres of the nerve.

Though the condition may occur at any age, it is most common in adults. It is usually unilateral but bilateral affections are seen, and in these

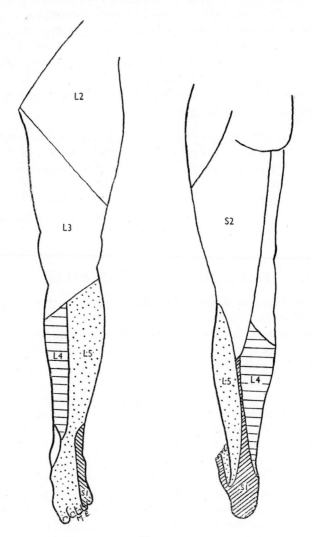

Fig. 12

cases the second side becomes paralysed about the fourth or fifth day after the first.

A sudden complete paralysis of all the muscles of expression of one side of the face, with consequent atonia, results in the absence of all expression, the forehead becomes smooth, the nasolabial fold obliterated and the cheek falls away from the teeth and gums. On attempt to close the eye the upper eyelid droops as a result of relaxation of the levator palpebrae superioris, but effective closure is impossible; the eye is therefore inadequately protected and conjunctivitis is a common complication. The lower eyelid sags and tears trickle over on to the face.

Lack of tone in the cheek and muscles of the mouth renders mastication difficult and fluid tends to dribble from the corner of the mouth. In a bilateral case speech is considerably affected. If the nerve is involved before the chorda tympani branch is given off, loss of taste in the anterior two-thirds of the tongue will result.

In most cases recovery commences in the frontalis muscle within two or three weeks and is complete by eight to twelve. Cases which show no recovery within four weeks are usually much slower and sometimes fail to recover completely. These cases often show fibrosis of the muscles and therefore contractures develop. These improve the appearance but not the voluntary power.

Except in the very early days, treatment will closely follow that for any lower motor neurone lesion, the same principles being considered.

In the first few days the main principle is to relieve congestion and promote absorption and one of the most satisfactory methods of physical treatment is the application of ultra-violet rays to the region of the pinna, styloid-mastoid foramen and mastoid, in such a way as to produce a third-degree erythema. Other methods which may be employed to achieve the same effects are the use of the constant-current or short-wave diathermy. Prevention of damage to the paralysed muscles may be obtained by the use of strapping or thin wire, enclosed in rubber tubing, hooked round the corner of the mouth and the ear. The circulation to the affected muscles is aided by the use of heat and very gentle massage, together with the interrupted galvanic current. Active re-education is necessary when recovery commences.

PART FIVE

DISEASES OF THE
CARDIO-VASCULAR SYSTEM

Chapter I

INTRODUCTION. HEART FAILURE.
CLASSIFICATION. CARDITIS

The heart may be said to show three components: the immediate covering the pericardium, the heart muscle or myocardium and the lining or endocardium. Any or all of these may be damaged by trauma or disease processes.

The myocardium consists of longitudinally and transversely striated muscle fibres. These fibres possess no sarcolemma but show branching processes which unite with other processes to form a syncytium. The muscular wall varies in thickness according to the work to be done, the left ventricular wall is consequently the thickest, while that of the auricles is the thinnest. The heart varies in size in different individuals according to the degree of activity followed during the period of growth. If a child is encouraged to lead an active life the myocardium grows in the number and size of its fibres, while if the individual is not allowed normal physical activity the musculature is poorly developed and the heart small. Under normal circumstances, by the time skeletal growth is complete, the cardiac muscle is so developed that it is capable of doing far more than is required of it in daily life. Thus a reserve is available for emergencies and for the wear and tear of advancing years. It is safe to say that the normal heart is capable of doing nine or ten times the amount it does under resting conditions. This is the 'cardiac reserve'.

Not only is there reserve, but if the myocardium is called upon to work harder for a continuous period, hypertrophy will occur just as it does in the voluntary, skeletal muscles. The increased work will arise either because there is a greater filling of the chambers or because increased resistance is met with in discharging the contents. The ability to contract more forcibly and so to hypertrophy cannot continue indefinitely and if the increased demand is not withdrawn the heart begins to fail. All the blood will not then be ejected at each beat and gradually dilatation of one or more chambers will occur.

313

The endocardium is a smooth lining continuous with that of the blood vessels. It not only lines the chambers of the heart but also, by reduplication it forms the valves guarding the orifices. In this situation it is strengthened by a small quantity of connective tissue.

The heart is provided with a special *conducting system* in which its beat is originated. In the process of development of the heart fusion of two longitudinal veins occurs. The walls of these vessels possess inherent excitable properties to a marked degree. The single vessel twists on itself and pouches gradually develop which eventually will form the chambers of the heart. As these chambers develop the special excitability is sacrificed in order to gain the property of contractibility. Eventually when the heart is fully developed, the greater part shows special contractile properties while a small amount, at the junctional areas where the pouches develop, retains its property of excitability. The most excitable of all is a little mass of tissue in the wall of the right auricle at the junction of the great veins This tissue discharges contraction waves and sets the pace of the heart. It is variously known as the sino-auricular node or the pace-maker. Similar, though less excitable tissue, is the auriculo-ventricular node which lies close to the coronary sinus and is continued around the right auriculo-ventricular orifice and into the interventricular septum where it divides to be distributed over the surface of both ventricles. Should the sino-auricular node lose its excitability, or some block occur between it and the auriculo-ventricular node, the latter will send out contraction waves but, being less excitable, these discharges will be at a slower rate.

The function of this conducting system is to initiate the heart beat, but alone it is unable to alter the rate to suit the needs of the body; for example a beat of seventy may be fast enough to supply an adequate quantity of oxygen and nutrition for ordinary activity, but is insufficient for unusual exercise. To enable necessary adjustments to be made the conducting system receives a double innervation from the autonomic nervous system (see Fig. 13), parasympathetic fibres decreasing the rate at which contraction waves are sent out, sympathetic stimuli increasing this rate. Thus during activity sympathetic stimuli cause increased heart rate, while during sleep the parasympathetic influences predominate and the heart slows down and is given a chance to recuperate. It will be readily understood that not only can the three component parts of the heart suffer from disease, but disturbances can also occur in the conducting system or in the autonomic innervation.

The heart is supplied with the necessary oxygen and nutrient products through the *coronary circulation*. There are two coronary arteries and together they are responsible for the entire supply of the heart since little

(a) AFFERENT FIBRES FROM THE HEART

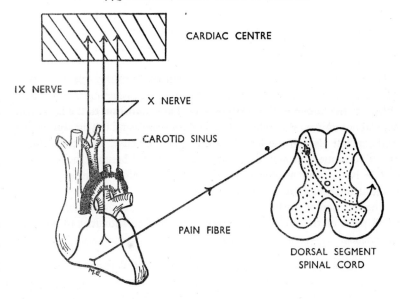

CARDIAC CENTRE

IX NERVE

X NERVE

CAROTID SINUS

PAIN FIBRE

DORSAL SEGMENT
SPINAL CORD

(b) EFFERENT FIBRES TO THE HEART

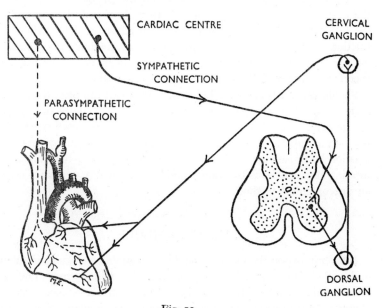

CARDIAC CENTRE

CERVICAL
GANGLION

SYMPATHETIC
CONNECTION

PARASYMPATHETIC
CONNECTION

DORSAL
GANGLION

Fig. 13

315

anastamosis occurs between the arteries and any other vessels. Only a limited anastamosis takes place between these two vessels, therefore sudden obstruction of a branch of a coronary artery may result in a complete cutting off from nutrition of part of the musculature. This results in an infarct and may be a major catastrophe.

Nutrition reaches the heart walls through the coronary vessels during cardiac diastole, since during systole the forcibly contracting muscle fibres obliterate the lumen of the small vessels. Thus, nutrition to the heart will depend not only on the state of the coronary vessels and the pressure within them, but also on the length of the diastolic pause. Increase of heart rate if continued for any length of time is harmful because the length of systole is uniform whatever the heart rate, therefore diastole must be reduced and nutrition proportionately decreased.

The function of the heart is to maintain an efficient circulation of blood to all parts of the body. This circulation must be sufficient to meet all exigencies.

Cardiac output, on which an efficient circulation depends, is itself dependent on the systemic venous return and the rate and force of cardiac contraction. The force of contraction varies with the initial length of the muscle fibres, the length of diastole or resting period, and with the quantity of oxygen and nutrition available. Increasing the rate of beat does not help the output eventually, since diastole is then shortened. This means that the heart has not time to recover from the effects of the previous contraction and the force of contraction is, therefore, diminished. A shortened diastole also means diminished filling of the chambers of the heart and therefore diminished force of subsequent contraction.

Should the needs of the body increase, the heart can meet them in two main ways: by increasing either the force or the rate of contraction. Usually the immediate reaction is to increase the rate, but increased resistance to the output rapidly results in increased force. Should the coronary circulation be impaired, greater force is less possible, and the only way of meeting emergencies is by a more rapid beat; but this, as already seen, is an uneconomical method.

CARDIAC FAILURE

If for any reason the heart is unable to maintain an efficient circulation under all circumstances the condition of cardiac failure arises. The cause of such failure will be either that there is too great a resistance to the discharge of blood into the systematic or pulmonary circulations, or that the beat is too weak to overcome the normal resistance. It may, in certain circumstances, be a combination of the two. Too great resistance in the systematic circulation may be the result of a high blood pressure, very strenuous exercise or stenosis of the aortic valve. High resistance in the pulmonary circulation may arise from diminution of the capillary bed as in emphysema or chronic fibrosis of the lungs, or from mitral stenosis. This increased resistance throws a continuous burden on the heart and eventually it begins to fail. A heart which is too weak may be the result of changes in the myocardial muscle. The muscle may be weakened as a result of coronary thrombosis and necrosis of areas of muscular tissue, or it may be weakened as the result of diminished nutrition in aortic incompetence. On the other hand, the weakness may be due to fatty degeneration as in pernicious anaemia, or degeneration may be caused by the toxins of acute infections such as diphtheria, pneumonia, influenza or scarlet fever.

Cardiac failure is a relative event, since though the heart may be unable to supply a sufficient circulation to meet the requirements of an emergency, it may be adequate to deal with the needs of ordinary life. If the heart is unable to maintain a circulation sufficient for the body at rest, then a serious situation has arisen. Cardiac failure is rarely sudden, except in cases of acute occlusion of coronary vessels or acute toxic dilatation.

The first symptom of a failing heart is *dyspnoea on exertion*. This breathlessness arises from the fact that an inadequate quantity of blood reaches the respiratory centre. This centre is thus stimulated and respiration increases in rate and depth. Naturally this is most felt on severe exertion. It is essential to remember that breathlessness is not necessarily a pathological phenomenon. It is the normal physiological result of severe exercise, but if an individual experiences breathlessness on exercise or activity which did not previously produce it, then a pathological condition is present.

The symptom of breathlessness will gradually increase in severity as the reserve is used up. At first, walking up a hill or walking quickly may produce it, later walking quickly along the flat may have the same effect, walking slowly a short distance may then produce the symptom, until eventually, breathlessness is present even at rest. At this stage the patient may only breathe in comfort in the sitting position.

In the later stages, to the inadequate quantity of blood reaching the respiratory centre, inadequate aeration of the blood will also be added. These two factors will lead to severe changes in respiratory rate and depth.

It is not always possible to rely on a patient's own account of this symptom. In such a case a simple test can be made. Provided the patient does not show dyspnoea at rest, he may be asked to walk up a flight of steps once or twice according to the number. The normal individual will not become dyspnoeic; the pulse will not rise more than ten and will return to normal within two minutes. The patient with diminished cardiac reserve will show some degree of breathlessness, a greater rise in pulse rate and a slower return to normal.

As increasing failure develops and the patient begins to suffer from dyspnoea while walking short distances on the flat, signs of venous congestion begin to appear and a condition of congestive cardiac failure exists. At this stage the heart is unable to discharge its contents fully and pressure therefore rises in the great veins. Sometimes it is the left ventricle which fails to do its job, possibly because a condition of hypertension throws too great a strain on it. Difficulty is then experienced in pumping blood from the left auricle into the congested left ventricle and congestion occurs in the pulmonary circulation. If there is a much diminished pulmonary capillary bed then the right ventricle may fail and congestion will first be seen in the systemic veins. In many cases bilateral failure occurs with pulmonary and systemic congestion.

Evidence of pulmonary congestion will be seen in extreme dyspnoea, oedema of the lungs, cyanosis, cough and often nocturnal dyspnoea, while in congestion of the systemic veins, pain, oedema, fatigue, abdominal visceral disturbances and some degree of breathlessness are the more noticeable symptoms.

Pulmonary congestion may arise not only as a result of failure of the left ventricular muscle but also through an advanced stenosis of the mitral valve causing an appreciable rise in pressure within the left auricle and consequently a rise in pressure in the pulmonary capillaries. Rise in the pressure of blood in the pulmonary capillaries results in increased exudate of tissue fluid, consequently the alveolar walls and interstitial tissue become oedematous. A certain amount of fluid passes into the alveoli displacing the alveolar air. Diminished gaseous interchange occurs and the blood returns to the left auricle insufficiently aerated, much reduced haemoglobin still being present. Deficiency of aeration stimulates the respiratory centre, and a severe degree of breathlessness may then be present even at rest. The patient breathes only with any degree of ease in the sitting position. A quantity of reduced haemoglobin in the blood causes cyanosis which is apparent generally in the face, hands, mucous membranes and even in the trunk.

In cases of pulmonary venous congestion, a cough is often present and it is accompanied by some sputum which occasionally may be blood-stained, since congested capillaries may rupture and minute haemorrhages occur into the alveoli. Not uncommonly the patient may suffer from attacks of nocturnal dyspnoea. These attacks may be the result of a sudden rise in pulmonary pressure, due to a failure of the left ventricle to cope with the extra blood entering the heart when the patient is in the recumbent position. This sudden rise in pressure causes a rapid oedema of the lungs and the patient wakes up with a feeling of suffocation. He sits up, clutches the nearest object in order to bring the accessory muscles of respiration into play, and fights for breath. There is usually a deep cyanosis and pro- fuse sweating. After some minutes the ventricle begins to deal with the blood and the attack subsides, the patient coughs up some frothy blood-stained sputum and is then left utterly exhausted.

Systemic venous congestion is less common but may be the result of fibrosis of the lung or of pulmonary stenosis. As venous pressure rises, congestion in the portal circulation results in enlargement of the liver, which becomes palpable below the costal margin. Tenderness and pain may then be present in the right hypochondrium and in the region of the sternum. Further portal congestion leads to digestive disturbances, and vomiting after food may occur.

A rise in venous pressure leads to a rise of pressure in the tiny venules and capillaries, increased exudate then occurs and in time a condition of cardiac oedema is seen. The increased fluid tends to collect in the sub-cutaneous tissues and may, after a time, be displaced by pressure. Pitting on pressure does not occur at once, though the limb will increase in volume and weight as the extra tissue fluid is absorbed into the cells and fibres. The fluid will collect in the dorsum of feet and round the ankles if the patient sits or stands for long, behind the malleoli or in the sacral region if the patient is in the lying position. Considerable discomfort may be experienced from this oedema. The limbs feel heavy and ache, movement is impeded, and nutrition of the tissues is impaired. Oedema may spread up the legs to the thighs, and may reach the abdomen and back, it rarely affects the arms. Occasionally fluid collects in the pleural and peritoneal cavities.

Patients with congestion of the systemic veins nearly all show breath-lessness, though it may not be so severe as in pulmonary congestion. The cause of this dyspnoea is a deficient quantity of blood reaching the respira-tory centre with resulting increase of messages to the muscles of inspira-tion. Other symptoms of cardiac disorders, such as fatigue, pain, variation in the pulse and palpitations, will be provoked increasingly easily. Fatigue is a natural concomitant of an inefficient circulation. Slowing of blood flow, and reduced haemoglobin, mean insufficient oxygen and nutrition to the tissues with impaired metabolism.

Cardiac pain is most often the result of a complete or relative ischaemia of the heart muscle, and is very similar to the cramp-like pains occurring in the calf muscles in arterio-sclerosis or Buerger's disease. Ischaemia of the muscle may be the result of coronary occlusion which is due to thrombosis or embolism cutting off the blood supply from an area of muscular tissue, or it may be due to a diminution in the lumen of the coronary vessels, as a result of sclerosis of the arteries, or a decreased pressure in the vessels due to an aortic regurgitation. In the first case ischaemia is complete and pain arises because the ischaemic muscle continues to work, fatigue products gather in the tissue spaces and cannot be swept away. In the other two cases ischaemia is relative, sufficient blood is probably available for the heart muscle during rest and mild activity, but when the heart beats more rapidly, as on exertion or emotion, then the blood supply is insufficient. Pain in this case has a rapid onset and disappears when the individual stands still. Pain due to either of these causes is most usually felt in the region of the sternum. In coronary occlusion it is more often in the lower sternal area and epigastrium, while in effort pain it is more often in the upper sternal segments. In both cases it may spread into left or right arms or neck. A dull aching in the precordial region is occasionally experienced in pericarditis and endocarditis, but is never so pronounced as in the preceding cases.

Palpitation, or a consciousness of the heart beat does not necessarily imply a cardiac lesion. Palpitations with a perfectly normal heart occur from overstimulation of the sympathetic innervation and may arise as a result of tobacco, alcohol, coffee and certain drugs. It also occurs in hysteria, anaemia and Grave's disease. Palpitation tends to occur in any minor irregularities of the heart's action as a change in the rhythm of the beat is liable to draw the patient's attention to the pulse. Thus palpitation is present in extra-systoles, particularly when a premature ventricular beat is too weak to eject enough blood into the aorta to cause a pulse wave and therefore an intermittent pulse is present. Again palpitation is present in aortic regurgitation because in this case an increased quantity of blood (the normal plus that regurgitated) is ejected on ventricular contraction. Systolic pressure is therefore very high though diastolic pressure is unduly low. The unusual momentum of the blood causes a feeling of 'shock' in the chest and throb in the neck and the beat can often be felt in the ears. Auricular fibrillation often provokes palpitation because it excites the ventricle to rapid and very irregular action. Again in cases of paroxysmal tachycardia, palpitation will occur.

CLASSIFICATION OF CARDIAC DISEASES

Cardiac diseases may be roughly divided into:

> Disturbances of rate and rhythm
> Carditis
> Chronic valvular lesions
> Chronic diseases of the myocardium
> Affections of the coronary vessels
> Effort syndrome
> Congenital cardiac disorders

Physiotherapy does not play a very great part in the treatment of these conditions, nevertheless it is exceedingly useful in some. These particular conditions will be more fully discussed here.

CARDITIS

Carditis, as the term implies, means inflammation of the heart. All coats are attacked; it is very rare for one to be involved alone. Though a pericarditis may predominate, there is inevitably some inflammation of the underlying myocardium, while the myocardium is also involved in an endocarditis.

The most common age for a carditis is during childhood or adolescence and the condition is often a rheumatic one, rather less often it is associated with diphtheria, scarlet fever or pneumonia. The symptoms are most markedly those of an infection, the heart involvement sometimes being masked by the symptoms of the primary disorder.

Pericarditis

Is nearly always part of an infective process, either rheumatic or pneumonic, though direct spread of infection from the pleura or through the diaphragm may occur. The pericardial membrane becomes hyperaemic and swollen, and fibrin is deposited on the surfaces, giving them a rough shaggy appearance. There may be much sero-fibrinous exudate if the origin of the condition is rheumatic, purulent if it is due to pneumonia. The symptoms are those of fever, malaise, raised temperature and pulse. Pain is not always present unless the extra-pericardial structures are involved; breathlessness may be due to obstruction to the venous return or to pressure on the lungs of a large effusion.

Occasionally, following a rheumatic pericarditis, thickening of the membrane occurs and the layers may become adherent; this appears, however, to produce few ill effects. Very uncommonly, gross thickening and fibrosis of the pericardium occurs, with the result that the heart is unable to expand adequately, or constriction of the great veins takes place; in this case marked venous congestion will arise with enlargement of the liver and ascites and some oedema of the legs.

Endocarditis

Rheumatic endocarditis may develop during an attack of rheumatic fever or chorea. The former disease is characterised by an inflammation of fibrous structures including the synovial membrane and periarticular structures of joints, the muscular and subcutaneous tissues, the serous membranes, and, most serious of all, the endocardium and, less frequently, the myocardium. In chorea the outstanding features are jerky, incoordinate movements and muscle weakness and hypotonia. This disease is closely allied to rheumatic fever; very probably both have the same cause.

Rheumatic fever is probably most dangerous in its subacute form. This type is most common in childhood and may show only vague pains in the legs and poor general health. The conditions may easily be missed, and the child may then be up and about with a smouldering process at work in the valves of the heart. In this way an endocarditis may not be detected and considerable damage may be done.

During the active process in the heart, the cusps of the valve become swollen and oedematous, the endothelium degenerates and therefore, along the line of apposition of the cusps, blood platelets are deposited layer upon layer. As thromboplastin is liberated by these platelets, a small amount of fibrin is formed and a number of firm pale thrombi result. In the course of time, fibroblasts and capillaries grow into these thrombi and they become converted into fibrous masses, firmly adherent to the edges of the cusps. In the meantime, inflammatory fibrous tissue forms in the underlying valve causing the cusps to thicken. During the acute stage, the edges of the cusps tend to become stuck together by the inflammatory exudate, then organisation occurs, firmly binding the edges together so that the valve does not open properly. The thickening cusp has a great tendency to shrink and should this occur, incompetence also will result. In some cases lime and calcium salts are deposited in the thickened cusps which therefore become calcified.

Although the endocardium is primarily affected some involvement of the myocardium nearly always occurs, fibrous nodules form in the interstitial tissue and often scarring tends to result.

As the rheumatic fever or chorea subside the inflammation of the endocardium becomes less marked though, without suitable treatment, it may continue in a chronic form for a long time. There is little evidence of this chronic lesion because the effect on the circulation through the heart of an incompetent or stenosed valve is overcome by hypertrophy of the heart muscle and a normal circulation is maintained. The real trouble lies in the fact that the hypertrophy cannot continue indefinitely and as the child grows older and more strains are thrown on the heart, eventually cardiac failure will occur. A further danger arises, in that a damaged valve is an area of lowered resistance and there is a possibility of bacterial invasion at a later date.

The essential treatment, therefore, of the child suffering from acute or subacute rheumatism or chorea is rest. This rest must be complete, and unless it is certain that the heart is not involved, it must be prolonged until all signs of activity have ceased. This is often a period of four to six weeks after the fever has completely subsided.

On the other hand, it is not desirable to prolong rest unnecessarily, since organisation of exudate and stenosis of the mitral valve are then more likely. In addition it will interfere with the development of the heart. Thus as soon as the physician is satisfied that the condition is no longer active the child should begin graded exercise under the care of a physiotherapist.

Subacute bacterial endocarditis. Acute bacterial endocarditis is rare and invariably fatal. The sub-acute condition is much more common. It occurs most often in young males between the ages of twenty and forty, as a result of invasion of a damaged valve by an organism of low virulence, nearly always the streptococcus viridans. This organism inhabits the mouth and throat and may invade the blood stream from decayed teeth. In practically every case there is already a defect which lowers the resistance to infection, it may be rheumatic carditis, congenital valvular defects, or patent ductus arteriosus. The changes which occur are not dissimilar to those of simple endocarditis, but the vegetations formed on the line of apposition of the cusps are larger, softer and contain bacteria. They are therefore much more easily broken up. More destruction of the underlying valve occurs, and the mural endocardium may also be involved.

The onset of the disease is nearly always insidious, often there is slight fever accompanied by malaise, lassitude, pains in the back and limbs and anorexia. Gradually an anaemic condition develops together with splenic enlargement, and a leucocytosis. These are all evidence of an infective condition. Signs of moderate enlargement of the heart, and murmurs, indicating aortic regurgitation or mitral stenosis, may be present. Usually the patient looks pale, and sometimes there is clubbing of the fingers; changes occur in the capillary endothelium, consequently minute skin haemorrhages—petechiae—may be seen. Emboli are very common since the vegetations are so friable, and as they are found most often on the mitral valve, they usually occur in the systemic system.

At one time the condition was invariably fatal within six or twelve months, death occurring partly as a result of infection and partly due to cardiac failure, occasionally as a result of embolism. With present-day treatment the future for these patients is brighter. The main object of treatment is to inhibit the growth of the bacteria before gross destruction of the valves has occurred, and as the streptococcus viridans is penicillin-sensitive, this is reasonably possible. Once the condition is diagnosed, these patients are usually treated by complete bed rest, and a course of systemic penicillin—injections four-hourly—over a period of at least six weeks. The actual length is, of course, determined by the repeated blood tests, and by pulse rate, temperature and cardiac signs. At the end of the course, rest is continued for a further week or ten days and graded activity is then started. A long period of complete rest means muscle weakness, and graduated exercise is required to restore muscle tone and power. These patients therefore require treatment by physiotherapy.

Myocarditis

Most commonly occurs as part of a rheumatic carditis but may occur in any acute infection. The inflamed muscle fibres dilate and gross enlargement of the heart takes place. The orifices are therefore widened, and the valves become relatively incompetent. In severe degrees of myocarditis sudden death may occur, or alternatively, symptoms of congestive failure will arise. Less commonly, if the causative infection is controlled, the heart may recover completely.

PRINCIPLES OF TREATMENT BY PHYSIOTHERAPY

Many eminent cardiologists consider that physiotherapy has no useful part to play in the treatment of cardiac disorders. There does, however, seem a point in the recovery from carditis at which physical measures, if not absolutely essential, are helpful. No claim is made that either massage or exercises aid the cure of the carditis, in fact so long as signs of an active condition of the heart are present, physiotherapy certainly should not be undertaken. But in all cases the patient will have been treated by complete bed rest for a comparatively long period, consequently reduction in muscle tone and some generalised disuse atrophy will be present. If the patient is allowed to resume graduated activity at this stage without re-educative exercise, postural defects will develop. Just as there is decreased tone in the general skeletal musculature, so there is also poor condition of the cardiac muscle. There has been inflammation resulting in weakening, even if the lesion has not been primarily of the myocardium. Reserve is still present, provided congestive failure has not occurred, and a heart with reserve, however poor its musculature, will not be damaged by exercise unless the exercise is excessive; rather, exercise will help to strengthen the heart muscle. The effect of exercise is not directly on the heart but on the blood pressure which rises, so throwing increased work on the left ventricle during systole only, while slight dilatation may occur during diastole to accommodate the increased venous input. Though the heart muscle cannot be entirely healthy following a pericarditis or endocarditis, it is unlikely to be damaged to the extent of loss of all reserve, and exercise, provided it does not make the patient breathless, will be beneficial in bringing about a little more work for the heart, and consequently an improvement in the condition of the muscle fibres. If, of course, too great a rise in pressure is produced, the weakened muscle might not be able to eject blood against this resistance, and dilatation with signs of failure might occur, consequently exercise has to be carefully chosen, controlled and graduated.

Two objects of physical treatment therefore emerge; the first is to build up the general musculature without throwing undue burden on the myocardium, the second is to increase very gradually the amount of work to be done by the cardiac muscle. These objects are fulfilled by graded active exercise. The usual medical and nursing procedure is to nurse the patient in the lying position, provided there is no dyspnoea. The patient is not allowed to undertake even the activities of feeding or washing himself until all evidence of an active lesion has disappeared. The first step in progress is an additional pillow, from this the patient progresses to sitting up to feed himself for one meal a day, then all meals. Next he is allowed to wash himself, then to shave; some days later he sits out of bed for twenty minutes, the time is then increased till he is allowed to walk a few steps.

Ideally, physical treatment begins when the patient is allowed his first additional pillow. Breathing exercises and muscular contractions are given. Breathing exercises are of value partly because of the increased oxygenation of the blood but also because they increase the venous input and so increase the work of the cardiac muscle. Because of this latter factor, they must be given with care. The choice of the amount of active contractions and movements depends on the level of the resting pulse, and on how long the patient has been resting. It is usual to find that contractions of all lower limb muscles, together with active movements of toes and feet, can be practised six to ten times with benefit. Further progression depends on the effects of these exercises. The only satisfactory way of testing the heart is by testing the exercise tolerance. Therefore three points stand out: How much has the exercise raised the heart rate? Has the pulse returned to resting level in under two minutes? Has the exercise made the patient breathless? Provided the pulse is not raised more than ten beats in the early days of treatment and that the pulse falls to resting level in two minutes, and the patient is not breathless or distressed, the amount of exercise is not too much, and progression may be made. Progression is made by the introduction of extra movements daily, adding first, exercise of the larger joints of the lower extremities, then contractions of trunk muscles, trunk exercises in sitting, exercises sitting on a chair beside the bed, standing correcting the posture, walking increasing distances and commencing stairs. At this stage the patient is usually discharged from hospital and attends as an out-patient, continuing with exercise.

Provided exercise does not make the patient breathless and the pulse returns to normal in the normal time, no fear need be felt when progressing to vigorous exercises.

Chapter II

CHRONIC VALVULAR DISORDERS. CORONARY OCCLUSION AND THROMBOSIS. ANGINA OF EFFORT. CONGENITAL ABNORMALITIES. EFFORT SYNDROME. HYPERTENSION

Disease of the cusps of the valves of the heart may be congenital but is more often acquired. Rheumatism is the most important factor, particularly tending to involve the mitral valve. Syphilis more often affects the aortic valve, while arterio-sclerosis of the aorta may spread to the cusps of this valve. Bacterial endocarditis attacks all the valves but more especially the mitral and aortic. In all chronic valvular diseases changes occur not only in the cusps but also in the myocardium. With the changes in the cusps we are already familiar (see preceding chapter). They lead either to a shrinking and puckering so that the cusps can no longer effect a complete closure of the orifice, or to a hardening and adherence of the edges so that the cusps fail to open properly and considerable force is needed to pump the blood through the narrowed orifice. In many cases the two changes occur together.

The changes in the myocardium are those of degeneration following the spread of inflammation from the endocardium, particularly is this so in rheumatic and bacterial endocarditis. Thus the cardiac muscle is not a normal healthy muscle and is eventually likely to show fibrillation and failure. It should be noted also that disease of the aortic valves may lead to pressure changes in the aorta and consequently in the coronary arteries and this reacts back on the myocardium and its efficiency.

The significance of a valvular disorder does not lie in the incompetence or stenosis, these can be readily overcome by a rather more forcible contraction of the muscular walls of the particular chamber involved, but in the progressive degeneration of the myocardium which gradually reduces the reserve. The additional strain of advancing years, rising blood pressure, and toxic illnesses will therefore lead to congestive failure far more readily than in those people who have a completely healthy musculature. The strain falls more on one part of the heart than another according to the valve affected; for example, a mitral stenosis involves harder work for the left auricle and right ventricle and pulmonary congestion arises first. Eventually, however, all parts of the heart are affected.

LESIONS OF THE AORTIC VALVE

The most usual lesion of this valve is a shrinkage and therefore incompetence. Stenosis is rare, since healing of the inflammation by organisation and binding of cusp edges together is unlikely where so much movement of the valve must occur.

In aortic incompetence blood regurgitates into the left ventricle on ventricular diastole. This blood, together with that normally in the ventricle, has to be ejected on each ventricular systole. The first effect is a slight dilatation of the left ventricle to accommodate the extra blood, the second is a stronger contraction in response to the greater initial length of the fibres. In time the stronger contraction leads to hypertrophy of the muscular fibres and the left ventricle is slightly enlarged. Therefore no ill effects of aortic regurgitation will be felt and, apart from diastolic murmur, high pulse pressure and altered pulse, no signs are present. The main symptom appreciable to the patient is the presence of palpitation. Due to regurgitation, the aorta is empty instead of full at the end of diastole, diastolic pressure is therefore very low. The ventricle pumps more than the usual quantity of blood into the empty vessel and systolic pressure is therefore unduly high. The consequent sudden expansion of the arteries and great momentum of the blood produces a large, strong and sudden pulse, which rapidly falls away.

Thus for a considerable time the systemic circulation remains efficient, ventricular hypertrophy having coped with aortic regurgitation. This, however, is unfortunately not the whole story. The coronary arteries open from two of the aortic pouches just distal to the cusps. As the aortic walls recoil on ventricular diastole, blood is pushed into the mouths of these vessels. The quantity and pressure of blood in the coronary circulation depends on the height and duration of arterial pressure in the aorta during ventricular diastole. As has already been seen, pressure drops rapidly in aortic regurgitation, consequently pressure in the coronary vessels is lowered, less exchange takes place through the coronary capillaries and reduced nutrition and oxygen eventually tells on the myocardial fibres, and so degeneration and fibrous replacement occurs. Thus a fibroid heart and a diminished reserve are gradually produced, till eventually, failure of the left ventricle to maintain an efficient output will give rise to pulmonary venous congestion.

We may say that 'compensation' has occurred when the left ventricle hypertrophies in response to increased work, in order to make the systemic circulation efficient. We speak of 'failing compensation' when failure occurs due to depletion of reserves. Neither term means a great deal; what really matters is that in the first case the patient is healthy with no harmful symptoms, in the second case breathlessness and venous congestion are appearing.

LESIONS OF THE MITRAL VALVE

Disease of the mitral valve is most often rheumatic in origin, later it is sometimes increased by bacterial infection. The lesion usually results in a severe degree of stenosis. Since the blood flows gently through this orifice, stenosis will more readily occur than in aortic valvular lesions. This hardening of the valve, and narrowing of its lumen, throws extra work on the left auricle, which therefore works harder to overcome the resistance and consequently shows hypertrophy. Since the muscular tissue of the auricles is not great, the left auricle may not be able to remedy the defect, and congestion therefore tends to occur in the pulmonary circulation. The right ventricle reacts to this, working harder to overcome the pulmonary resistance, with consequent hypertrophy and enlargement. Many cases of mitral stenosis show no symptoms, since a normal pulmonary circulation is maintained by the right ventricle. Altered heart sounds are the only certain signs of such a lesion. The significance of the lesion again lies in the effect it has on the cardiac reserve. In times of increased activity or emotion, a greater cardiac input, plus a rise in resistance to output due to raised blood pressure, brings about a more forcible contraction of the left ventricle and a greater output. This cannot be achieved, however, in a severe mitral stenosis, since the mitral orifice is unable to allow the extra blood to pass into the ventricle. The ventricle, without increased input, is unable to respond by stronger beats and can only provide the increased quantity of blood needed by beating more quickly. Tachycardia results, and, if this is long continued, the nutrition to the musculature is impaired and the muscle, which is probably already unhealthy due to the original rheumatic lesion, cannot withstand the strain. Cardiac failure therefore occurs. Supposing a prolonged strain such as that imposed by pregnancy and parturition is imposed, then reserves will be depleted and failure is liable to occur.

The presence of valvular lesion does not therefore necessitate the appearance of any symptoms and the patient may lead a perfectly healthy normal life and eventually die of some intercurrent disease. On the other hand, a time may come when due to the gradual depletion of reserves the heart begins to be unable to supply an efficient circulation in times of emergency. Breathlessness on some exertion makes its appearance, gradually increasing until the patient is breathless on walking slowly on the flat. At this stage other symptoms of congestive failure are evident, according to the area of the heart most affected.

PRINCIPLES OF TREATMENT BY PHYSIOTHERAPY

It is at the stage of congestive cardiac failure that patients suffering from chronic valvular lesions often attend for treatment.

Many of these patients are treated conservatively by rest, oxygen, cardiac stimulants, diuretics and by tapping if oedema is excessive and threatening to involve the abdominal cavity. Others may undergo surgical treatment. Both groups of patients benefit, at some period in their treatment, by physiotherapy.

PHYSIOTHERAPY FOR THE PATIENTS UNDERGOING MEDICAL TREATMENT

Five main principles underlie the physical treatment of these patients.

Firstly—since pulmonary congestion leads to a rise of pressure within the small vessels, oedema of the lungs will develop. There will, therefore, be a loss of aerating surface and diminished vital capacity. Chronic bronchitis will be a characteristic feature and cough and expectoration will be present leading to further strain on the heart.

Breathing exercises are, therefore, an essential part of the treatment of these patients. Expectoration may be made easier by gentle percussion on the chest wall and the patient may be turned from side to side though 'tipping' is usually difficult and rarely possible. It has been suggested that breathing exercises serve only to increase pulmonary congestion but this has not been found to be correct. The patient is not told to take deep breaths in and out but, in time to his present respiratory rate, he is encouraged to try to think of emptying the lungs of air and of using the bases of the lungs more fully. Gradually the length of expiration naturally increases and respiratory rate slows. Coughing is made easier by gentle chest clapping and shaking and, as the chest clears, dyspnoea is lessened.

Secondly—as the patient has probably undergone a period of four to six weeks of almost complete bed rest the condition of the cardiac and voluntary heart musculature is likely to have deteriorated considerably. The patient should resume activity only gradually. Carefully graded active exercises are, therefore, valuable. These, while progressively introducing all muscle groups, should be particularly directed to the strengthening of the postural muscles. Exercises should not make the patient dyspnoeic, hence a careful watch must be kept during their performance.

Thirdly—in chronic cardiac disease, owing to the slowing of blood flow and relative inactivity of the patient, there is a tendency towards the development of thrombosis. During the period of bed rest, therefore, massage and passive movements of the legs serve to hasten the superficial blood flow and lessen this danger. These should be started as soon as the physician considers the patient is able to tolerate them, probably three to four weeks after the commencement of medical treatment.

Fourthly—these patients are nearly all tense and frightened. Many are very anxious about the future. This state of anxiety is detrimental to the condition of the heart and blood vessels and much can be done to reduce tension by training the patient to relax. General relaxation is begun as soon as the physician allows the patient to commence physical treatment.

Fifthly—as soon as the patient is allowed to resume activity it is important to show him what exercise he can take with safety. Some patients are nervous and fail to do enough, others try to do too much. The patient is, therefore, encouraged to do a little more each day but it is carefully pointed out that exercise should not make his breathing difficult and that if this does occur then he is doing too much.

One or two points should be borne in mind when commencing physical treatment. It is usually begun one to two weeks after signs and symptoms of congestive cardiac failure have disappeared while the patient is at rest. The patient will be found in bed, usually propped up in the half lying position. The position of the head and shoulders should not be lowered since breathing then becomes more difficult. Too much pulse taking is unwise because the patient is already over-anxious about his heart. The best way of judging the suitability of a scheme of physical treatment is the effect it has on the respiratory rate, though other changes such as cyanosis, irritability, inability to concentrate may all be noted. Exercise should not be pressed too far since, after congestive cardiac failure, the patient is unlikely to be able ever to return to full normal activity, although he will probably be able to walk comfortably on the flat and resume a sedentary occupation.

PHYSIOTHERAPY FOR PATIENTS UNDERGOING SURGICAL TREATMENT

Some patients are found suitable for a valvotomy. The operation is one in which the commissures of the valve are split, thus lessening the resistance offered by stenosed valves to the flow of blood through the heart. Patients are very carefully selected for this operation. They are most often those suffering from mitral stenosis with a minimum amount of incompetence, since the procedure cannot correct any incompetence. The most suitable age group is that between twenty and fifty since for those younger than this it cannot be certain that any rheumatic condition, responsible for the stenosis, is completely inactive. The operation has spectacular results, because once the commissures are split an immediate relief of obstruction is obtained. Cyanosis therefore disappears, the limbs become warmer, the sense of constriction in the chest is no longer present and breathing is easier. Often patients who have not previously been able to lie down are now able to sleep in the recumbent position and sometimes they are able to return to quite heavy work.

Both pre- and post-operative treatment are valuable. As has already been seen these patients are liable to chest complications and to thrombosis and embolism. Pre-operative breathing exercises both general and local, coughing and percussion, relaxation, and simple leg exercises are, therefore, essential. Post-operatively the objects of physical treatment are to prevent lung collapse, to avoid thrombosis and embolism, to train to the gradual resumption of activity and to prevent faults in posture and limitation of arm movements.

CORONARY OCCLUSION

Occlusion of a coronary artery or its branches may be sudden or gradual. Sudden occlusion is due to an embolus, probably from a vegetation on one of the cusps of the aortic valve, or to thrombosis in arteries already diseased. Gradual occlusion arises as a result either of arteriosclerosis of the coronary arteries, or is due to the same condition affecting the aorta and giving rise to a thickening which blocks the mouths of the coronary vessels. If the condition occurs in elderly people it is often due to arteriosclerosis which is part of a generalised disease of the arteries. When arteriosclerosis occurs in young adults it appears to attack the coronary vessels particularly, probably because the intima seems to be much thicker in these vessels than in any other arteries of similar size.

CORONARY THROMBOSIS

Occlusion occurs most commonly from thrombosis of the descending branch of the left coronary artery, which supplies the anterior surface of the left ventricle, much of the interventricular septum and the apex of the heart. This area is cut off from its nutrition and consequently necroses, an infarct being formed. Gradually the necrosed area is replaced by fibrous tissue forming a weak spot in the wall of the ventricle. If the area of necrosis arises on the endocardial surface of the muscle, a large thrombus will form; should it occur on the pericardial surface an area of pericarditis results. Gradual occlusion has the same final result but necrosis does not occur, fibrous replacement of cardiac cells taking place over a long period.

An occlusion due to thrombosis most often occurs when the individual is at rest, often when he is asleep. If the main artery is involved death will occur at once; if a smaller branch, pain is a most characteristic feature. This pain, which is the result of complete ischaemia, starts behind the lower segment of the sternum, and becomes more widespread as it increases in intensity. It lasts for an hour or more, since the ischaemic muscle goes on working, and then the pain gradually subsides, possibly over several days. The patient is usually restless or may roll about in agony, movement does not appear to affect the pain. During the attack the patient looks pale and anxious, sweats profusely, is deeply cyanosed. The blood pressure drops, and the pulse is feeble or impalpable. Breathlessness may be present. Owing to the development of an area of necrosis the patient becomes febrile the same or the following day, the rise of temperature lasting a day or two and being accompanied by a leucocytosis.

Two particular dangers arise; one is a rupture of the heart, occurring about the second week when infarction is present and firm fibrous tissue has not taken its place; the second is an embolus from the thrombosis on the endocardium.

The ultimate condition depends upon the extent of damage to the heart muscle and the original state of that muscle. Coronary thrombosis occurring in those who have already suffered from heart failure, or angina, is likely to result in permanent limitation of activity. If thrombosis is small, and the patient previously healthy, recovery may be complete and the patient may have many years of active life ahead.

Sometimes the physiotherapist is asked to treat these patients following a long period of complete rest in bed. The object of prolonged and complete rest is to ensure firm scarring of the necrotic tissue. Towards the end of this period of rest physical treatment should be given on the same lines

333

as that for carditis. Since there is good hope of the patient being able to return to full activity, limited only by the onset of breathlessness on exertion, carefully graded active exercises should be given.

ANGINA OF EFFORT

This is a condition of pain in the chest making its appearance on exercise or emotion. While there may be no pathological explanation of the condition it is often the result of arteriosclerosis of the coronary arteries, syphilitic aortitis or aortic stenosis. Whatever the cause, there is a relative ischaemia, and insufficient blood is available for the myocardium when the heart is called upon for extra effort. The first attack usually occurs during the performance of some ordinary activity, the patient experiencing discomfort or pain in the region of the upper half of the sternum. He immediately stands immobile and within a moment or two the pain subsides. In time, the attacks tend to become more frequent and severe, pain spreads into the neck and down the medial side of the left forearm. The patient appears terrified and often sweats profusely and the attack leaves him weak and exhausted. Through fear of pain the patient gradually limits his own activities and eventually, after perhaps ten years or more, he will die, either from coronary thrombosis or cardiac failure.

The main principle of treatment is the regulation of activity in relation to the pain, therefore rest is not complete, but exercise is limited to that which does not produce angina. On the other hand exercise should certainly not be cut out, provided it does not produce pain it is beneficial and increases the strength of the cardiac muscle. Since these patients set and limit their own exercise, they are rarely treated by physical measures. The use of short-wave diathermy to the chest has been advocated to improve the coronary circulation. No marked effect, however, has been proved.

CONGENITAL ABNORMALITIES

Congenital disorders of the heart and great vessels are of considerable interest to the physiotherapist, since it may be her function to give pre- and post-operative treatment, or she may be called upon to give exercise tolerance tests when the value of operative procedure is being considered.

The commonest defects in development are defects in the interventricular septum and pulmonary stenosis, coarctation of the aorta, persistent ductus arteriosus and patent foramen ovale.

CONGENITAL ABNORMALITIES

Pulmonary Stenosis and Interventricular Septum Defects—Fallot's Tetralogy.

About eighty per cent of all congenital abnormalities consist of a group of four defects described by Fallot and now known as Fallot's Tetralogy. These defects comprise an imperfect interventricular septum, an aorta arising from both ventricles, a pulmonary artery grossly stenosed and the right ventricle much hypertrophied. The result is a mixing of arterial and venous blood, since with each ventricular contraction blood passes from right to left ventricle. Much blood therefore by-passes the pulmonary circulation. The patient shows deep cyanosis, becoming increasingly blue on any exercise. There is marked dyspnoea, the fingers are clubbed, the number of red blood corpuscles may be as high as eight million per cubic millimetre of blood. Reduced oxygenation of the blood will cause reduced rate of mental and physical growth. The child invariably looks many years younger than his age. Unless something can be done the expectation of life is poor. In 1944 Professor Blalock of Baltimore devised an operation in which an anastomosis was made between the left subclavian and left pulmonary arteries. Since that time various other procedures have been tried out but all aim at the same object—increasing the quantity of blood passing into the pulmonary circulation.

Coarctation of the Aorta

During foetal life a communication exists between the aorta and the pulmonary artery just beyond the origin of the subclavian artery. This vessel is known as the ductus arteriosus. At birth this closes and atrophies. Occasionally when the ductus shrinks the aorta becomes severely constricted just beyond its attachment. This does not, as might be expected, completely cut off the arterial circulation to the lower extremities, since dilatation and hypertrophy of collateral vessels occurs. Blood is carried into the areas below the constriction by an anastamosis between the sub-scapular and intercostal arteries and the internal mammary and inferior epigastric vessels. These collateral vessels grow in length, and in the size and strength of their walls. The condition may be detected by the presence of a high blood pressure in the carotid and upper extremity vessels, while the pulse in the lower extremities may be less full or absent.

The condition produces no immediate ill-effects, and the expectation of life is reasonably good, but there is always danger of rupture of the aorta, infective endocarditis, or death from cerebral haemorrhage which in its turn is the result of high carotid pressure. In some cases to avoid these dangers the constricted section of the aorta is excised.

PERSISTENT DUCTUS ARTERIOSUS

Occasionally the ductus arteriosus fails to close at birth; this has serious consequences because blood will pass from the aorta into the pulmonary artery (see Fig. 14). At least half, if not more of the blood, takes this

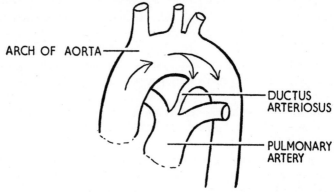

ARCH OF AORTA

DUCTUS ARTERIOSUS

PULMONARY ARTERY

Fig. 14. Diagram showing patent Ductus Arteriosus and direction of bloodflow.

pathway. There is, therefore, a considerable rise of pressure in the pulmonary capillaries. The greater quantity of blood in the pulmonary circulation means a greater filling of the left auricle and this in its turn means a larger amount of blood in the left ventricle. Considerable hypertrophy of the left side of the heart follows the increased filling and, if the condition is allowed to persist, dilatation and failure must eventually occur.

Cyanosis does not occur because there is no mixing of arterial or venous blood; systolic blood pressure is not greatly raised because no ventricular systole blood is passing from the aorta to the pulmonary artery, but diastolic pressure will fall as there is less blood in the aorta. The pulse pressure is therefore high and the pulse is of the water-hammer type, characteristic of aortic incompetence (see page 328).

This condition requires treatment largely because of the certainty of later cardiac failure and also because it predisposes towards a bacterial endocarditis. The treatment is surgical, the patent vessel being ligatured at either end.

Patent Foramen Ovale

In a few cases defects occur in the development of the inter-auricular septum or the foramen ovale fails to close. Provided the defect is not too great no ill-effects result.

336

PRINCIPLES OF TREATMENT OF CONGENITAL ABNOR-MALITIES BY PHYSIOTHERAPY

Details of physical treatment will be found in textbooks dealing with surgical chest conditions. The principles are those underlying the treatment of valvotomy, but, in addition, in congenital cyanotic disease (Fallot's Tetralogy), it has to be borne in mind that these children have often been kept at home, allowed little exercise because exertion results in increased dyspnoea and cyanosis, and have, therefore, had little contact with the outside world. It is, therefore, essential to gain the child's confidence prior to the operation, to increase the exercise tolerance and find out of what the child really is capable.

EFFORT SYNDROME

Some patients who are not in good health complain of a group of symptoms which occur on mild degrees of exercise. Fairly severe exercise is normally followed by certain physical signs and symptoms, thus a man undertaking reasonably hard work may suffer from breathlessness, which only subsides gradually when the activity is completed. He may feel giddy or faint, he may become conscious of his heart beat and feel exhausted. His blood pressure and pulse will both be considerably raised, but these will fall rapidly at the end of the exercise. The patient suffering from effort syndrome has exactly this set of symptoms, but they arise much sooner than would be expected, a mild degree of exercise, sometimes very slight indeed, produces them. They lead the patient to the erroneous belief that the heart is diseased.

The condition occurs most often in young people, though it can occur at any age. In some, it is the result of infection from some toxic focus, in others it occurs after a severe infection such as influenza or pneumonia. It sometimes occurs in early cases of tuberculosis. Occasionally it is seen in young men who are called on to undertake strenuous physical exertion when their normal occupation is a sedentary one. Some cases show none of these causes, but in these a psychological factor may be present. Such a patient may be unsuitably placed in his work, unhappy at home, or undergoing some emotional crisis.

In most patients the signs and symptoms arise gradually. The patient complains of becoming breathless very readily, of having palpitations, of fainting on sudden change of posture, of suffering from extreme fatigue and a sense of exhaustion following quite light exercise. This patient is often 'heart conscious', he takes his own pulse and may find it fast or irregular.

If this patient is given a simple endurance test, such as hopping on one foot a certain number of times, it will be found that the pulse, which, in the normal individual, would rise only ten or fifteen beats, may rise to 120 or more, and may take five, ten or fifteen minutes to fall to its normal level. The resting pulse is also unduly high. The same test which would not be likely to alter the normal young adult's respiratory rate or depth will make this patient dyspnoeic.

Other signs of autonomic instability are usually present, the patient sweats profusely, the feet and hands are cold, the face and neck flush easily and the patient is unduly emotional.

No evidence of organic lesion of the heart is present. The heart is not enlarged, the normal cardiac impulse is present, the pulse and respiratory rates are normal during sleep. It would seem that there is some over-stimulation of the sympathetic cardiac nerves. Treatment for these cases is on rather different lines from that used for the organic cardiac lesion. Usually the first step taken by the physician is a thorough examination and testing of the heart to exclude the presence of any organic lesion. A more general examination is also carried out to search for any evidence of chronic infection in tonsils, antra, sinuses or for early tuberculosis. If no organic lesion is present, the physician reassures the patient as to the condition of his heart and explains the symptoms to him. If any area of infection is discovered this is dealt with. In some cases it may be necessary to give psychiatric treatment. Change from work and home surroundings usually proves helpful.

OUTLINE OF TREATMENT BY PHYSIOTHERAPY

These patients are best treated in a rehabilitation centre where full attention can be given to adequate rest, satisfactory diet, fresh air and reasonable occupation and entertainment. Ideally, the physiotherapist should be part of the team undertaking the rehabilitation of this patient. The general health may be improved by a course of artificial sunlight and relaxation exercises. General exercises are most valuable because they improve the condition of both skeletal and cardiac musculature, their object also is to increase the patient's exercise tolerance. The exercises used for these patients differ from those used for cardiac diseases in that they may make the patient slightly breathless provided they do not produce real distress. They may send the pulse up to 150 or more provided it falls below 100 two minutes after the exercise is completed. Work consists, therefore, of a light scheme of general exercises, carried out twice a day in the open air if possible, and including plenty of breathing exercises to increase oxygenation and vital capacity. The scheme should be progressed to the point of increasing appreciably the rate and depth of respiration. Many of these patients show marked improvement in two or three months and are able to return to their employment. Usually by the end of two or three years the symptoms have completely disappeared.

HYPERTENSION

A condition of hypertension is one in which there is a persistent elevation of the blood pressure above the normal. Two main types are recognised: Primary or Essential Hypertension in which no inflammation of the kidneys can be detected, and Secondary, in which an acute or chronic nephritis is present.

In both cases the cause of the high blood pressure is due to increased tone in the peripheral blood vessels. In essential hypertension no explanation of this increased tone can be given but in the secondary condition it is the result of liberation of pressor substances by the damaged kidney.

The age of onset varies with the type; essential hypertension is characteristic of elderly people usually between fifty and seventy, while secondary hypertension nearly always makes its appearance before forty. In many cases the patient is obese but this is not by any means invariably so. Both men and women are affected, and when women are involved essential hypertension often makes its appearance just after the menopause.

Pathological changes occur both in the heart and in the blood vessels. The left ventricle is subjected to a much increased strain since resistance to its output is raised. The result is a great increase in its size due to hypertrophy of the muscular fibres. Though the right ventricle shows some hypertrophy, the left is particularly involved. Eventually the time will come when the strain is too great and signs of cardiac failure will begin to appear. Not only is there continuous extra work for the heart but in addition the persistent high pressure exerts a strain on the blood vessels and arterio-sclerotic changes are liable to occur. These changes result in thickening of the vessel walls and narrowing of the lumen, consequently blood flow is impaired and nutrition to the tissues reduced. Visceral vessels appear to be particularly involved and visceral complications are liable to arise.

Signs and symptoms are not necessarily present. Many a patient leads a healthy active life totally unaware that he has an unduly high blood pressure. Hypertension may be accidentally discovered when the patient is being medically examined for a life insurance firm or for a new post.

Where symptoms do arise they are nearly always due to the ischaemia resulting from the arterio-sclerotic changes. Often the cerebral vessels are affected and the patient may complain of headaches, severe after exercise or on getting up in the morning. Sometimes minor attacks of giddiness occur, the patient is restless and irritable and sleeps badly. Later he may find difficulty in concentrating and may suffer from lapses of memory. Lack of energy and general fatigue are common later symptoms. When cardiac failure begins, breathlessness on exertion is seen, this becomes increasingly marked until signs of congestive failure appear. In the later stages cardiac asthma may be a feature.

Rupture of the arterio-sclerotic vessels sometimes occurs; this accounts for the retinal and petechial haemorrhages which are a feature of hypertension. Thrombosis or rupture of cerebral vessels may produce a hemiplegia.

Owing to defective circulation and nutrition these patients are particularly liable to develop respiratory conditions and bronchitis and pneumonia are not uncommon complications.

OUTLINE OF TREATMENT BY PHYSIOTHERAPY

These patients mainly require medical treatment in the form of drugs, diet, attention to adequate rest and sleep. In some cases a bilateral thoraco-lumbar sympathectomy is performed and pre- and post-operative breathing exercises and general active exercises are ordered. Physiotherapy for the actual lowering of blood pressure could at best be only a very temporary measure. General massage and passive movements, together with a course of general diathermy, will in many cases produce a temporary lowering of the pressure, by producing a reduction in vascular tone, but no permanent effect is obtained. On the other hand physical measures will help in the relief of certain of the symptoms.

Adequate rest and plenty of sleep is an essential for these patients and these can be better obtained if the patient is taught relaxation. Occasionally the patient may acquire a better habit of sleep if deep rhythmical general massage is given, together with relaxation, for a week or two, prior to settling down at night.

A certain amount of active work is good for the heart and blood vessels, especially if taken in the fresh air. This may be graded and supervised by the physiotherapist who keeps it well within the level at which it causes any distress. If the patient is overweight and cannot, by means of exercise, help himself to reduce weight then massage combined with strict dieting and drugs will help. These patients are sometimes ordered physiotherapy for the complications which arise—for example a hemiplegia. In carrying out suitable physical treatment the hypertension should be remembered; suitable positions with the head and shoulders raised should be chosen and care should be taken to keep exercise within the limit of the patient's capabilities.

Chapter III

DISEASES OF THE BLOOD VESSELS.
ANAEMIA

The physiotherapist is mainly concerned with those diseases which affect the limb vessels. Each limb is supplied by a main artery and its terminal branches. In addition, at various points in the course of the artery, subsidiary branches are given off which join one another according to a definite plan to form a collateral circulation. This collateral circulation is capable of carrying sufficient blood to maintain the life of the tissues if the main artery is obstructed.

The quantity of arterial blood in the limb as a whole is mainly regulated by the vaso-motor centre in the floor of the fourth ventricle. Fibres from the cells of this centre travel down the cervical region of the spinal cord to form a synapse with the cells of the lateral horn of the dorsal and first two lumbar segments. Medullated pre-ganglionic fibres leave the lateral horn, pass through the anterior nerve root to enter the white ramus and so reach the sympathetic trunk. Nerve fibres to the large vessels such as the aorta, subclavian and iliac vessels are supplied from sympathetic ganglia directly. Fibres to the limb vessels, the femoral and axillary, travel via the spinal nerves, particularly in the median and ulnar nerves in the arm and the sciatic nerve in the leg. Nerve fibres are eventually distributed to arteries, arterioles, capillaries and veins. The vaso-motor centre continuously discharges impulses which maintain the blood vessels in a degree of contraction or tone. The centre itself is stimulated by higher centres, by increased carbon-dioxide content of the blood and by messages from the respiratory centre, while it is depressed by messages from the sinus and aortic nerves and by even a slight rise in the temperature of the blood (see Figs. 15 and 16).

The local regulation of the vascular tone is mainly brought about by chemical substances liberated by the tissues themselves. Active tissues liberate more products of metabolism (metabolites) and these act directly on arteriole and capillary walls, producing vaso-dilatation. In addition, increased activity means increased heat production and a rise of temperature in the tissues acts directly on the vessel walls, producing dilatation.

342

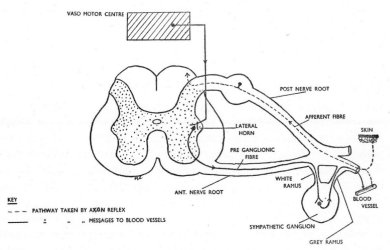

KEY

- - - PATHWAY TAKEN BY AXON REFLEX

———— :. " " MESSAGES TO BLOOD VESSELS

Fig. 15

FACTORS INFLUENCING VASCULAR TONE

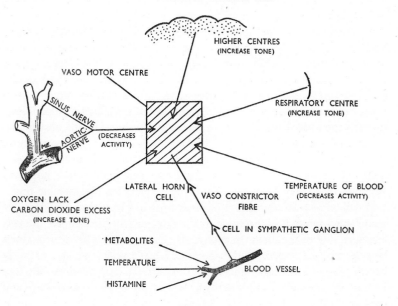

Fig. 16

343

In this way the active tissues gain greater nutrition. When the tissues become less active their temperature falls, less metabolites are produced, consequently blood vessels shrink.

EFFECTS OF CIRCULATORY OBSTRUCTION

If the limb circulation is completely obstructed the pulse disappears, the temperature falls and skin becomes deeply cyanotic. Within twenty or thirty minutes nerves and muscles become ischaemic. If muscles are exercised, pain occurs, since metabolites accumulate and irritate the sensory nerve endings. As nerves become ischaemic, numbness is followed by increasing sensory loss, muscle weakness commences at the periphery and spreads up the limb until complete paralysis is present. Provided the period of obstruction is brief, complete recovery is rapid and is characterised by hyperaemia, as the blood vessels dilate in response to the accumulated metabolites, and tingling, due to changes in the nerves. If, however, obstruction is prolonged to several hours, permanent damage results. If ischaemia persists for six hours, necrosis of muscle and fibrous replacement will develop, while if it is slightly more prolonged degeneration of nerve occurs. Skin first shows wealing and blistering, while if ischaemia extends beyond twenty-four hours ulceration will occur.

Obstruction of a main limb artery does not produce such severe changes because there will be dilatation of the collateral vessels. This is due to the accumulation of metabolites in the area supplied by the blocked vessel. Should the obstruction persist, the walls of the collateral vessels gradually lengthen and thicken, and the lumen is increased. This alteration is probably the direct result of the stimulating effect of the increased blood flow, through the dilated vessels. The immediate symptoms of the obstruction are loss of the pulses below the level of the lesion, fall in temperature, cyanosis of the limb and pain on attempted exercise of the part. Within a short time, however, the temperature rises again and colour improves although there may be obliteration of the pulse for a considerable time.

It will be realised that conditions may arise in which gradually developing changes result in diminution in the lumen of all the arteries, the collateral as well as the main. In such a case less symptoms arise than would be expected, partly because the process is usually very gradual, and partly because an enormous number of tiny arterial anastamoses develop. Eventually, however, ischaemic pain, loss of pulse, low temperature and gangrene will develop.

Circulatory obstruction may be the result of three main factors: thrombosis or embolism; organic changes in the vessel walls; and vaso-motor spasm. The first two of these, though seen separately, often occur together. Arterial obstruction due to organic changes in vessel walls is most commonly seen in the physiotherapy department in cases of thrombo-angiitis obliterans and arteriosclerosis; while Raynaud's disease is a common example of vaso-motor spasm.

THROMBO-ANGIITIS OBLITERANS (Buerger's Disease)

This is a disease of arteries occurring in young males almost exclusively. It attacks the vessels of the lower extremities particularly, though those of the arms may also be affected. The cause of the condition is unknown; it has, however, been suggested that there is an inherited hyper-sensitiveness to tobacco proteins and that this factor, together with sex and age, predisposes the vessels to attack by some micro-organism.

The condition is an inflammatory one attacking all the coats of long or short segments of the arteries. It is not the main artery only which is affected, the collateral vessels are also involved in the process. During the acute phase the walls and the perivascular tissues are invaded by inflammatory cells, thrombosis occurs on the inflamed endothelium and the lumen of the affected segment is obliterated. Gradually inflammation subsides but it leaves the arteries, veins and nerves within the vascular sheath matted together in fibrous tissue. The organised clot turns the vessels into fibrous cords. Occasionally tiny vessels are formed in the fibrous tissue as blood gradually works its way through.

Not only is the lumen of the affected vessels narrowed or lost as a result of the inflammatory changes, but in addition some element of spasm may be present due to trapping of vaso-motor nerves in the fibrous tissue.

The symptoms develop due to the diminution of blood, and therefore of nutrition to the tissues. In the acute stage no symptoms are present with the exception of red tender spots which may arise as a result of phlebitis of superficial veins. The most usual symptom in the chronic stage is that of intermittent claudication. This is the condition in which there is sudden onset of pain in the calf on walking, which may be so severe that it may bring the patient to an abrupt standstill. When the activity ceases the pain passes off. This sudden onset of severe pain which passes off on rest is explained by the fact that the circulation is inadequate to meet the demands of the contracting muscles, while it is adequate for the muscles at rest. The result is that metabolites rapidly accumulate in the tissues on activity, irritation of sensory nerve endings results and pain arises. As the disease progresses the amount of walking possible before the onset of pain decreases and the pain is slower to subside when the patient stands still.

As time passes other symptoms develop, the dorsalis pedis and posterior tibial pulses disappear, the foot blanches very rapidly if it is elevated and becomes unduly red and throbs painfully if the leg is allowed to hang down. This is probably the result of the loss of vaso-motor control since the sympathetic nerves in the connective sheath of the blood vessels are involved in the inflammatory process and fibrosis. Pain comes on without activity, often being noticeable in the toes and ball of the foot, especially when the foot becomes warm at night; the patient only then finds comfort if the leg is removed from under the bedclothes. In time trophic changes tend to take place in the skin and if care is not taken slight abrasions will be followed by ulceration. Dry gangrene is likely then to develop. In many cases amputation is eventually necessary.

ARTERIOSCLEROSIS

Arteriosclerosis is the term applied to the condition in which changes occur in the arterial walls leading to loss of elasticity, thickening of the intima and narrowing of the lumen. There are several varieties of arteriosclerosis, but it is when it affects the limb arteries that the patient reaches the department of physical medicine.

There is a proliferation of the elastic and fibrous elements of the tunica intima and often thrombus formation. These changes lead to narrowing of the lumen and sometimes to complete obliteration of the vessel. In some cases degenerative changes arise also in the tunica media and calcium is deposited in the muscular coat. This type of sclerosis is known as Monckeborg's sclerosis and is found in the arteries of the lower extremities of elderly people.

The cause of these changes is uncertain. They occur most often in old age and men are more affected than women. It is common in diabetic patients and in association with high blood pressure. Unlike thromboangiitis obliterans it is the whole length of the arteries which is involved.

Since signs and symptoms are due to the gradual reduction in the supply of blood to the extremities, they are very similar to those of the preceding condition. The first complaints may be of a feeling of coldness and numbness in the feet, and frequent cramp. Later there may be pain in the foot and leg and ischaemic pain on walking, leading to intermittent claudication. Discoloration of the skin is often seen. Oedema may be present since the endothelium becomes more permeable as the oxygen tension falls with slowing of blood flow. The pulse in the main vessels will eventually be lost and gradually necrotic changes and gangrene make their appearance. Necrosis usually begins round the nail of the great toe due to some slight trauma such as might occur from an ingrowing nail. The devitalised tissues fail to heal and ulceration spreads; infection readily occurs. Gradually the tissues change colour and become black, a clear line of demarcation appears between healthy and unhealthy tissue and eventually the necrosed area may shrivel and fall off.

RAYNAUD'S DISEASE

This disease is a paroxysmal spasm of the digital arteries and capillaries occurring far more often in the fingers than in the toes. It tends to occur in women more commonly than men and usually in adolescence or early adult life. It is symmetrical and bilateral.

The cause of the spasm is uncertain, but it appears to be an abnormal sensitiveness of the small vessels to cold, so that on exposure they develop an abnormally high degree of tone. Thus an attack may easily be precipitated by swimming in cold water, by washing the hands in cold water, and in more severe cases even by exposure of the hands to cold environmental temperature. The fault does not lie, as was at one time thought, in the vaso-motor centre but in the small blood vessels themselves. In some cases the tunica intima is thickened and the vessels are therefore unable to expand completely, but whether this is the cause or the result of the spasm is uncertain. In mild cases during an attack the fingers become slightly pale, then greyish as oxygen is lost to the tissues, after a few moments the whole finger may be dead white. Recovery rapidly occurs, the vessels relaxing and the finger becoming red from base to tip.

In more severe cases, instead of recovery, the capillaries may relax while the arterioles remain constricted, venous blood therefore flows back into the capillaries and the fingers become deeply cyanotic. In these cases there is usually numbness and pain.

Slight cases of Raynaud's disease rarely progress but more severe cases will progress until full recovery from an attack does not occur. Marked nutritional changes will then appear, the fingers atrophy, the pads flattening, the nails becoming more curved and ridged, the bones rarefied. Often some loss of elasticity in the skin results in stiffness of the fingers. In many cases necrosis occurs at the tip of the fingers. Blisters form which burst and scabs result; these eventually fall off, leaving scars or tiny unhealed ulcers. Over a long period of time gradual loss of substance from the finger tips often takes place. Fingers which show this necrosis are painful, and use of the hands is much impaired.

TREATMENT

The main object of treatment for these conditions is to increase the quantity of blood in the limb and so to raise the nutrition and relieve the symptoms. How the quantity of blood can be increased depends on whether there is any element of vaso-motor spasm or whether the condition is entirely due to changes in the vessel walls. The first step, therefore, is to examine the vessels to estimate their condition and their capacity to dilate. Various tests may be made. The simplest is a palpation of the artery to detect changes in its wall or the presence or absence of a pulse wave. If the pulse cannot be detected one of the three preceding conditions is probably present. A temperature test is most commonly used to detect capacity to dilate. The limbs are exposed to room temperature for twenty minutes, the temperature of the tip of each toe being taken by a skin thermometer. One or both arms (where lower limb vessels are to be tested) are then immersed in warm water baths for three-quarters of an hour. The temperature of each toe is taken at intervals of five minutes during this time. The warmed blood in the upper extremities will circulate to the vaso-motor centre and reduce its activity; in this case tone in the blood vessels should drop. If the constriction in the vessels of the lower extremity is due to spasm the vessels will dilate. If, on the other hand, there is little or no element of spasm, little dilatation can occur. If the vessels dilate, the skin will become warmer and the temperature will rise steeply. If no rise of skin temperature occurs it may be considered that no element of spasm exists. If a rise of 4° C. takes place some spasm is probably present, while a rise of 6° or more indicates a considerable element of spasm.

Another simple test is to note the appearance of the limb in different positions. If arterial obstruction is present, when the limb is elevated it will blanch very readily and when it is suspended over the edge of the bed the foot will become very congested. This test does not, of course, detect shades of spasm, it simply gives an idea of degrees of obstruction. An X-ray photograph will show the presence or absence of calcification of arteries. The injection of radio-opaque substance into the blood stream and subsequent X-ray photograph will show the site of obstruction and the condition of the collateral circulation.

Surgical treatment. In cases in which the heat test shows a rise of more than 4°C., if the patient is willing and his physical condition is suitable a sympathectomy may be performed. This cuts off the normal tonic impulses from the blood vessels and relaxation of the walls occurs. A cervical sympathectomy is the most frequent method of treatment for Raynaud's disease. A lumbar sympathectomy is not uncommonly advocated in Buerger's disease, since there may be some element of spasm and, in addition, those vessels which do not show organic changes will lose their tone, dilate and offer less resistance to blood flow. A sympathectomy is rarely of value for cases of arterio-sclerosis, since there is little element of spasm and the patients are elderly and often unsuitable for operative procedures.

In some cases in which there is a gross narrowing of the lumen of a segment of an artery, an arterial graft may be attempted.

Medical treatment. For those patients who are unwilling or unsuitable for sympathectomy, medical treatment consists of the use of vaso-dilator drugs such as nicotinic acid, training the patient to live within the limits of his arteries, protecting the tissues from injuries, and dealing with such complications as thrombosis and incipient gangrene.

PRINCIPLES OF TREATMENT BY PHYSIOTHERAPY

The object of any physical treatment is to improve the circulation to the limbs and so to relieve symptoms. There are two main ways in which circulation may be improved. In those cases in which spasm is the main element, attention is directed towards relief of this spasm; in those cases in which organic changes are present, attempt is made to assist the collateral circulation to develop as fully as possible. Even when all the vessels are affected, it has been seen how surprisingly few are the symptoms over a long period because smaller arterial anastamoses develop. Though it is clear that in certain cases amputation will eventually be necessary, the longer this can be delayed the better and therefore all that can should be done to aid the establishment of these small anastamoses. In addition all measures possible should be taken to prevent abrasions and avoid skin ulceration and gangrene.

Relief of Spasm. In order to relieve spasm in the blood vessels and to reduce tone in other unaffected vessels heat may be applied by the use of a tunnel radiant heat bath, or by inductothermy or short-wave therapy. The principle is that the trunk should be heated, not the affected limbs. If the trunk is heated, the blood in the splanchnic area is warmed and carried to the vaso-motor centre. The activity of this centre is depressed by the raised temperature of the blood, and there will be a drop in the tone of the blood vessels throughout the body, with consequent increased blood flow to the extremities. If, on the other hand, the affected limbs are heated, their metabolism is increased, a greater number of metabolites are produced; there is, therefore, a greater need for blood which cannot be met. General heat to the trunk should ideally be given daily over a period of four to six weeks. By this means the blood supply to the extremities is often improved sufficiently to prevent, at least temporarily, the onset of gangrene or to allow a small area of gangrene to separate, and thus for a time delay the necessity for amputation.

Massage may temporarily relieve spasm in Raynaud's disease and active exercises are sometimes useful, since the warming of the tissues may aid in relaxation of the spasm.

Particularly in cases of Raynaud's disease should the patient be kept warm. Exposure to cold may provoke an attack of vascular spasm. For this reason the patient will have been advised to wear warm clothing and to cover the hands and feet warmly; this must be borne in mind when administering any form of physical treatment.

Improvement of the collateral circulation. Buerger's exercises, either given alone or as an adjunct to other measures, often prove very successful. They are particularly useful for those cases suffering from intermittent claudication, in which gangrene has not developed. It is not clear exactly how these exercises obtain their effects. It is probable that the alterations in pressure, obtained by variations in posture, have a suction and stimulating effect on the blood flow in the limbs, and encourage the development of a more efficient collateral circulation. The limb is elevated until the skin blanches, it is then kept dependent until congestion occurs, when it is allowed to lie flat until normal colour returns. This series of positions may be repeated for one hour several times a day. This method of treatment is often combined with the use of suction and pressure. In this method the limb is encased in an airtight chamber and by means of a motor subjected to alternate negative and positive pressure, causing blood to be alternately sucked into the vessels of the lower extremity and then driven out.

A similar method is that of intermittent venous occlusion by means of a cuff wrapped round the upper extremity of the thigh and alternate inflation and deflation of this cuff by a small electric motor. This method may be used continuously for the greater part of the day over a period of three weeks, being taken off twice a day while Buerger's exercises are performed.

Contrast baths are often most effective, and in a modified form may be practised at home. They should not be used for cases of Raynaud's disease. From time to time ionisation with vaso-dilator drugs has been advocated, and has had a fair measure of success.

Sinusoidal baths sometimes prove effective. By stimulating the cutaneous nerve endings the axon reflex may be set in action and vaso-dilatation results. These baths should not be used in severe cases or in cases of incipient gangrene, since they are valueless where vaso-dilatation has become impossible.

Relief of oedema, stiffness and trophic changes. Massage will be found of use to disperse oedema in advanced cases of arterio-sclerosis and to hasten the removal of metabolites from the muscle groups by the blood and lymph stream in cases of ischaemic pain. Active exercises will help to relieve the stiffness which arises from trophic changes and fibrosis, but they must not produce pain.

Care of the skin. Special precautions should be observed whenever physical measures are applied in cases of defective circulation. Scrupulous care must be taken to avoid the slightest damage to the skin. The patient will have received adequate warning by the physician, but the physiotherapist must take great care both in the application of heat or other electrical treatments, and in attention to any abrasions which may be present. In cases where ulcers have developed treatment by artificial sunlight or heat rays may be ordered but these should be given with care and using strict aseptic precautions.

ESTIMATION OF THE VALUE OF PHYSICAL MEASURES

The questions as to the real value of physical treatment in diseases of the arteries is often raised. The effectiveness of treatment actually depends upon whether there is any possibility of improving the circulation to the legs. The great feature of a permanent diminution of the arterial supply is intermittent claudication.

There are three stages of progression of this symptom. Stage one occurs when there is pain on walking, but the pain passes off if walking is continued. Here the blood vessels are able to adapt to the increased demand for blood but they adapt less readily and a greater stimulus is required. In stage two there is pain on walking which only passes off on rest. The blood vessels are not able to adapt to the increased demands and help is needed to develop collateral vessels. In stage three, pain does not pass off immediately on resting, and there is also pain at rest when the limb becomes warm. In this stage, the blood vessels can no longer adapt at all, they cannot provide sufficient blood even at rest, such collateral circulation as is possible will have already developed and there is no hope of improvement.

In stage one, the treatment of the patient is exercise which he is able to carry out for himself. Physical treatment is, therefore, of little importance.

In stage two, there is still ability to adapt but not to such a great extent as under normal circumstances. Help may be given in two ways: by relaxing any spasm, and by stimulating the collateral vessels. This, therefore, is the stage in which the various physical methods are of most value.

In stage three, there is no ability to adapt and, therefore, there is nothing that physiotherapy can do. The patient has simply to learn to live within the limits of his arteries. Any exercise which brings on pain must be avoided. Pain at rest can only be relieved by keeping the temperature of the limb low.

The only possible value of physiotherapy is to relieve oedema and treat sores, but both of these would have to be carried out very carefully.

CONDITIONS AFFECTING VEINS

There are two conditions of veins for which physiotherapy is of some value. These are venous thrombosis and varicose veins.

THROMBOSIS IN VEINS

If thrombosis is accompanied by inflammation of the vein wall (phlebitis), the condition is usually referred to as a thrombo-phlebitis. If it occurs in the absence of inflammation it is known as a phlebo-thrombosis. Since the precipitating factors, signs and symptoms and relative dangers of these types are different, they will be considered separately.

THROMBO-PHLEBITIS

Any vein may be affected but the superficial veins are probably more often involved than the deep and, of these, the long saphenous vein is a common site partly because it is so often used for intravenous-drip therapy, and partly because it is so often varicose.

As a result of the liberation of considerable quantities of thromboplastin from the inflamed endothelium, extensive clotting of blood within the affected segment of the vein rapidly occurs and the lumen of the vessel is occluded.

Precipitating factors. Inflammation of the vein wall may be caused by trauma, by toxins, by spread of inflammation from the surrounding tissues, and by infection. Varicose veins being particularly liable to trauma, are the frequent site of thrombo-phlebitis. One of the most common factors in this condition is the introduction of chemical irritants into the vein. This may be done deliberately in the treatment of varicose veins, when sclerosing agents are used to obliterate the vein, or it may occur unavoidably if saline, glucose, or glucose-saline infusions are necessary. It also occurs, however, where other substances are used in intravenous-drip therapy. The reason for this is as yet unexplained, but there is a theory that a chemical substance in the rubber tubing of the apparatus may be the offending agent.

The signs and symptoms. General and local symptoms usually accompany a thrombo-phlebitis, although their severity varies with the extent and often the cause of the condition. They are less severe in the case of a thrombo-phlebitis of a superficial varicose vein and well-marked if the precipitating factor is an intravenous-drip. There is usually a rise in the temperature and pulse rate and the patient feels unwell. Locally the patient complains of pain and extreme tenderness in the region of the affected vein. If the vein is superficial there will be an area of oedema and redness, and it may be possible to feel the hardened vein running through this area. The temperature usually falls within a few days and with suitable treatment the local symptoms tend to disappear within three to ten days.

Principles of Treatment by Physiotherapy

With the removal or treatment of the cause, thrombo-phlebitis usually clears rapidly. The main object of physiotherapy, therefore, is the relief of symptoms. Relief of pain is obtained by the application of a not too intensive form of heat, by elevation of the limb and light non-weight-bearing exercise. Inductothermy often proves most successful both in the relief of pain and in promoting the absorption of the oedema.

If the thrombo-phlebitis is situated in the deep veins, it presents a somewhat different problem since blocking of these veins is liable to add to oedema, and deep thrombosis is more likely to give rise to embolism. For these cases, therefore, anti-coagulant therapy is usually employed and a few days' complete rest for the limb is advocated. After a period of about three days when the clot should be firmly adherent, the object of physiotherapy will be to relieve oedema by measures directed towards the establishment of a good collateral circulation. Active exercises are the chief means available to fulfil this object.

PHLEBO-THROMBOSIS

The deep veins of the legs are by far the most common site of this type of thrombosis though the condition also occurs in the abdominal veins including the inferior vena cava and in the subclavian and axillary veins.

Probably as a combined result of slight roughening of the vessel wall, slowing of the circulation, and increased coagulability of the blood plate-lets, which adhere to the vessel wall, fibrin is formed and a small thrombus develops. This gradually increases in size (see page 37) until it sufficiently occludes the lumen of the vein to cause stagnation of the blood distal to the block. Clotting then occurs.

Embolism is far more liable to occur than in thrombosis of inflammatory origin because the thrombus and clot are only adherent to a small area of the vessel wall, the point at which the platelets were first deposited. The increasing mass extends back into the blood stream and fragments may be broken off and swept into the blood stream until such time as the vessel is almost completely obstructed.

This type of thrombosis is particularly liable to occur in post-operation states, following child-birth, in prolonged illness and in cardiac failure, since in all these some or all of these factors are probably present. After abdominal surgery the circulation is slowed, not only as a result of in-activity, but also because the presence of an abdominal, or thoraco-abdominal incision, causes reflex and voluntary inhibition of the dia-phragm through fear and pain. The diaphragm plays an effective part in venous return because as it descends it draws out the walls of the inferior vena cava at the point at which they are blended with the central tendon, and it causes a drop in intra-thoracic pressure and a rise in intra-abdominal pressure so exerting a suction effect on the blood in the great veins of the abdomen. This effect is very much reduced by diminished diaphragmatic excursion.

The signs and symptoms. Most cases of phlebo-thrombosis are insidious in onset and are, therefore, accompanied by few, if any, symptoms. A pulmonary embolism may be the first warning of a thrombus of this type. With a careful check, however, certain signs may often be detected. Slight swelling gradually develops and usually is first seen, in the leg, as a masking of the extensor tendons on the dorsum of the foot. Later it may extend around the ankle and up the calf so that it is appreciable on measurement. Should a deep femoral thrombosis occur suddenly, without time for the establishment of a collateral circulation, oedema is marked, extending to the groin. Such an oedema is often accompanied by arterio-spasm and the leg will then be cold and white. Usually there is a slight fullness of the superficial veins in the area. This may be seen on the dorsum of the foot in a thrombosis of the deep calf veins or on the chest and medial aspect of the arm in an axillary thrombosis.

Palpation will elicit tenderness in the centre of the calf, the popliteal fossa, or the groin, according to the site of thrombosis and the patient may complain of pain in these areas, increased by stretching of the vein. Passive dorsiflexion of the foot with the knee held extended will produce pain if the deep veins of the calf are involved. Sometimes there is a slight rise in the body temperature, but constitutional symptoms are rarely marked.

Principles of Treatment by Physiotherapy

If one of the main factors concerned in the onset of thrombosis is circulatory stasis, treatment is obviously preventative rather than therapeutic and any measures which can be safely used to keep the circulation satisfactory should be applied in cases in which thrombosis is known to be a possibility. Obviously such measures are not applicable in cases of sudden onset without obvious cause. Preventative measures are, therefore, chiefly of value immediately before and after surgery, in cardiac failure, and for patients suffering from medical illnesses necessitating prolonged recumbency.

Massage and passive movements, breathing exercises, active leg and trunk exercises, early ambulation, relaxation, and training the patient to move freely about the bed are all possible means.

Massage. This has a mechanical effect on the blood flow in the veins, pressing the blood centripetally, while back flow is prevented by the presence of valves. It has its greatest value for patients who are unable to perform active exercise and is, therefore, useful for patients who are too ill to be disturbed by active work, for those suffering from heart failure and who are being treated by rest, and for the first few days after valvotomy. Passive movements are also of value for these patients since they have a pumping effect on the veins and do not demand any active work.

Breathing exercises. These stimulate venous return and are of value in all patients but particularly following thoracic and abdominal surgery. Since it is uncomfortable for the patient to use the diaphragm fully, diaphragmatic breathing must be taught, if possible, before the operation and practised as soon as the patient recovers consciousness. This type of breathing should be taught until it becomes a habit not only to those confined to bed for a long period but also to those suffering from cardiac failure (see page 330).

z*

Active exercises. These are the most important means of stimulating the circulation. Foot, knee and hip exercises can be carried out in full range vigorously, provided that double hip work is avoided. The addition of trunk exercises depends on the condition of the patient.

While practising active exercises the patient is taught to relax and to move about the bed freely, because the majority of ill patients are tense and worried, and those who have a recent incision are afraid that movement may strain the sutures or cause pain. Tense muscles impede rather than aid the circulation.

The question of early ambulation following operation is still a debatable one. Surgeons who favour it, do so because the upright position stimulates venous return and overcomes the kinking in the femoral vein produced by the half lying position. If early ambulation is ordered the physiotherapist will help the patient and watch for signs of faintness and giddiness. In addition it is important to check the tendency to stoop, so common in patients who have an abdominal incision.

Therapeutic treatment. Once the onset of thrombosis has been recognised, the main object is to prevent the process spreading and to lessen the danger of embolism. Anti-coagulant therapy is, therefore, begun at once, unless there are any special contra-indications. It is important during this stage that the circulation should be maintained and all physical measures previously used should be continued, with the exception of massage. This is better omitted since there may be thrombi present elsewhere and undetected and it is just possible that massage might dislodge these. Ambulation may also be omitted until the thrombus has become firmly adherent to the vessel wall, probably a period of about three days.

In cases of thrombosis of sudden onset in which the thrombus may be developed before it is detected, and a free 'tail' is therefore present, active exercises may be contra-indicated since they may possibly increase the tendency to embolism. The limb is usually then elevated and protected from pressure for a period of approximately seven to ten days, when exercises may be begun. If oedema persists in these cases, as it sometimes does for months or longer, physical treatment will be necessary to assist in the establishment of a collateral circulation (see obstructive oedema, page 45).

Detection of the Onset of Non-inflammatory Thrombosis

While preventative physical treatment is being carried out a careful watch must always be kept, since in spite of all treatment thrombosis can develop. The foot should be examined for masking of the extensor tendons and fullness of the veins. Gentle passive dorsiflexion of the feet, with the knees extended may be carried out and careful palpation of the calf, popliteal space and medial side of the thigh should be undertaken. Daily measurement of the calves is advisable. If any of these signs or tests are positive or the patient complains of pain in the legs, a report to the sister in charge of the ward should be made at once so that immediate treatment can, if necessary, be undertaken.

VARICOSE VEINS

Veins which are varicose are dilated, lengthened, and usually tortuous in their course. The veins commonly affected are those which either have a long column of blood to support, such as the long saphenous vein, or those which have little muscular support, such as the haemorrhoidal veins. In nearly all patients who suffer from this condition there is an inherited weakness of the vein walls and its valves. Varicosity may then develop as a result of various factors. A severe obstruction to venous return will cause congestion in the veins and lead to dilatation, if the tone is already poor. Such an obstruction might be a general one, the result of mitral stenosis or emphysema; on the other hand it might be a local obstruction due to the pressure of scar tissue, tumours, an over-loaded rectum, or the foetal head during pregnancy. Prolonged standing may be the cause of varicose veins, since in standing muscle tone gradually lessens and muscular support to the veins is lost.

At first, due to strain, the muscular layer hypertrophies, but in time hypertrophy changes to atrophy and the vein then dilates. As the vein dilates the valves become relatively insufficient and regurgitation of blood tends to occur. Blood stagnates in the pouches just proximal to the valve cusps, thrombosis is consequently a common complication.

These changes in the veins lead to a variety of symptoms. The appearance of the vein is, of course, diagnostic if the affected veins are superficial. Chronic congestion and tendency to regurgitation lead to disturbance of the circulation, muscles and ligaments become hypotonic and lax, the skin becomes oedematous, devitalised, and very readily breaks down. Patches of dark pigmentation are often seen, since repeated small haemorrhages occur from the small distended veins. As a result of poor nutrition, the legs feel heavy and there is complaint of aching and discomfort.

Several complications arise from the condition of varicosity; haemorrhage may be severe from a rupture of a superficial dilated vein, phlebitis is very common, thrombosis readily occurs in the pouches proximal to the valves, ulcer and eczema are due to the poor atrophic condition of the skin.

OUTLINE OF TREATMENT BY PHYSIOTHERAPY

The object of any form of treatment is the obliteration of the vein and so the prevention of these complications.

This obliteration may be obtained in one of two ways. Firstly, the vein may be subjected to continuous external pressure by means of a special elastic bandage. Secondly, the vein may be ligatured or injected. Whichever of these two procedures is undertaken the result is the same. In the first case, the flow of blood is arrested, venous return is obtained through collateral vessels and any blood in the vein clots. In the second case a chemical phlebitis is produced, thrombosis occurs, thrombus will organise and the vein become converted into a fibrous cord.

Physiotherapy is rarely ordered for the condition itself, but sometimes the physiotherapist is asked to apply the bandage or to instruct the patient in its application or use.

Physiotherapy has its greatest practical value in the treatment of the complications, particularly where ulcers have formed or where there is much oedema and induration and the skin is softened and atrophic. In these cases the main object of treatment is to clean and aid healing of infected or indolent ulcers, to relieve oedema and soften indurated areas, to stimulate the circulation and strengthen the muscles.

Various methods are available for the treatment of varicose ulcers. Some ulcers yield to one form, others to other methods and no adequate explanation of this fact can be given. Many respond well to zinc ionisation while septic, and to chlorine when clean, the latter drug stimulating the healing process. Others respond better to ultra-violet irradiation. While the surface is discharging the short abiotic rays may be used for their destructive properties; when the ulcer is clean, then stimulating treatment to the raw surface and the unhealthy sluggish skin will be given, cutting out the abiotic rays. Some ulcers respond well to the application twice daily of infra-red rays; others do well with a combination of infra-red and ultra-violet irradiation. The most useful measures are massage and exercises. Special massage to relieve oedema is essential and a deep massage to the whole of the thickened indurated area should be combined with this. To protect the skin some form of inunction, such as lanoline or olive oil, may be used during the application of the massage. Exercises will be vigorous to stimulate the circulation and resistance will be added when possible to strengthen the muscles to form a better support for the veins. These exercises will be non-weight bearing. Breathing exercises and light trunk exercises performed while the legs are elevated are valuable to aid venous return.

The Bisgaard method is today widely used in the treatment of varicose ulcers. In principle it consists of deep massage, given with special pastes, to the indurated area around the ulcer and to the oedematous foot and ankle. In addition an elastic bandage is applied giving firm even pressure. In this the patient performs vigorous active exercises, stands and walks.

DISEASES OF THE BLOOD

While treating patients for other conditions the physiotherapist will often come across the condition of anaemia. For this reason, though physical treatment is rarely directed towards the anaemia, it is necessary to know something of the condition and its dangers.

ANAEMIA

Anaemia is the result either of interference with the normal formation of blood or is due to loss or too rapid blood destruction.

Interference with the formation of blood arises either from defective action of the bone marrow or from an absence of an essential factor such as iron or the liver principle. The different types of anaemia can therefore be classified according to their cause into deficiency anaemia, aplastic anaemia, and haemolytic anaemia.

DEFICIENCY ANAEMIA

Two main varieties of deficiency anaemia are seen, pernicious and simple achlorhydric; a third type, chlorosis or Green Sickness, is rarely met today.

Pernicious Anaemia (Addison's Disease)

This type of anaemia is characterised by an inability to obtain full maturation of the red blood corpuscles. It occurs in men rather more commonly than in women and its onset is usually in early middle age.

It will be remembered that the healthy gastric mucous membrane produces an enzyme which interacts with a protein substance found in meat in the diet (probably vitamin B_2) to form an anti-anaemic factor which is absorbed from the alimentary tract and stored in the liver. Liberated by the liver, it travels in the blood stream to the red bone marrow and stimulates it to produce red blood corpuscles. Absence of a sufficient number of red cells in the blood might therefore be due to a failure on the part of the bone marrow to react to this anti-anaemic factor; it might be due to failure of the stomach to produce the enzyme, or to absence of the necessary factor in the diet, or to failure in absorption or storage. In practice it appears that nearly always it is absence of the intrinsic factor produced by the gastric mucous membrane which is the cause. Changes occur in the blood, bone marrow, heart and other organs when this condition develops.

Changes in the blood. A very great drop in the number of normal red blood corpuscles occurs, often as low as one or one-and-a-half million per cubic millimetre of blood. In addition, there is a rise in the number of reticulocytes (the precursors of mature red cells) and a flooding of the blood with many abnormally small red corpuscles. The numbers of blood platelets and polymorphonuclear leucocytes are also reduced.

The bone marrow becomes increasingly active and consequently more vascular. Yellow marrow in the shafts of the long bones is replaced by red in an effort to meet the blood requirements.

The organs show fatty degeneration, typical of an oxygen deprivation. The heart becomes flabby and shows fatty infiltration; the liver is enlarged and fatty; the alimentary tract shows inflammatory changes and there is an absence of hydrochloric acid and enzymes in the gastric juice. Fatty degeneration of the blood vessels leads to easy rupture and petechial haemorrhages.

The voluntary muscles are weak and flabby.

Degenerative changes occur in the spinal nerves and in addition demyelination and destruction of the fibres in the posterior and lateral column of the spinal cord is a common accompaniment, though it is not clear that this last change is due to the condition of the blood.

The signs and symptoms may be divided into those present in any anaemia and those which are peculiar to this special type. In all anaemia there is breathlessness on exertion since there is insufficient oxygenation of the blood; palpitation is common, as is also muscular weakness and fatigue. Oedema of the ankles may be seen. Symptoms peculiar to the pernicious type of anaemia are the vomiting and diarrhoea due to the inflammation of the alimentary tract, petechial haemorrhages, the result of degenerative changes in the blood vessels, and the peculiar lemon yellow tint of the skin. In addition there is often tingling, numbness, paraesthesia and weakness of the limbs resulting from degenerative changes in the peripheral nerves, while, either before the onset of pernicious anaemia, or soon after, signs of changes in the spinal cord may be detected.

Simple Achlorhydric Anaemia

This type of anaemia chiefly affects middle-aged women. The deficiency is one of iron, either because it is lacking in the diet or because there is some impairment in its absorption. The result is a deficient quantity of haemoglobin in the red blood cells, consequently less oxygen is conveyed round the body and general metabolism is impaired. In these cases there is always an absence of hydrochloric acid in the gastric juice. The symptoms are those associated with all anaemias and in addition there is usually anorexia and dyspepsia.

APLASTIC ANAEMIA

In this type of anaemia the bone marrow is at fault. It fails to produce the red corpuscles, platelets and polymorphs for which it is responsible. Changes occur in the red marrow; it becomes more yellow because its fat content increases, and it diminishes in quantity.

For some cases there is no apparent cause, in others it is thought to be the result of the toxic effect on the marrow of arsenic, radium or X-rays.

In this type a very severe anaemia is produced. Since platelets are reduced, haemorrhages are common. Due to the reduced white cell count the resistance of the patient is low and he readily succumbs to some intercurrent infection. These patients show a very rapid progress of the disease. Though life may be prolonged for a short time by repeated blood transfusions, death will ensue fairly soon.

ANAEMIA DUE TO BLOOD LOSS

Anaemia may be the result of repeated mild haemorrhages or of a very severe single haemorrhage. Such an anaemia is readily diagnosed and successfully treated.

HAEMOLYTIC ANAEMIA

Occasionally a too rapid destruction of red blood cells occurs. This may be the result of an increased fragility of the corpuscles of unknown origin. The cells are rapidly broken up in the spleen, and as haemoglobin is liberated the pigments are turned into bile pigments, and absorbed into the blood stream, so causing jaundice. In addition to the symptoms of anaemia the spleen will usually be found to be much enlarged. The most successful treatment for these patients is splenectomy.

PHYSICAL MEASURES

There is not a great deal of real value to be gained from physical treatment for the anaemias. For simple achlorhydric anaemia and anaemia due to blood loss, a course of ultra-violet light is beneficial since it increases the quantity of red cells in the blood, and acts as a tonic. Breathing exercises are also valuable in order to get the maximum possible aeration of the blood. As the anaemia decreases with medical treatment, progressive exercises will help to build up the skeletal and cardiac musculature.

In cases of pernicious anaemia, massage and exercises may be helpful in dealing with weakness due to changes in the peripheral nerves. Treatment will also be necessary in cases complicated by subacute combined degeneration of the cord.

When any physical treatment is being given to anaemic patients it is well to bear in mind that the heart muscle is suffering from the effects of oxygen shortage. Strenuous exercises are to be avoided and sudden changes of posture are unwise since they are liable to result in attacks of fainting or giddiness.

PART SIX

SOME COMMON DISEASES OF THE SKIN AND ITS APPENDAGES

SOME COMMON DISEASES OF THE SKIN
AND ITS APPENDAGES

Not very many of the common cutaneous diseases are suitable for treatment by physiotherapy. Probably acne, psoriasis, alopecia and staphylococcal infections obtain most benefit from physical measures and in addition some cases of lupus vulgaris are sometimes sent to the department. The measures which are usually most beneficial are relaxation, light, general exercises and actinotherapy.

Relaxation deserves a special word here because it is so seldom employed in the treatment of skin diseases and yet it is of such supreme importance. In the majority of diseases of the skin there is a marked psychological factor. Ingram points out that there is a very close link between the skin and the nervous system since the central nervous system is developed as an infolding of the ectoderm of the embryo. Maladjustments, emotional disturbances, anxieties, are all reflected in the skin. Many cutaneous diseases appear at times of physiological nervous instability, at puberty, pregnancy and the menopause. This element in the development of skin diseases is particularly marked in alopecia, psoriasis and eczema.

In the treatment of patients suffering from these diseases at least a small part, therefore, can be played by the physiotherapist. The patient who is usually tense and nervous is taught to relax. It may take a long time to gain relaxation of the whole body but as the patient attains some degree of relaxation there is a greater ability to sleep and the skin condition often begins to improve.

STAPHYLOCOCCAL SKIN INFECTIONS

Staphylococci are always found in great numbers on the skin but if, owing to trauma or lowered resistance, they are allowed to multiply, then pus formation and necrosis of tissue is likely to result. The common conditions which may arise are: furunculosis, carbunculosis and sycosis.

FURUNCULOSIS

A furuncle or boil is a small round inflammatory lesion which has a central core of pus.

Two things appear to be necessary for the development of boils; a general lowered resistance such as might be due to anaemia, diabetes or some toxic focus, and a local irritation, the result perhaps of pressure, friction or scratching. There are cases in which the patient appears in otherwise perfect health but these are less common.

The staphylococci multiply as a rule in the hair follicle and set up an inflammatory reaction. They become surrounded by inflammatory cells, and their toxins, spreading into the neighbouring tissues, cause stimulation of the connective tissue cells. Considerable necrosis takes place. Usually the leucocytes, which invade the area, separate the necrosed from the healthy tissue so that a core is formed. Gradually by phagocytic action the core is softened, the epidermis breaks down and the soft core, now pus, is discharged.

A boil, therefore, starts as a small red spot. Gradually redness and swelling spread peripherally, while the centre rises above the surrounding tissue and becomes hard and purplish in colour. As the core is softened the centre becomes yellow and then discharges.

The treatment, like that of other skin conditions, is two-fold; first to build up the patient's general health and resistance, and secondly to destroy the bacteria and heal the local lesion.

Among other measures suitable for restoring the patient's general health and resistance, general ultra-violet irradiation is effective. While the local condition is often entirely treated by penicillin therapy, beneficial results can always be obtained by the use of short-wave diathermy. This is best applied in sub-thermal doses. In this way a better circulation to the area is produced without increasing the activity of the bacteria. By increasing the circulation more leucocytes are brought to the area to separate the core and to promote absorption without pus formation.

CARBUNCULOSIS

A carbuncle is similar to a boil but much more extensive, often considerably deeper and usually accompanied by pain and constitutional symptoms. Several hair follicles are involved, inflammation spreads to the subcutaneous tissue and widespread necrosis occurs. Should the carbuncle remain superficial, the skin over it rapidly reddens and breaks down at several points. A deep carbuncle after separating leaves a deep cavity which will take some time to heal and will result in scarring.

In these cases as in furunculosis, treatment is usually by means of systemic and local penicillin, but here also short-wave therapy and, in addition, local ultra-violet and infra-red rays prove effective.

The object is to promote the circulation without increasing the activity of the staphylococci and for this reason sub-thermal doses are most suitable. Usually separation then occurs much more quickly, and when it is complete a strong dose of ultra-violet rays will help to clear the remaining slough. Subsequently, to promote more rapid healing of the cavity with less scarring, ultra-violet and infra-red irradiation may be used. General sunlight is also administered when pyrexia is no longer present.

SYCOSIS

This condition, sometimes known as 'Barber's rash', is characterised by the formation of small pustules in the openings of the hair follicles. It particularly occurs in the region of the upper lip, chin and side of cheek, but may also occur on the eyebrows, axillae, pubis and the back of the neck. The pustules break easily on washing the skin or on shaving, leaving behind a reddened area of skin on which more pustules form. The condition if untreated is very liable to remain a chronic one over a period of years. It is most satisfactorily treated by X-ray therapy and physiotherapy is rarely called for. Occasionally a course of general ultra-violet light may be found helpful. If local ultra-violet light is ordered its object will be to destroy bacteria and provide a marked vaso-dilatation, hence strong doses will be needed.

ACNE VULGARIS

This is a chronic inflammatory condition of the sebaceous glands opening into the hair follicles, and is characterised by the formation of comedones (blackheads), pustules and nodules. It occurs most often at puberty or in adolescence, though it may be seen at any age. Acne develops in the 'seborrhoeic' subject, that is, the patient in whom there is an increased secretion of sebum and a greasy condition of the skin. Usually, this patient is of the rather lethargic sluggish type, and the skin has a low resistance to infection. The lesions are most noticeable on the face, the cheeks and chin being more affected than elsewhere. They are, however, also fairly common on the back and chest. The cause is not certain but it is quite probable that the increased activity of the endocrine glands at puberty may influence the sebaceous glands. In addition, the condition is invariably worse if there are local sources of infection, or if the patient eats too much, particularly of carbohydrate foods. Many of these patients take too little exercise, indulge too much in cakes, sweets and pastries and are often constipated.

The condition is one of increased formation of sebum of a very oily consistency, with the resulting difficulty in discharging it on to the surface of the skin. Either a retention cyst is formed or the upper part of the hair follicle becomes blocked. Many acne bacilli are found in the retained sebum, and partly owing to this, and partly due to dirt and oxidation processes, the distal end of the plug changes colour and becomes black. This is the stage of comedone formation. The inflammation of the hair follicle and skin is followed by the appearance of a raised purplish-red papule, usually with a tiny yellow centre which breaks down and discharges pus. When the pus is evacuated the papule may disappear or it may simply shrink to reoccur later. Sometimes several of these papules coalesce and a large pustule is formed. In this chronic form, when healing eventually occurs, it does so by fibrous tissue formation and pitting and scarring result, leading to permanent deformity of the skin.

PRINCIPLES OF TREATMENT BY PHYSIOTHERAPY

Treatment aims at obtaining a good desquamation of the skin so that the hair follicles are opened and the contents can be discharged. Bacteria may also be destroyed. Attempts are made to increase the vascularity of the skin so that resistance is raised and the sebaceous glands function normally. Further it is essential to improve the patient's general health and general skin activity.

The local effects may well be obtained by the use of X-ray therapy but this is not suitable for acute lesions or necessary for superficial ones. These latter two types are ideally treated by local ultra-violet light. Since desquamation and strong erythema are required, the best results will be obtained by the application of third-degree doses if the patient is willing to tolerate the discomfort and unsightly appearance. These should rapidly clear all but deep lesions and where these are present the sunlight prepares the way for the application of X-rays. For those cases in which scarring and pitting have already occurred, similar applications are most helpful, since the inflammatory reaction helps, by production of granulation tissue, to fill in the depressions, while desquamation aids the removal of superficial scars.

Improvement of the general health of the body and of the skin will be considerably aided by the general sunlight; the carbon arc lamp has the advantage of stimulating elimination by the skin, the mercury vapour lamp the advantage of more abiotic rays. Either lamp may therefore be used.

These patients also derive benefit from a course of general exercises to stimulate circulation and metabolism. Where possible these exercises should be given in the open air.

PSORIASIS

This is an inflammatory condition of the skin characterised by the formation of raised, rounded, salmon-red patches covered by dry silvery scales.

The actual changes in the skin consist of a dilatation of the capillaries in the dermis and oedema and hypertrophy of the epidermis. The fluid in the epidermis appears to cause increased activity on the part of the stratum germinatum. Multiplication and production of new cells, therefore, occurs and the new cells are pushed to the surface too rapidly to become completely changed into horny scales. The result of this is that the cells do not rub off but tend to adhere, become desiccated and tiny spaces which reflect the light occur between them, giving a silvery scale-like appearance. The scales are adherent at the centre of the patch, loose at the circumference and when removed tend to leave small bleeding points. In the case of old-standing chronic patches the skin is thick and tough and covered by many layers of scales.

Males are more often affected than females and the condition tends to make its first appearance about puberty. It varies in its mode of onset, but commonly commences with small patches on the scalp or extensor surfaces of the knees and elbows which may remain localised for a long period or may disappear, to reappear again later. Occasionally there may be a sudden onset with a wide spread.

The areas most often affected are the elbows, knees, extensor surfaces of legs and forearms, lower back, and gluteal and adductor region of thighs, but no area is immune.

The cause of this condition is unknown. There appears to be an inherited tendency and it is often associated with rheumatic conditions. An attack seems often to be precipitated by nervous shock, general debility or some illness.

The appearance is quite characteristic, as is the distribution. The patches are usually oval or round with a clear edge. At first each is only about half an inch in diameter but it tends to increase to about two inches and then to be arrested, though if many patches are present they may fuse to cover a wide area. The patches have a tendency to heal at the centre and to leave rings. Some irritation is often associated with the condition.

PRINCIPLES OF TREATMENT BY PHYSIOTHERAPY

The main objects of treatment are to improve the physical and mental health of the patient, to cure the attack, and to prevent its recurrence. Many different measures have been advocated and no certain cure as yet exists. Naturally those who come for treatment in a first attack are most likely to have a successful result. To attain these objects the treatment is usually a combination of relaxation exercises, tar baths, the application of cignolin paste and general and local sunlight.

A very usual method is to give the patient a tar bath for ten to fifteen minutes each morning. While in the bath, provided the areas of psoriasis are not acute, the patient scrubs the patches to remove the scales. A sub-erythematous dose of general sunlight is then given, most often using the mercury vapour lamp. Very often the patient is provided with an ointment of salicylic acid, mercury and tar to apply at night.

Alternatively, all patches are covered twice daily with cignolin paste; this is washed off in the morning and a sub-erythematous dose of general ultra-violet light is given. Thick, tough, chronic patches are often cleared by local doses of sunlight obtaining a strong erythematous reaction. It is essential to remove the scales by a spirit soap before the local dose is administered, if a good counter-irritant effect is to be obtained.

A combination of baths, ointment, general and local sunlight usually provides temporary relief. It has been found that the most satisfactory way to prevent a recurrence is by a course of ultra-violet light each autumn and winter.

ALOPECIA

This is a condition in which the hair is deficient. It is usually an acquired condition, and may be temporary or permanent. Many factors enter into its development. There is in many cases an hereditary tendency. Some cases follow severe illnesses, particularly acute infections such as typhoid fever and influenza. Others may be due to disease of the hair follicles or trauma to the scalp resulting in scarring, while yet others are thought to be the result of disturbances of the sympathetic nerve supply to the blood vessels and hair follicles of the scalp.

The hereditary type is seen in the premature baldness of men, in which no regrowth of hair is possible. A milder form is seen in women, especially those with fine hair, who show a falling out of hair chiefly near the vertex; this never becomes complete as it does in men but the hair which disappears is not replaced. For those patients whose alopecia follows severe infections, the hair loss usually starts about six weeks after the illness, progresses slowly for a subsequent six weeks, until the patient is completely bald, and then regrows again, slowly, but usually completely. The new growth starts as a fine yellowish downy hair which is later replaced by normal hair, at first white but soon becoming normally pigmented.

Certain patients show a rapid loss of hair in patches until, in some cases, complete loss has occurred. This is known as alopecia areata and its cause is unknown, though the general health is often poor, and it is thought that these are cases in which there is disturbance of the sympathetic nervous supply. When first seen, these patients usually present one or more circumscribed circular, smooth, bald patches but these increase rapidly in numbers and often coalesce.

PRINCIPLES OF TREATMENT BY PHYSIOTHERAPY

The underlying rationale of treatment lies in the fact that the hair grows from the hair follicle which is richly supplied with blood vessels and with nerves from the sympathetic system. If the hair follicle atrophies, as is probable in the hereditary alopecias, or if it is destroyed as in scarring, then regrowth is impossible. Provided the follicle is intact, regrowth will depend on the nerve fibres and the vascularity. Obviously, therefore, if the blood supply to the follicle is increased and the nerve is stimulated, growth should be more rapid. A second factor to remember is that of general health and sympathetic disturbance. If the health is improved and better nervous stability is obtained, regrowth of hair, provided the follicle is intact, should be stimulated. Treatment is therefore likely to be necessary and effective for those who suffer from alopecia areata, whether it is in the form of patches or complete.

General health is improved by medical measures but relaxation and general ultra-violet light are most effective in improving the condition of the blood, stimulating the appetite and generally acting as a tonic.

Local treatment may be carried out by counter-irritant applications, high-frequency currents of high voltage and low amperage, or massage; but far more effective in obtaining an erythema of the scalp, and much more lasting in its effects, is the erythema obtained by local applications of ultra-violet rays. Ultra-violet rays should be used in such a way as to produce a really well-marked erythema. Individual patches may be treated, but if the whole scalp is affected it is treated in several sections on different days. Since the reaction obtained should be just short of blistering, the dose is not repeated for a week or ten days but it is then reapplied, treatment being continued until the area is covered with normal hair.

TUBERCULOUS DISEASE OF THE SKIN

There are certain skin diseases such as lupus vulgaris and scrofuloderma in which the tubercle bacilli can actually be found in the affected skin. In other conditions, such as Bazin's disease, the tubercle bacilli are not found but certain facts, such as the type of lesion and its association with other tubercular conditions, suggest a tuberculous origin. These conditions are known as tuberculides.

Invasion of the tissues by any micro-organism sets up an inflammatory reaction but the exact nature of this reaction varies with the causative agent; thus the tubercle bacilli produce their own type of reaction whatever tissue they invade.

When they enter the tissues they multiply and secrete toxic substances which destroy the tissue cells. The response to this is a movement of polymorphonuclear leucocytes into the area, many of which are destroyed. The reaction to dead polymorphs is a further invasion by a variety of mononuclear cells known as macrophages which probably originate from the tissue spaces, the blood and the endothelial cells of the blood and lymph vessels. These cells interlock with one another and form a network around the tubercle bacilli, dead and living polymorphs, and tissue cells. Usually around this is found an irregular wall of lymphocytes. The whole mass of cells forms a microscopic tuberculous follicle. Often this increases in size or others coalesce with it until a larger mass is formed, sometimes a millimetre in diameter. This mass is known as a miliary tubercle. One interesting feature of the tubercle is an absence of blood vessels, and this, together with the effect of toxic substances, causes necrosis of the centre of the tubercle with coagulation of the cells. This process is termed caseation. As the miliary tubercles multiply in number and coalesce, caseated nodules are formed. Usually the surrounding tissue reacts to these by the formation of a fibrous tissue envelope. The presence of several nodules, therefore, accounts for the fibrous induration of the surrounding tissue.

Tuberculous skin disease and tuberculides are characterised by tubercles or nodules or both. But as they form in the dermis or subcutaneous tissue the epidermis over them tends to become atrophic or infiltrated, and often eventually breaks down, resulting in ulceration.

The extent of spread of a tuberculous lesion in any tissue depends very largely on the general and local resistance of the patient and his tissues. If the resistance is high the spread is likely to be quickly checked, the tubercles become walled off in fibrous tissue, and healing results. If the resistance is low more tubercles are formed and there is less encapsulation.

Quite often when the skin is affected the centre of the affected area heals by scarring while more tubercles form at the edge; thus destruction and scarring go on at the same time.

The main object in the treatment of all tuberculous conditions is to improve the patient's general health so that the defensive mechanism can be mobilised to fight the disease. In the skin condition it is also sometimes possible to destroy the bacilli and the tubercles because they are superficial.

With the introduction of calciferol (Vitamin D) therapy combined with suitable diet and adequate rest, fresh air and sunlight, the skin lesions often subside without local treatment and patients suffering from tuberculosis of the skin rarely reach the physiotherapy department. There are, however, two particular lesions which do sometimes require physical treatment, particularly if they do not respond well to calciferol. These two conditions are lupus vulgaris and Bazin's disease.

LUPUS VULGARIS

This is a chronic inflammatory tuberculous lesion in which tubercle bacilli are actually found in the affected skin. It is characterised by the development of brownish-red patches on which scabs may form and in which, on deep pressure with a glass slide, tubercles can be seen, looking a yellowish-brown like apple-jelly. Sometimes the skin breaks down over the patches, causing ulceration. These patches are very much more common on the face, though they can occur elsewhere, and they often begin by direct spread from the mucous membrane of the nasal cavity or mouth.

The age is quite characteristic of the condition, since it begins almost always under the age of twenty—often well before this. Girls are much more often affected than boys and it is usually the child who is living in unhygienic surroundings, who is inadequately fed and who gets little natural sunlight who is affected by the condition.

It is not certain how the bacilli reach the skin; they may do so via the lymph stream from a primary source elsewhere—often lymphatic glands; they may enter from the hands through a break in the skin; or they may spread direct from the mucous membrane. Once in the skin they cause the familiar reaction, tubercles form, destruction of tissue takes place and there is considerable fibrous tissue formation. Sometimes the epidermis becomes atrophic and breaks down. If the condition spreads, it does so by the formation of more tubercles, healing by scarring often occurring at the earliest site of infection. Sometimes much destruction takes place, the soft tissues of the nose and the lobes of the ears being completely destroyed. Gross disfigurement will be the result of destruction and scarring.

The main objects of treatment are to raise the general resistance and to destroy the local lesion, bacilli and tubercles, with the least possible damage to healthy tissue, and therefore with minimal scarring. Treatment is therefore general and local. As previously seen, diet, rest, good food, fresh air and calciferol are the most usual measures and with this treatment alone the tubercles gradually disappear and healing occurs. Sometimes, however, the response is slow and general sunlight baths are a most useful adjunct, partly for their tonic effect and partly because ultra-violet light increases the haemoglobin, calcium, vitamin D, and white cells in the blood. It also increases the bactericidal action of the blood. The tubercle bacilli and the tubercles themselves may be destroyed by chemical caustics or by excision, but the disadvantage is the scarring which is a result, and which is undesirable on the face. Sometimes, therefore, no local treatment is given and reliance is placed on calciferol therapy. If the local lesions do not respond to this their destruction can definitely be obtained by the use of the ultra-violet rays and the resultant scar is soft and smooth. The physiotherapist may, therefore, be asked to treat the lupus patch. Since the object is to destroy, the dose must be a very strong one producing acute inflammation and therefore intense hyperaemia which will have a bactericidal effect. To obtain this very strong reaction contact must be given, and for this reason all heat rays must be absorbed and a water-cooled lamp such as the kromayer, or a water-cooled applicator used with the Finsen-Lomholt lamp, must be employed. In order to concentrate the effect, the part should be exsanguinated so that the products of tissue destruction will not be carried away. For this reason, not only must there be contact but a convex quartz applicator must be used and pressed firmly over the area to be treated. This serves also to press the tissues together so that the rays penetrate further. Owing to the fact that the condition spreads by the production of new follicles and these are microscopic, an apparently healthy area of skin must be included in each treatment. It is usual to treat an area, of about the size of a shilling, at the circumference of the patch and to work round the edge at successive treatments, exposing an area of healthy tissue beyond the edge at the same time. The same area may be treated again when the reaction from the preceding application has subsided after approximately two to three weeks.

Since such a strong reaction is required it is necessary to give about five or more times the dose required to produce a fourth-degree erythema on normal skin. One precaution should always be taken when treating patients suffering from lupus vulgaris. There is a possibility of phthisis, though this is uncommon, and it must be ascertained before general sunlight is given that the chest is quite clear.

BAZIN'S DISEASE

The tubercle bacilli are not actually found in the affected skin in this condition but the nodules formed closely resemble in type those produced by the tubercle bacilli and a tuberculous infection of lymph glands is often present.

The condition attacks young girls and affects the lower part of the calves symmetrically. It is characterised by the development of purplish red patches, beneath which nodules can be felt. There is usually considerable induration of the tissues around. The nodules tend to soften as a result of central necrosis and sometimes the skin over them breaks down and deep ulcers are formed. These are invariably slow to heal. In all cases of Bazin's disease the circulation is poor and the legs are often cold and blue; it would appear, therefore, that a deficient circulation plays some part in the development of the disease. This is confirmed by the fact that the lesions usually first appear during the winter and gradually clear up in the summer, to reoccur the next winter. As they heal slowly much scar tissue is formed in the process and white depressed scars are nearly always found on the legs.

The objects of treatment are to raise the patient's resistance, and to promote resolution of the patches and healing of the ulcers. Calciferol again plays a very important part and it may alone be successful, but any measures which improve the circulation in the legs are a valuable adjunct. Physiotherapy, therefore, is of value to help the patient's general condition by a tonic course of artificial sunlight baths. It can also be used to aid the peripheral circulation. One of the most useful measures to fulfil this second object is local ultra-violet light. The whole of the back of the legs below the knee may be treated by a dose sufficient to produce a second-degree erythema reaction. Diathermy is also of value to achieve the same object. It would be applied by the longitudinal method, or the inductothermy cable may be used. General exercises are also of value to stimulate venous return. Sometimes strong local doses of abiotic rays are helpful in hastening the healing of the ulcers.

ECZEMA

Eczema is not a condition often treated in a department of physical medicine but it is sometimes seen when a patient suffering from it attends for physical treatment for some other condition. Its presence in these cases indicates that care should be taken not to apply heat, massage or any form of electrotherapy to that area.

It has certain characteristic features which may make it possible for it to be recognised or at least to suspect that it is present and to take precautions accordingly. The lesion consists of groups of tiny red spots, vesicles or papules each about the size of a pin's head. Sometimes the area shows fine scales or crusts or is weeping. In chronic cases there may be much 'leathery' thickening of the skin. These are explained by the changes which take place. The capillary loops of the papillae in the dermis dilate and therefore there is exudation of serous fluid sometimes containing fibrin. This finds its way into the epidermis where the layers of epidermal cells are separated and minute vesicles form. The patient then scratches the skin and the vesicles break and as they dry up tiny yellowish crusts are formed. Sometimes the epidermis becomes oedematous and a considerable amount of desquamation occurs.

In chronic cases the epidermis thickens probably partly as the result of continuous scratching. In other cases the vesicles become infected and there is a discharge of pus.

The cause of this condition may not be obvious, though there are certain predisposing factors. A skin which is excessively dry or very moist or one which has a poor circulation is liable to be affected. There is no doubt that anxiety, general fatigue, nervous debility, all predispose to it and the disease particularly tends to develop at puberty, pregnancy and the menopause when the nervous system is unstable. There may be some definite exciting factor such as an external irritant.

It will be clear that the treatment of these patients is general rather than local, while soothing applications are necessary for the actual patch of eczema. Most physical measures have a stimulating effect and should not therefore be used. There have been occasions when actinotherapy has been ordered but it can only be given if all the irritating short rays are cut out by use of a blue uviol filter. Even general sunlight baths are better avoided.

Should the patient suffering from eczema be sent for physical treatment, a course of relaxation exercises is the method of choice and usually proves most helpful.

SCLERODERMA

This is a condition of uncertain cause in which the skin and subcutaneous tissues become hard and adherent to the underlying tissues. There are different types, but the underlying changes are the same. The blood vessels dilate and there is proliferation of the connective tissue cells and fibres. Gradually the fibres contract and the blood vessels are obliterated. Later the epidermis becomes thin and atrophic and glands and hairs are obliterated. In some cases the disease spreads to involve the underlying muscles which become atrophied and fibrotic. Whether the condition spreads to the muscles or not, there is gradually an increasing limitation of movement of the area. If it involves the neck, face and chest, eating, swallowing and breathing may become difficult. If it involves the limbs, contractures and deformities may develop. The condition may be generalised but it is more common in a localised form known as morphoea. In this case, small patches or bands of hardening develop which appear suddenly as thick hard pinkish patches. These gradually become yellowish and eventually form depressed white atrophic areas. There is little treatment of any value but sometimes massage with oil or cream may help to prevent further hardening of a local patch, and movements may help to prevent contractures. It has been suggested that some improvement might be gained by driving in the ions of hyaluronidase. It is thought that there may be a deficiency of this substance so that hyaluronic acid, which exists as a gel in many of the body tissues, is in excess and there is therefore a resistance to fluid absorption.

IMPETIGO CONTAGIOSA

This is an acute inflammation of the skin caused by pyogenic organisms. It occurs most commonly in children and is contagious, so tends to spread rapidly from one child to another.

The capillaries of the skin dilate and exudation of fluid takes place to such an extent that the layers of the epidermis are separated and blisters formed. Since the organism is pus-producing, the fluid in the vesicle rapidly becomes purulent. The vesicle usually quickly ruptures and the fluid or pus dries up and leaves a thick yellow crust which adheres to the underlying moist surface, from which it is difficult to separate it. The vesicles and surrounding inflammatory areas itch and when the child scratches them he tends to carry the infection in his finger-nails to another area, near or far away; hence there is often a rapid and patchy spread.

While any area of the body may be attacked, the exposed areas are most likely to be infected, and particularly areas to which a child so often takes the hands, such as the corners of the mouth, the nostrils and the ears.

Treatment is entirely medical and is quickly successful provided the child can be encouraged not to scratch and spread the infection. Penicillin powder or cream are often used and various forms of pastes applied.

Should a patient attend the physiotherapy department for some other ailment while suffering from this condition, it has to be remembered that it is contagious and great care must be taken to ensure that the child is kept away from other patients and that anything that is handled is disinfected. Should the physiotherapist fail to recognise the condition and be unfortunate enough to become infected, she must take the precaution not to re-infect herself by auto-inoculation, and she must take equal care not to infect others. It is wiser, if possible, to use paper towels and handkerchiefs, to avoid make-up and destroy old 'make-up' equipment. Sheets and pillowcases must be disinfected and boiled. For this reason it is important to have some knowledge of the condition. An attempt to recognise it should be made by noting the thick yellow adherent crusts, the size of the lesion (much larger than in eczema, often the size of a pea or larger) and the patchiness and site of the distribution. If its presence is suspected the patient should be referred to the physician.

BIBLIOGRAPHY

DISEASES OF THE CARDIO-VASCULAR SYSTEM

'Arterial Supply to the Extremities' by Sir James Learmonth (*Physiotherapy*, February 1948).

Diseases of the Heart by Sir Thomas Lewis (Macmillan, 1933, 1937, 1942, 1946).

'The Diagnosis and Treatment of Chronic Obliterative Arterial Diseases of the Extremities' by Richard Warren (*The Practitioner*, September 1955).

A Practice of Thoracic Surgery by A. L. d'Abreu (Edward Arnold, 1953).

'The Prevention and Treatment of Thrombophlebitis' by R. I. S. Bayliss (*The Practitioner*, September 1955).

'The Treatment of Varicose Veins' by Ian Fraser (*The Practitioner*, September 1955).

Vascular Disorders of the Limbs by Sir Thomas Lewis (Macmillan, 1936, 1946).

DISEASES OF THE NERVOUS SYSTEM

Diseases of the Nervous System by W. R. Brain (Oxford University Press, 1931, 1945, 1948, 1951).

Diseases of the Nervous System by F. M. R. Walshe (Livingstone, 1943, 1945, 1947, 1952, 1955).

Introduction to Clinical Neurology by Gordon Holmes (Livingstone, 1946, 1952).

Peripheral Nerve Injuries by Haymaker and Woodall (W. B. Saunders, 1945, 1953).

Poliomyelitis by W. Ritchie Russell (Edward Arnold, 1952).

A Way of Life for the Handicapped Child by Eirene Collis (Faber & Faber).

Physical Rehabilitation for Daily Living, edited by Edith Buchwald (McGraw-Hill Book Company, 1952).

Ambulation by Dening, Deyoe and Ellison (Funk and Wagnalls, 1951).

Muscle Testing and Function by Henry O. Kendall and Florence P. Kendall (The Williams and Wilkins Company, 1949).

BIBLIOGRAPHY

Orthopaedic Surgery by Walter Mercer (Edward Arnold, 1932, 1936, 1944, 1950).

Essentials of Orthopaedics by Philip Wiles (Churchill, 1949, 1955).

Outline of Orthopaedics by John Crawford Adams (Livingstone, 1956).

'The Principles of Physiotherapy in the Treatment of Spinal Paraplegia' by L. Guttmann (*Physiotherapy*, October 1949).

'Restoration of Function through Neuromuscular Re-education in Traumatic Paraplegia' by H. Kabat (*Archives of Neurology and Psychiatry*, June 1952).

Infantile Cerebral Palsy

'Some Observations on Treatment' by C. D. S. Agassiz.

'Pathology and its Bearing on Treatment' by W. F. Dunham.

'The Basis of Treatment' by Eirene Collis.

(All the above three articles appeared in *Physiotherapy*, September 1949.)

'The Treatment of Cerebral Palsy' by G. A. Pollock (*The Spastics' Quarterly*, September 1953).

'A Study of Abnormal Postural Reflex Activity in Patients with Lesions of the Central Nervous System' by Berta Bobath (*Physiotherapy*, September, October, November, December, 1954).

'The Importance of the Reduction of Muscle Tone and the Control of Mass Reflex Action in the Treatment of Spasticity' by Berta Bobath (*Occupational Therapy and Rehabilitation*, October 1948).

'A Treatment of Cerebral Palsy' by Karel Bobath and Berta Bobath (*British Journal of Physical Medicine*, May 1952).

'Patterns of Motion for Proprioceptive Neuro-Muscular Facilitation' by Dorothy E. Voss and Margaret Knott (*The British Journal of Physical Medicine*, September 1954).

'Studies of Neuro-Muscular Dysfunction', X, XI, XII, XIII, XIV, by H. Kabat (reprinted from the *Permanente Fondation Medical Bulletins*).

'Peripheral Nerve Injuries, their Diagnosis, Prognosis and Treatment' by R. E. M. Bowden (*Physiotherapy*, July 1946).

'Physical Methods Used in the Diagnosis and Treatment of Neuro-Muscular Disorders' by R. E. M. Bowden in *Physical Medicine and Rehabilitation*, edited by B. Kiernander (Blackwell, 1953).

'Symposium of Peripheral Nerve Injuries' by R. E. M. Bowden and J. R. Napier (*British Journal of Physical Medicine*, December 1951).

DISEASES OF THE RESPIRATORY SYSTEM

Chest Surgery for Nurses by J. Leigh Collis and L. E. Mabbitt (Bailliere, Tindall and Cox, 1944, 1946, 1951).

The Anatomy of the Bronchial Tree by R. C. Brock (Oxford University Press, 1947, 1954).

Diseases of the Chest by R. Coope (Livingstone, 1944, 1948).

A Practice of Thoracic Surgery by A. L. d'Abreu (Edward Arnold, 1953).

An Introduction to Diseases of the Chest by John Maxwell (Hodder and Stoughton, 2nd edition, 1945).

'Chronic Respiratory Disease' by H. J. Anderson and G. M. Storey (*Physiotherapy*, December 1955).

Physiotherapy in the Treatment of Pulmonary Tuberculosis by Thoracoplasty by Lois Caink (Chartered Society of Physiotherapy, 1952).

Physical Exercises for Asthma (8th edition, 1949). (Published in aid of the funds of the Asthma Research Council, c/o King's College, Strand, London, W.C.2.)

DISEASES OF THE SKIN

Diseases of the Skin by John T. Ingram and Reginald T. Brain (Churchill, 1911, 1915, 1919, 1927, 1936, 1947).

Gardiner's Handbook of Skin Diseases, revised by John Kinnear (Livingstone, 1919, 1924, 1931, 1939, 1948).

'Cortisone and Corticotrophin in Dermatology' by W. N. Goldsmith (*The Practitioner*, November 1955).

'Advances in the Treatment of Skin Diseases' by Brian Russell (*The Practitioner*, October 1955).

'Use of Hyaluronidase in Iontophoresis, in the Treatment of Generalised Scleroderma' by Roy J. Popkin (*Journal of Investigative Dermatology*, Vol. 16, 1951).

PATHOLOGY

Pathology by J. Henry Dible and Thomas B. Davie (Churchill, 1939, 1945, 1950).

An Introduction to Pathology by G. Payling Wright (Longmans Green, 1950).

Textbook of Pathology by William Boyd (Kimpton, 1932, 1934, 1938, 1943, 1947, 1953).

RHEUMATIC DISEASES

Ankylosing Spondylitis by F. Hernaman-Johnson and W. Alexander Law (Butterworth, 1949).

Comroe's Arthritis, edited by Joseph Lee Hollander (Kimpton, 5th edition, 1953).

Diseases of the Joints and Rheumatism by Kenneth Stone (Heinemann, 1947).

Rheumatism and Soft Tissue Injuries by J. Cyriax (Hamish Hamilton Medical Books, 1947).

Rheumatoid Arthritis—A Handbook for Patients, published by the Empire Rheumatism Council).

Textbook of the Rheumatic Diseases, edited by W. S. C. Copeman (Livingstone, 1948, 1955).

The Rheumatic Diseases by G. D. Kersley (Heinemann, 1950).

Textbook of Orthopaedic Medicine by J. Cyriax (Cassell, 1954).

Fracture and Joint Injuries by Sir Reginald Watson-Jones (Livingstone. 1940, 1941, 1943; 1st volume 1952, 2nd volume 1955).

'Citrate Iontophoresis in Rheumatoid Arthritis of the Hands' by A. B. Coyer (*Annals of Physical Medicine*, January 1954).

'Cortisone and Corticotrophin in Chronic Rheumatic Diseases and Gout' by Stanley J. Hartfall (*The Practitioner*, November 1955).

'The Dangers and Complications of Cortisone and Corticotrophin Therapy', by E. J. Wayne (*The Practitioner*, November 1955).

Rheumatoid Arthritis' by W. S. Tegner (*British Journal of Physical Medicine*, February 1949).

'Rehabilitation of the Disabled Housewife' by R. Harris and J. B. Millard (*Annals of Physical Medicine*, April 1955).

'Osteo-Arthritis and its Treatment' by Ernest Fletcher (*British Journal of Physical Medicine*, September–October 1948).

'The Management of the Rheumatic Patient' by Francis Bach (*The British Journal of Physical Medicine*, September 1955).

'The Value of Physiotherapy in Rheumatic Diseases' by J. S. Lawrence and R. J. Sladden (*Annals of Physical Medicine*, October 1955, Volume II, No. 8).

INDEX